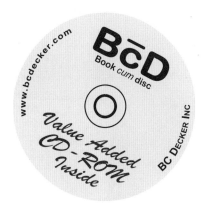

Ask for the accompanying software at
the circulation desk in this Library

DATE DUE	

American Cancer Society
Atlas of
Clinical Oncology

Published

Blumgart, Fong, Jarnagin	*Hepatobiliary Cancer (2001)*
Cameron	*Pancreatic Cancer (2001)*
Carroll, Grossfeld	*Prostate Cancer (2002)*
Char	*Tumors of the Eye and Ocular Adnexa (2001)*
Clark, Duh, Jahan, Perrier	*Endocrine Tumors (2003)*
Droller	*Urothelial Tumors (2004)*
Eifel, Levenback	*Cancer of the Female Lower Genital Tract (2001)*
Fuller, Seiden, Young	*Uterine Cancer (2004)*
Ginsberg	*Lung Cancer (2002)*
Grossbard	*Malignant Lymphomas (2002)*
Ozols	*Ovarian Cancer (2003)*
Pollock	*Soft Tissue Sarcomas (2002)*
Posner, Vokes, Weichselbaum	*Cancer of the Upper Gastrointestinal Tract (2002)*
Prados	*Brain Cancer (2002)*
Raghavan	*Germ Cell Tumors (2003)*
Shah	*Cancer of the Head and Neck (2001)*
Silverman	*Oral Cancer 5th Edition (2003)*
Sober, Haluska	*Skin Cancer (2001)*
Wiernik	*Adult Leukemias (2001)*
Willett	*Cancer of Lower Gastrointestinal Tract (2001)*
Winchester, Winchester	*Breast Cancer (2000)*

Forthcoming

Richie, Steele	*Kidney Tumors (2004)*
Volberding, Palefsky	*Viral and Immunological Malignancies (2004)*
Yasko	*Bone Tumors (2004)*

American Cancer Society
Atlas of
Clinical Oncology

Editors

GLENN D. STEELE JR, MD
Geisinger Health System

THEODORE L. PHILLIPS, MD
University of California

BRUCE A. CHABNER, MD
Harvard Medical School

Managing Editor

TED S. GANSLER, MD, MBA
Director of Health Content, American Cancer Society

American Cancer Society
Atlas of
Clinical Oncology

Uterine Cancer

Arlan F. Fuller Jr, MD

Associate Professor
Harvard Medical School
Chief, Gynecologic Oncology Service
Massachusetts General Hospital
Boston, Massachusetts

Michael V. Seiden, MD, PhD

Associate Professor of Medicine
Harvard Medical School
Associate Physician
Massachusetts General Hospital
Boston, Massachusetts

Robert H. Young, MD, FRCPath

Professor of Pathology
Harvard Medical School
Director of Anatomic Pathology
Massachusetts General Hospital
Boston, Massachusetts

2004
BC Decker Inc
Hamilton • London

BC Decker Inc
P.O. Box 620, LCD 1
Hamilton, Ontario L8N 3K7
Tel: 905-522-7017; 1-800-568-7281
Fax: 905-522-7839; 1-888-311-4987
E-mail: info@bcdecker.com
www.bcdecker.com

ISBN 1–55009–163–8
Printed in Spain

Sales and Distribution

United States
BC Decker Inc
P.O. Box 785
Lewiston, NY 14092-0785
Tel: 905-522-7017; 800-568-7281
Fax: 905-522-7839; 888-311-4987
E-mail: info@bcdecker.com
www.bcdecker.com

Canada
BC Decker Inc
20 Hughson Street South
P.O. Box 620, LCD 1
Hamilton, Ontario L8N 3K7
Tel: 905-522-7017; 800-568-7281
Fax: 905-522-7839; 888-311-4987
E-mail: info@bcdecker.com
www.bcdecker.com

Foreign Rights
John Scott & Company
International Publishers' Agency
P.O. Box 878
Kimberton, PA 19442
Tel: 610-827-1640; Fax: 610-827-1671
E-mail: jsco@voicenet.com

Japan
Igaku-Shoin Ltd.
Foreign Publications Department
3-24-17 Hongo
Bunkyo-ku, Tokyo, Japan 113-8719
Tel: 3 3817 5680; Fax: 3 3815 6776
E-mail: fd@igaku-shoin.co.jp

UK, Europe, Scandinavia, Middle East
Elsevier Science
Customer Service Department
Foots Cray High Street
Sidcup, Kent
DA14 5HP, UK
Tel: 44 (0) 208 308 5760
Fax: 44 (0) 181 308 5702
E-mail: cservice@harcourt.com

Singapore, Malaysia,Thailand,
Philippines, Indonesia, Vietnam,
Pacific Rim, Korea
Elsevier Science Asia
583 Orchard Road
#09/01, Forum
Singapore 238884
Tel: 65-737-3593; Fax: 65-753-2145

Australia, New Zealand
Elsevier Science Australia
Customer Service Department
STM Division
Locked Bag 16
St. Peters, New South Wales, 2044
Australia
Tel: 61 02 9517-8999
Fax: 61 02 9517-2249
E-mail: stmp@harcourt.com.au
www.harcourt.com.au

Mexico and Central America
ETM SA de CV
Calle de Tula 59
Colonia Condesa
06140 Mexico DF, Mexico
Tel: 52-5-5553-6657
Fax: 52-5-5211-8468
E-mail: editoresdetextosmex@prodigy.net.mx

Brazil
Tecmedd
Av. Maurílio Biagi, 2850
City Ribeirão Preto – SP – CEP: 14021-000
Tel: 0800 992236
Fax: (16) 3993-9000
E-mail: tecmedd@tecmedd.com.br

India, Bangladesh, Pakistan, Sri Lanka
Elsevier Health Sciences Division
Customer Service Department
17A/1, Main Ring Road
Lajpat Nagar IV
New Delhi – 110024, India
Tel: 91 11 2644 7160-64
Fax: 91 11 2644 7156
E-mail: esindia@vsnl.net

Contents

Preface

Tumors of the uterine corpus include endometrial carcinoma, the most frequent gynecologic malignancy in the developed countries, as well as a wide collection of mesenchymal tumors. Advances in classical and molecular pathology now provide a more consistent structured approach to classifying and studying of these tumors. This volume of the American Cancer Society's, Atlas of Clinical Oncology, focusing on cancers of the uterus is meant to provide a comprehensive overview of epidemiologic, pathologic, biologic, and treatment paradigms relevant to both epithelial cancers and mesenchymal tumors of the uterine corpus. In addition, a series of current controversies are reviewed, including the role of hormone replacement therapy in patients with a history of endometrial cancer, and the appropriate surgical management in women who present with what appears to be early clinical stage endometrial carcinoma. The book includes a comprehensive and liberally illustrated description of the pathology of endometrial and mesenchymal tumors, which form the basis for appropriate management. In addition, a contemporary overview of the molecular pathology, which underpins early endometrial carcinogenesis, is reviewed. Epithelial tumors are also discussed in the context of epidemiologic associations, as well as germline mutations which may predispose individuals or families to the early onset of endometrial carcinoma. Clinical management issues, including surgical staging, prognostic factors, indications for radiation therapy in the postoperative management of endometrial cancer, and the roles of hormonal and systemic chemotherapy in the treatment of this disease, are discussed in detail. Special clinical situations, such as the evaluation of women on tamoxifen or treatment of low-stage, low-grade endometrial carcinoma in women who desire to preserve their uterus, receive special and detailed attention in dedicated chapter. Expanded discussions on the treatment of uncommon but important histological subtype of endometrial carcinomas (serous plus clear cell and mesenchymal tumors) are also reviewed in dedicated chapters. Edited by experts in surgery, medical oncology, and pathology, the text provides a comprehensive mult-disciplinary review of this common malignancy.

The editors would like to thank each of the authors for their fine contribution and Linda Dell'Olio for her editorial assistance.

Arlan F. Fuller, MD
Michael V. Seiden, MD, PhD
Robert H. Young, MD

Contributors

Ross S. Berkowitz, MD
Department of Obstetrics and Gynecology
Harvard Medical School
Boston, Massachusetts
Evaluation of Uterine Smooth Muscle, Stromal, and Malignant Mixed Müllerian Neoplasms: Symptoms, Radiologic, Evaluation, and Diagnostic Techniques

Edmund S. Cibas, MD
Department of Pathology
Harvard Medical School
Boston, Massachusetts
Positive Peritoneal Cytology in Women With Endometrial Cancer

Philip B. Clement, MD
Department of Pathology
University of British Columbia
Vancouver, British Columbia
Pathology of Endometrial Carcinoma

Daniel W. Cramer, MD, ScD
Department of Obstetrics and Gynecology
Harvard Medical School
Boston, Massachusetts
Epidemiology of Endometrial Cancer

Thomas F. Delaney, MD
Department of Radiation Oncology
Harvard Medical School
Boston, Massachusetts
Radiotherapy and Postsurgical Management of Endometrial Cancer

Linda R. Duska, MD
Department of Obstetrics, Gynecology, and Reproductive Biology
Harvard Medical School
Boston, Massachusetts
Primary Hormonal Therapy for Endometrial Carcinoma

Arlan F. Fuller Jr, MD
Department of Obstetrics and Gynecology
Harvard Medical School
Boston, Massachusetts
Diagnosis, Screening, and Staging of Endometrial Carcinoma and *Prognostic and Predictive Factors in the Management of Endometrial Carcinoma*

Annekathryn Goodman, MD
Department of Obstetrics and Gynecology
Harvard Medical School
Boston, Massachusetts
Estrogen Replacement Therapy after Endometrial Cancer and *Endometrial Hyperplasia and Management of the Endometrium for Women on Tamoxifen*

Karen A. Gronau, MD, MSc
Department of Obstetrics and Gynecology
University of Toronto
Toronto, Ontario
Familial Endometrial Cancer

Tan A. Ince, MD, PhD
Department of Pathology
Harvard Medical School
Boston, Massachusetts
Molecular Pathogenesis of Endometrial Cancer

CAROLYN KRASNER, MD
Department of Medicine
Harvard Medical School
Boston, Massachusetts
Treatment of Uterine Sarcomas

SUSANNA I. LEE, MD, PHD
Department of Radiology
Harvard Medical School
Boston, Massachusetts
*Evaluation of Uterine Smooth Muscle, Stromal,
    and Malignant Mixed Müllerian Neoplasms:
    Symptoms, Radiologic, Evaluation, and
    Diagnostic Techniques*

URSULA MATULONIS, MD
Department of Medicine
Harvard Medical School
Boston, Massachusetts
*Positive Peritoneal Cytology in Women With
    Endometrial Cancer*

JOAN MURPHY, MD, FRCSC
Department of Obstetrics and Gynecology
University of Toronto
Toronto, Ontario
Familial Endometrial Cancer

GEORGE L. MUTTER, MD
Department of Pathology
Harvard Medical School
Boston, Massachusetts
Molecular Pathogenesis of Endometrial Cancer

NAJMOSAMA NIKRUI, MD
Department of Obstetrics and Gynecology,
    and Reproductive Biology
Harvard Medical School
Boston, Massachusetts
*Papillary Serous, Clear Cell, and Small Cell
    Carcinomas of the Endometrium*

ESTHER OLIVA, MD
Department of Pathology
Harvard Medical School
Boston, Massachusetts
*Pathology of Sarcomas and Mixed Müllerian
    Tumors of the Uterine Corpus*

B. HANNAH ORTIZ, MD
Department of Gynecologic Oncology
Florida Hospital Cancer Institute
Orlando, Florida
*Evaluation of Uterine Smooth Muscle, Stromal,
    and Malignant Mixed Müllerian Neoplasms:
    Symptoms, Radiologic Evaluation, and
    Diagnostic Techniques*

RICHARD T. PENSON, MD, MRCP
Department of Medicine
Harvard Medical School
Boston, Massachusetts
*Radiotherapy and Post-Surgical Management of
    Endometrial Cancer*

BARRY ROSEN, MD, FRCSC
Department of Obstetrics and Gynecology
University of Toronto
Toronto, Ontario
Familial Endometrial Cancer

BO R. RUEDA, PHD
Department of Obstetrics, Gynecology, and
    Reproductive Biology
Harvard Medical School
Boston, Massachusetts
*Primary Hormonal Therapy for Endometrial
    Carcinoma*

MICHAEL V. SEIDEN, MD, PHD
Department of Hematology/Oncology
Harvard University
Boston, Massachusetts
*Management of Recurrent or Metastatic
    Endometrial Carcinoma* and *Papillary Serous,
    Clear Cell, and Small Cell Carcinomas of the
    Endometrium,* and *Treatment of Uterine
    Sarcomas*

ROBERT H. YOUNG, MD, FRCPATH
Department of Pathology
Harvard Medical School
Boston, Massachusetts
Pathology of Endometrial Carcinoma and
    *Pathology of Sarcomas and Mixed Müllerian
    Tumors of the Uterine Corpus*

Epidemiology of Endometrial Cancer

DANIEL W. CRAMER, MD, ScD

Uterine corpus cancer is the fourth most common cancer among American women and the most common of the gynecologic malignancies, with an estimated 40,100 new cases in the year 2003.[1] However, it accounts for disproportionally fewer cancer deaths, about 6,800, making it about the eighth most common cause of cancer deaths among women and second to ovarian cancer among the gynecologic cancers. Many statistics about endometrial cancer are reported within the broader category "cancers of the uterine corpus," which includes the relatively rare sarcomas. However, because adenocarcinomas comprise the vast majority of cancers of the uterine corpus, this chapter focuses on endometrial cancer, even though some studies reviewed in this chapter may not have specifically excluded sarcomas.

Endometrial adenocarcinomas may be further subdivided by histologic type, with endometrioid cancers accounting for about 85%, the remainder being of various other cell types as discussed in Chapters 5 and 11. It should be noted that endometrioid cancers may be preceded by endometrial hyperplasia, especially with atypia, making factors related to hyperplasia also relevant to the epidemiology of endometrial cancer. Many of the studies cited heredo not distinguish among histologic subtypes of endometrial cancer, and, as a general rule, the term "endometrial cancer" in this review should be equated to the endometrioid subtype. Whether epidemiologic factors for endometrial cancer contribute equally to nonendometrioid cancer is unclear.

Studies support the role of demographics and medical conditions (such as obesity), reproductive factors, contraception, hormone replacement therapy and other medications, lifestyle factors, and heredity in the risk of developing endometrial cancer. A theme, which will become apparent early in the discussion, is that the epidemiology of endometrial cancer appears to be largely explained by conditions which lead to an excess of estrogen relative to progesterone, hence it is no surprise that many of these epidemiologic factors may be related to the development of endometrial hyperplasia.

DEMOGRAPHIC DIFFERENCES AND TEMPORAL TRENDS

Figure 1–1 shows the age-specific incidence and mortality rates for endometrial cancer in White and Black females in the United States over the years 1994 to 1998.[2] Endometrial cancer is rare in White females under age 40 years, but the incidence sharply increases around the time of menopause and peaks between 70 and 79 years at approximately 110 cases per 100,000 annually. The pattern is more irregular in Black females but shows the same perimenopausal increase with annual rates peaking at about 85 per 100,000. Although incidence rates, overall, are about 30% higher for Whites, this excess incidence does not translate into higher mortality rates. At all ages, Blacks have greater mortality rates for endometrial cancer than Whites. The survival disadvantage of Blacks compared with Whites may be due not only to the occurrence of less favorable histologic types and more advanced stages at presentation[3,4] but also to less

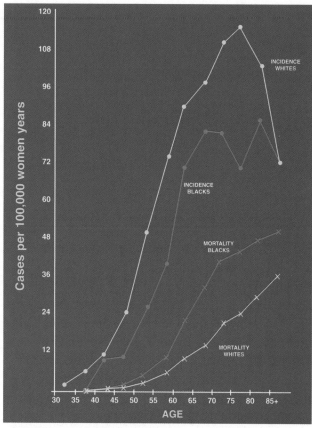

Figure 1–1. Age-specific incidence and mortality rates for endometrial cancer in the United States (1994–1998). Reproduced with permission from Ries LAG et al.[2]

during the early 1970s and mortality rates have shown gradual improvement since 1973.

OBESITY AND MEDICAL CONDITIONS

Even in the earliest clinical and epidemiologic studies, some dating back half a century, obesity, hypertension, and diabetes have been recognized as strong risk factors for endometrial cancer.[8–10] Research since then has confirmed the importance of obesity, examined whether diabetes or hypertension are risk factors independent of obesity, and sought to clarify the likely biologic explanation for the importance of obesity.

Table 1–1 illustrates the effect of body habitus, as determined by various anthropometric measures, and risk of endometrial cancer. In a large study in Sweden, Weiderpass and colleagues found a convincing dose-response relationship in the risk of endometrial cancer with an increasing body mass index (BMI), such that relative risk increased 9% with each kg/m^2 BMI unit.[11] Compared with women with a BMI less than 22.5, women with a BMI between 30 and 34 have about a 3-fold increase in risk of endometrial cancer; and the risk increases about 5-fold for women with a BMI greater than 34. In the same study, weight gain

aggressive treatments offered to Blacks.[5] (See Chapter 6 for further discussion.)

Figure 1–2 shows time trends between 1973 and 1998 for endometrial cancer incidence and mortality (on a log scale) in White and Black females, age 50 years and older.[2] Apparent for White (but not Black) females was a sharp rise and fall in the incidence of endometrial cancer that occurred approximately between 1973 and 1980. Correlational studies done in individual communities or within health maintenance organizations suggested that this "epidemic" of endometrial cancers likely related to a dramatic increase in the use of unopposed estrogen for menopausal treatment that occurred in the late 1960s and early 1970s.[6] Conversely, more recent data from health maintenance organizations suggest that the decline in endometrial cancer occurrence in the 1980s tracked well with the increasing use of menopausal hormone regimens that included a progestogen.[7] No increase in mortality was apparent

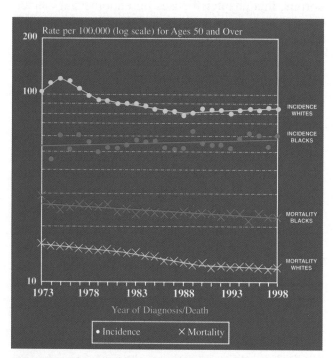

Figure 1–2. Time trends for endometrial cancer in the United States between 1973 and 1998. Reproduced with permission from Ries LAG et al.[2]

Table 1–1. ANTHROPOMETRIC VARIABLES AND RISK OF ENDOMETRIAL CANCER			
Study	Meaures/Units	Cases/Controls	RR (95% CI)
Weiderpass et al[11]	BMI (kg/m^2)		
	< 22.5	117/772	1.0 referent
	22.5–24.9	154/929	1.1 (0.8–1.4)
	25.0–27.9	144/894	1.0 (0.8–1.3)
	28–29.9	89/348	1.6 (1.2–2.2)
	30–33.9	120/268	2.8 (1.4–3.2)
	34+	85/112	4.8 (3.4–6.8)
Weiderpass et al[11]	Weight gain since age 18 (kg)		
	< 0	36/248	0.8 (0.5–1.2)
	0–9	134/757	1.0 referent
	10–19	183/895	1.2 (0.9–1.5)
	20–29	106/362	1.6 (1.2–2.2)
	30+	101/152	3.7 (2.7–5.0)
Swanson et al[12]	Waist-to-thigh ratio		
	< 1.62	45/68	1.0 referent
	1.62–1.78	81/71	1.5 (0.8–2.5)
	1.79–1.99	105/69	1.8 (1.1–3.2)
	> 1.99	147/70	2.6 (1.5–4.5)

BMI = body mass index; CI = confidence interval; RR = relative risk.

after age 18 years also produced a strong and consistent trend such that the relative risk increased about 3% with each kilogram increase in weight postadolescence. In another large study, the dose response was less consistent for current weight, although women above 78 kg had a significant increase in risk of endometrial cancer of about 2.3-fold.[12] This same study found a strong trend for increasing upper body obesity as measured by waist-to-thigh circumference ratios (see Table 1–1). No consistent trend has been found for height.[11,12] A biologic explanation for the long-appreciated link between obesity and endometrial cancer was suggested when endocrine studies established that fat possesses aromatase enzymes capable of converting androstenedione into estrone, a biologically active estrogen.[13,14]

Considerable interest has focused on whether the classic link between endometrial cancer and diabetes varies by type of diabetes or is independent of obesity. Regarding the former issue, the literature is not entirely consistent. Weiderpass and colleagues found an association with both type I and type II diabetes,[11] whereas Parazzini and colleagues found no association with diabetes, which was likely to be insulin dependent, diagnosed before the age 40 years.[15] Regarding the interaction between weight and diabetes, two studies found no increased risk

with diabetes in women who were of normal weight, but the combination of both diabetes and obesity gave the highest risk.[16,17] The possible "synergistic" effect between obesity and diabetes has been interpreted to indicate that besides estrogen, there may be an added importance of insulin or insulin-like growth factor for endometrial cancer because these endocrine factors have been hypothesized to play a role in other hormonally related cancers.[15,18] In contrast, hypertension does not appear to be an independent risk factor for endometrial cancer and may only increase risk among those who are obese.[11]

In contrast to diabetes, a medical condition associated with a decreased risk of endometrial cancer is bone fracture.[19,20] The inverse association with fracture appears to be explained by the well-described link between osteoporosis and low estrogen levels.[21] There are other medical conditions that are linked to endometrial cancer but only through case reports. Although such reports do not allow formal estimates of risk, these reports are of interest because they provide additional support for the "unopposed estrogen" theory. Thus, case reports link endometrial cancer with cirrhosis, where there is decreased clearance of estrogen, and with estrogen-producing tumors of the ovary, where there is excessive estrogen production.[22,23]

REPRODUCTIVE FACTORS AND CONTRACEPTION

Two reproductive factors, which are also "classic," include nulliparity, especially among married women, and a late age at menopause.[8] Both these risk factors would appear to fit with the unopposed estrogen theory. Married women who remain nulliparous might have fertility problems, such as anovulatory cycles, which may be associated with chronic estrogen exposure and lack of luteal phase progesterone. Indeed, a review of papers addressing cancer risk among women attending fertility clinics described an excess number of endometrial cancers in the group with ovulatory causes for their infertility.[24] Late age at menopause is likely to be explained by the fact that anovulatory cycles are known to be associated with the transition to menopause. Women who take a longer time to make their transition to the menopause may have a longer exposure to anovulatory cycles without progesterone "rescue" of the endometrium and periodic sloughing.

In addition to nulliparity increasing risk, Table 1–2 illustrates that with each additional pregnancy, there is a further decrease in risk.[25,26] Also, the later the age of the last pregnancy the lower the risk of endometrial cancer.[26] An interpretation involving unopposed estrogen is perhaps less clear for the added protection with more than one pregnancy or for pregnancy at a late age. Investigators have speculated that the endometrial "exfoliation" that occurs with delivery of the placenta serves to remove abnormal precursor cells.[26] Beyond the effect of pregnancy, there also appears to be additional protection with the number of years a women has breast fed her children.[27,28] This would also be consistent with the estrogen theory because lactation is associated with low estrogen levels.[29]

There is consistent evidence that use of oral contraceptives decreases the risk of endometrial cancer in a dose-dependent manner; that is, the longer the period of use, the lower the risk (see Table 1–2).[30–32] It should be emphasized that this protection pertains to combination oral contraceptives where each pill contains estrogen and progesterone but not to the now-discontinued sequential preparations. The latter preparations contained estrogen-only pills in

Table 1–2. REPRODUCTIVE FACTORS AND ENDOMETRIAL CANCER RISK			
Study	Number of Pregnancies	Cases/Controls	RR (95% CI)
Lambe et al[26]	0	1,057/3,305	1.4 (1.2–1.5)
	1	1,086/4,679	1.0
	2	1,640/8,765	0.8 (0.7–0.9)
	3	739/4,768	0.6 (0.6–0.7)
	4	212/1,755	0.5 (0.4–0.6)
	5	71/1,543	0.5 (0.4–0.7)
	≥ 6	34/368	0.4 (0.2–0.5)
Lambe et al[26]	Age at last birth		
	< 25	476/2,791	1.0
	25–29	1,296/7,724	0.9 (0.8–1.1)
	30–34	740/4,444	0.8 (0.7–0.9)
	35–39	166/1,004	0.6 (0.5–0.7)
	≥ 40	181/156	0.5 (0.4–0.7)
Rosenblatt and Thomas[27]	Months breast fed		
	None	15/69	1.0
	1–12	50/203	1.0 (0.5–2.1)
	13–36	34/245	0.6 (0.3–1.3)
	37–72	30/231	0.7 (0.3–1.4)
	> 72	71/185	0.2 (0.1–0.7)
Weiderpass et al[32]	Years of OC use		
	Never	551/2,252	1.0
	< 1	63/245	1.2 (0.9–1.6)
	1–4	47/292	0.7 (0.5–1.0)
	5–9	20/190	0.5 (0.3–0.8)
	≥ 10	6/212	0.1 (0.1–0.3)

CI = confidence interval; OC = oral contraceptive; RR = relative risk.

the first half of the cycle with a progestogen added to the pills in the second half, making sequential preparations estrogen dominant. Reports of endometrial cancer in young women taking sequential oral contraceptives provided another example of the harmful effect of (relatively) unopposed exogenous estrogen.[33] These preparations were removed from the market in the United States around the same time that the menopausal hormone association with endometrial cancer became clear.

Regarding the protection associated with combination birth control pills, it should be noted that the protective effect is not confined to the period of use but may persist for many years after use is discontinued.[32] This suggests that chronic exposure to an estrogen/progesterone combination may have long-term effects on the endometrium. Protection has also been observed with depot-medroxyprogesterone acetate.[34] Other contraceptive practices investigated in relation to endometrial cancer have included tubal ligation and the use of an intrauterine device (IUD).[35–37] There are no biologic reasons to link these practices to endometrial cancer nor have any consistent associations been found.

HORMONAL REPLACEMENT THERAPY

The "epidemic" of endometrial cancers occurring in the 1970s was likely due to the increasing use of unopposed estrogen for menopausal therapy. Data from numerous case-control and cohort studies support this link. According to a meta-analysis by Grady and colleagues, there were 37 epidemiologic studies of hormone replacement therapy (HRT) and endometrial cancer published between 1970 and 1994, a positive association was found in all but two of these. [38] The summary relative risk (*rr*) and 95% confidence interval for "ever use" of HRT was 2.3 (2.1–2.5). A dose response was evident in the combined summary estimates with an *rr* of 1.4 (1.0–1.8) for less than one year of use and 9.5 (7.4–12.3) for 9 to 10 years of use. It has been argued that the relationship between menopausal estrogen and endometrial cancer was due to a "surveillance" bias, that is, physicians were more likely to perform a biopsy on women with irregular bleeding who were taking hormones.[39] However, given the strength and consistency of the

association, there now seems little doubt that a real and, likely, causal association exists between unopposed HRT and endometrial cancer risk.

Risk may also occur with the use of unopposed regimens of "weak" estrogens, such as estriol, and low-dose menopausal hormones, such as 0.3 mg of conjugated equine estrogens.[40,41] These observations raise concern that women taking unopposed plant estrogens in the form of herbal supplements may also face an increased risk of endometrial cancer.[42] Physicians should inquire about the use of such supplements in their peri- or postmenopausal patients and take this into consideration in deciding when endometrial screening might be necessary (see Chapter 4).

Data suggest that a decline in endometrial cancer occurrence appeared to follow the introduction of combined estrogen plus progesterone HRT regimens.[7] Is there additional epidemiologic evidence to support this? In studies that had the opportunity to compare risk of endometrial cancer in various unopposed and opposed regimens, a trend was seen for the risk to weaken with greater use (duration of use) of a progestogen during the cycle (Table 1–3).[43–45] Thus, no significantly increased risk was found for endometrial cancer when a progestin was used for more than 10 days during a month of treatment—generally 10 mg of medroxyprogesterone acetate (MPA) per day. In the study by Weiderpass and colleagues, the use of progesterone on a daily (continuous) basis was actually associated with a decreased risk of endometrial cancer.[45]

The conclusions of these observational epidemiologic studies are supported by prospective studies that have monitored rates of endometrial hyperplasia in women receiving various HRT regimens. Whitehead and colleagues confirmed that at least 10 days of opposed therapy per month was required to reduce the risk of hyperplasia.[46] In a randomized controlled study known as the PEPI trial (Postmenopausal Estrogen/Progestin Interventions), the occurrence of simple, complex, or atypical hyperplasia occurred almost exclusively in women assigned to the unopposed estrogen regimen.[47] Over the three years of follow-up, about 62% of the subjects receiving unopposed therapy developed hyperplasia, compared with about 5% of women who received 10 mg of MPA or 200 mg of

Table 1–3.   RISK OF ENDOMETRIAL CANCER WITH DIFFERENT ESTROGEN AND MPA COMBINATIONS

Study	Unopposed ERT	Sequential < 10 d	Sequential > 10 d	Continuous Combined
Beresford et al[43]	4.0 (3.1–5.1)	3.1 (1.7–5.7)	1.3 (0.8–2.2)	
Pike et al[44]	2.17 (1.91–2.47)	1.87 (1.32–2.65)	1.07 (0.82–1.41)	1.07 (0.80–1.43)
Weiderpass et al[45]	6.6 (3.6–12.0)	2.9 (1.8–4.6)		0.2 (0.1–0.8)

ERT = estrogen replacement therapy; MPA = medroxyprogesterone acetate.

micronized progesterone for 12 days per month. Notably, only one (1%) of the women assigned to continuous therapy with 2.5 mg of MPA daily developed hyperplasia, and this was characterized as simple. Thus, continuous estrogen plus progesterone combinations carry the least risk for the development of hyperplasia and, by inference, provide the greatest protection against endometrial cancer.

OTHER MEDICATIONS

Tamoxifen is a selective estrogen receptor modulator (SERM) that appears to have estrogen antagonist effects in the breast but estrogen agonist effects in the uterus. In their review of numerous case-control and cohort studies addressing the association between tamoxifen and endometrial cancer, the International Agency for Research on Cancer concluded that tamoxifen increases the risk of endometrial cancer.[48] In a recent review of four breast cancer chemoprevention trials, endometrial cancer risk was found to be significantly increased by two- to 3-fold when tamoxifen was used for five years.[49] No increased risk is expected, and none has been found, with raloxifene, a SERM that appears to be an estrogen antagonist in both the breast and the uterus.[50] Finally, one report suggested that the use of psychotropic medications, including major and minor tranquilizers, led to a modest increase in the risk of endometrial cancer that was of borderline statistical significance.[51]

LIFESTYLE FACTORS

A number of lifestyle factors have been investigated in relation to endometrial cancer including diet, exercise, alcohol use, and smoking. In view of the strong association between obesity and endometrial cancer, it could be predicted, and has been found, that simple caloric excess is a risk factor for endometrial cancer.[52–54] It is also possible that there is a greater risk

associated with calories from fat than with calories from protein or carbohydrates.[52,55] Two studies also suggest that the consumption of vegetables, especially those high in carotenoids, may decrease risk.[54,55] Many studies have found a decreased risk of endometrial cancers associated with increased physical activity.[56–59] The effect appears to be largely related to current and not past levels of activity. Once again, this observation is compatible with the "estrogen hypothesis" in that physical activity is associated with lower endogenous estrogen levels.[60]

Other lifestyle factors that have been investigated in relation to endometrial cancer include alcohol and smoking. In view of the evidence that alcohol may increase estrogen levels and the link between alcohol and breast cancer, it might be predicted that alcohol would increase endometrial cancer risk. However, several studies investigating alcohol use in relation to endometrial cancer have been negative.[61–65] Conversely, there is some evidence that smoking may decrease estrogen levels, perhaps by blocking aromatase action.[66] This habit would be predicted to decrease the risk of endometrial cancer; and, indeed, several studies investigating the exposure have reported a modest decrease in the risk of endometrial cancer associated with smoking even after adjustment for weight or controlled for weight.[67–69] Although one study has suggested coffee consumption might lead to increased serum estradiol, two recent epidemiological studies found that coffee consumption might actually be associated with a slight decrease in risk for endometrial cancer.[70–72]

HEREDITY

Endometrial cancer may occur as part of hereditary nonpolyposis colorectal cancer (HNPCC) and this will be addressed in Chapter 3. Here, we address whether a family history of endometrial cancer, even if it cannot be linked to a predisposition syndrome, increases the risk of endometrial cancer. Overall, a modest increased risk of endometrial cancer, about 1.5-fold, was associated with a family history of endometrial cancer in a first-degree relative.[73] The risk associated with family history may be higher, about 3-fold, for endometrial cancers arising in younger women age 20 to 54 years.[74] Undoubtedly some degree of recall bias could affect this association in case control studies. Often, women may simply know that a "uterine" cancer occurred in a relative and be uncertain whether it arose from the cervix or endometrium. Women with endometrial cancer might be more likely to report that such relatives had endometrial cancer.

CONCLUSION

As a generalization, the woman who gets endometrial cancer is overweight, has had menopause at a late age, may be nulliparous, may have had little use of oral contraceptives, and may have used unopposed estrogen or tamoxifen. Again as a generalization, most risk factors for endometrial cancer appear to be mediated by conditions that lead to an excess of estrogen relative to progesterone. Although this theory may not explain all cases and has not yet been translated into a strategy for complete control of endometrial cancer, a few suggestions seem clear. Maintenance of a healthy diet and ideal body weight as well as the use of a continuous estrogen/progesterone regimen for the woman who decides to use replacement therapy are important measures. Physicians should have a low threshold for endometrial sampling in women with irregular bleeding patterns or risk factors, such as obesity, late menopause, use of unopposed estrogen regimens or tamoxifen, and a family history of the disease.

From a public health standpoint, there are several areas needing further investigation. First, we need to identify and address factors contributing to the poorer survival of Black women with the disease (see Chapter 6). Second, we need to refine the description of risk factors for women with the most unfavorable forms of endometrial cancer (such as papillary serous or clear cell) to see if more specific preventive strategies could be developed for these more lethal types of endometrial cancer. Finally, any

inconsistencies with "unopposed estrogen" as the key underpinning theory for the pathogenesis of endometrial cancer need to be explained or alternative theories proposed.

REFERENCES

1. Jemal A, Murray T, Samuels A, et al. Cancer statistics, 2003. Ca Cancer J Clin 2003;53:5–26.
2. Ries LAG, Eisner MD, Kosary CL, et al, editors. SEER cancer statistics review, 1973–1998. Bethesda MD: National Cancer Institute; 2001.
3. Connell PP, Rotmensch J, Waggoner SE, Mundt AJ. Race and clinical outcome in endometrial carcinoma. Obstet Gynecol 1999;94:713–20.
4. Aziz H, Rotman M, Hussain F, et al. Poor survival of black patients in carcinoma of the endometrium. Int J Radiat Oncol Biol Phys 1993;27:293–301.
5. Hicks ML, Phillips JL, Parham G, et al. The National Cancer Data Base report on endometrial carcinoma in African-American women. Cancer 1998;83:2629–37.
6. Weiss NS, Szekely DR, Austin DF. Increasing incidence of endometrial cancer in the United States. N Engl J Med 1976;294:1259–62.
7. Ziel HK, Finkle WD, Greenland S. Decline in incidence of endometrial cancer following increase in prescriptions for opposed conjugated estrogens in a prepaid health plan. Gynecol Oncol 1998;68:253–5.
8. Corscaden JA, Gusberg SB. The background of cancer of the corpus. Am J Obstet Gynecol 1947;53:419–29.
9. Damon A. Host factors in cancer of the breast and uterine cervix and corpus. J Natl Cancer Inst 1960;24:483–516.
10. Fox H, Sen DK. A controlled study of the constitutional stigmata of endometrial adenocarcinoma. Br J Cancer 1970;24:30–6.
11. Weiderpass E, Persson I, Adami HO, et al. Body size in different periods of life, diabetes mellitus, hypertension and risk of postmenopausal endometrial cancer (Sweden). Cancer Causes Control 2000;11:185–92.
12. Swanson CA, Potischman N, Wilbanks GD, et al. Relation of endometrial cancer risk to past and contemporary body size and body fat distribution. Cancer Epidemiol Biomarkers Prev 1993;2:321–7.
13. MacDonald PC, Siiteri PK. The relationship between the extra glandular production of estrone and the occurrence of endometrial neoplasia. Gynecol Oncol 1974;2:259–63.
14. Rizkallah TH, Tovell NM, Kelly WG. Production of estrone and fractional conversion of circulating androstenedione to estrone in women with endometrial carcinoma. J Clin Endocrinol Metab 1975;40:1045–51.
15. Parazzini F, La Vecchia C, Negri E, et al. Diabetes and endometrial cancer; an Italian case-control study. Int J Cancer 1999;81:539–42.
16. Shoff SM, Newcomb PA. Diabetes, body size, and risk of endometrial cancer. Am J Epidemiol 1998;148:234–40.
17. Anderson KE, Anderson E, Mink PJ, et al. Diabetes and endometrial cancer in the Iowa women's health study. Cancer Epidemiol Biomarkers Prev 2001;10:611–6.

18. Kazer RR. Insulin resistance, insulin-like growth factor I and breast cancer: a hypothesis. Int J Cancer 1995;62: 403–6.

19. Persson I, Adami HO, McLaughlin JK, et al. Reduced risk of breast and endometrial cancer among women with hip fractures. Cancer Causes Control 1994;5:523–8.

20. Newcomb PA, Trentham-Dietz A, Egan KM, et al. Fracture history and risk of breast and endometrial cancer. Am J Epidemiol 2001;153:1071–8.

21. Richelson LS, Wahner HW, Melton LJ, Riggs BL. Relative contributions of aging and estrogen deficiency to postmenopausal bone loss. N Engl J Med 1984;311:1273–5.

22. Speert H. Endometrial cancer and hepatic cirrhosis. Cancer 1949;2:597–603.

23. Salerno W. Feminizing mesenchymomas of the ovary: an analysis of 28 ganulosa-theca cell tumors and their relationship to co-existent carcinoma. Am J Obstet Gynecol 1962;84:731–8.

24. Klip H, Burger CW, Kenemans P, van Leeuwen FE. Cancer risk associated with subfertility and ovulation induction: a review. Cancer Causes Control 2000;11:319–44.

25. Salazar-Martinez E, Lazcano-Ponce EC, Gonzalez Lira-Lira G, et al. Reproductive factors of ovarian and endometrial cancer risk in a high fertility population in Mexico. Cancer Res 1999;59:3658–62.

26. Lambe M, Wuu J, Weiderpass E, Hsieh CC. Childbearing at older age and endometrial cancer risk (Sweden). Cancer Causes Control 1999;10:43–9.

27. Rosenblatt KA, Thomas DB. Prolonged lactation and endometrial cancer. WHO Collaborative Study of Neoplasia and Steroid Contraceptives. Int J Epidemiol 1995;24:499–503.

28. Newcomb PA, Trentham-Dietz A. Breast feeding practices in relation to endometrial cancer risk, USA. Cancer Causes Control 2000;11:663–7.

29. Petrakis NL, Wrensch MR, Ernster VL, et al. Influence of pregnancy and lactation on serum and breast fluid estrogen levels: implications for breast cancer risk. Int J Cancer 1987;40:587–91.

30. Voigt LF, Deng Q, Weiss NS. Recency, duration, and progestin content of oral contraceptives in relation to the incidence of endometrial cancer (Washington, USA). Cancer Causes Control 1994;5:227–33.

31. Vessey MP, Painter R. Endometrial and ovarian cancer and oral contraceptives—findings in a large cohort study. Br J Cancer 1995;71:1340–2.

32. Weiderpass E, Adami HO, Baron JA, et al. Use of oral contraceptives and endometrial cancer risk (Sweden). Cancer Causes Control 1999;10:277–84.

33. Silverberg SG, Makowski EL. Endometrial carcinoma in young women taking oral contraceptive agents. Obstet Gynecol 1975;46:503–6.

34. Lumbiganon P. Depot-medroxyprogesterone acetate (DMPA) and cancer of the endometrium and ovary. Contraception 1994;49:203–9.

35. Castellsauge X, Thompson WD, Dubrow R. Tubal sterilization and the risk of endometrial cancer. Int J Cancer 1996; 65:607–12.

36. Lacey JV Jr, Brinton LA, Mortel R, et al. Tubal sterilization and risk of cancer of the endometrium. Gynecol Oncol 2000; 79:482–4.

37. Sturgeon SR, Brinton LA, Berman ML, et al. Intrauterine device use and endometrial cancer risk. Int J Epidemiol 1997;26:496–500.

38. Grady D, Gebretsadik T, Kerlikowske K, et al. Hormone replacement therapy and endometrial cancer risk: a meta-analysis. Obstet Gynecol 1995;85:304–13.

39. Horwitz R, Feinsterin A. Alternative analytic methods for case-control studies of estrogens and endometrial cancer. N Engl J Med 1978;299:1089–94.

40. Weiderpass E, Baron JA, Adami HO, et al. Low-potency oestrogen and risk of endometrial cancer: a case-control study. Lancet 1999;353:1824–8.

41. Cushing KL, Weiss NS, Voigt LF, et al. Risk of endometrial cancer in relation to use of low-dose, unopposed estrogens. Obstet Gynecol 1998;91:35–9.

42. Johnson EB, Muto MG, Yanushpolsky EH, Mutter GL. Phytoestrogen supplementation and endometrial cancer. Obstet Gynecol 2001;98:947–50.

43. Beresford SAA, Weiss NS, Voigt LF, McKnight B. Risk of endometrial cancer in relation to use of oestrogen combined with cyclic progestogen therapy in postmenopausal women. Lancet 1997;349:458–61.

44. Pike MC, Peters RK, Cozen W, et al. Estrogen-progestin replacement therapy and endometrial cancer. J Natl Cancer Inst 1997;89:1110–6.

45. Weiderpass E, Adami HO, Baron JA, et al. Risk of endometrial cancer following estrogen replacement with and without progestins. J Natl Cancer Inst 1999;91:1131–7.

46. Whitehead MI, Townsend PT, Pryse-Davies J, et al. Effects of estrogens and progestins on the biochemistry and morphology of the postmenopausal endometrium. N Engl J Med 1981;305:1599–605.

47. The Writing Group for the PEPI Trial. Effects of hormone replacement therapy on endometrial histology in postmenopausal women. JAMA 1996;275:370–5.

48. IARC Working Group on the Evaluation of Carcinogenic Risks to Humans. Some pharmaceutical drugs. IARC monographs on the evaluation of carcinogenic risks to humans. Vol 66, 253. Lyon: World Health Organization, International Agency for Research on Cancer, 1996.

49. Cuzick J. A brief review of the current breast cancer prevention trials and proposals for future trials. Eur J Cancer 2000;36:1298–302.

50. Cummings SR, Eckert S, Krueger KA, et al. The effect of raloxifene on risk of breast cancer in postmenopausal women: results from the MORE randomized trial. Multiple Outcomes of Raloxifene Evaluation. JAMA 1999; 281:2189–97.

51. Kato I, Zeleniuch-Jacquotte A, Toniolo PG, et al. Psychotropic medication use and risk of hormone-related cancers: the New York University Women's Health Study. J Public Health Med 2000;22:155–60.

52. Potischman N, Swanson CA, Brinton LA, et al. Dietary associations in a case-control study of endometrial cancer. Cancer Causes Control 1993;4:239–50.

53. Shu XO, Zheng W, Potischman N, et al. A population-based case-control study of dietary factors and endometrial cancer in Shanghai, People's Republic of China. Am J Epidemiol 1993;137:155–65.

54. Negri E, La Vecchia C, Franceschi S, et al. Intake of selected

micronutrients and the risk of endometrial carcinoma. Cancer 1996;77:917–23.

55. Barbone F, Austin H, Partridge EE. Diet and endometrial cancer: a case-control study. Am J Epidemiol 1993;137: 393–403.

56. Levi F, La Vecchia C, Negri E, Franceschi S. Selected physical activities and the risk of endometrial cancer. Br J Cancer 1993;67:846–51.

57. Sturgeon SR, Brinton LA, Berman ML, et al. Past and present physical activity and endometrial cancer risk. Br J Cancer 1993;68:584–9.

58. Olson SH, Vena JE, Dorn JP, et al. Exercise, occupational activity and risk of endometrial cancer. Ann Epidemiol 1997;7:46–53.

59. Moradi T, Nyren O, Bergstrom R, et al. Risk for endometrial cancer in relation to occupational physical activity: a nationwide cohort study in Sweden. Int J Cancer 1998;76: 665–70.

60. Boyden TW, Pamenter RW, Stanforth P, et al. Sex steroids and endurance running in women. Fertil Steril 1983;39:629–32.

61. Reichman ME, Judd JT, Longcope C, et al. Effects of alcohol consumption on plasma and urinary hormone concentrations in premenopausal women. J Natl Cancer Inst 1993; 85:722–7.

62. Longnecker MP. Alcoholic beverage consumption in relation to risk of breast cancer; meta-analysis and review. Cancer Causes Control 1994;5:73–82.

63. Gapstur SM, Potter JD, Sellers TA, et al. Alcohol consumption and postmenopausal endometrial cancer: results from the Iowa Women's Health Study. Cancer Causes Control 1993;4:323–9.

64. Parazzini F, La Vecchia C, D'Avanzo B, et al. Alcohol and endometrial cancer risk: findings from an Italian case-control study. Nutr Cancer 1995;23:55–62.

65. Newcomb PA, Trentham-Dietz A, Storer BE. Alcohol consumption in relation to endometrial cancer risk. Cancer Epidemiol Biomarkers Prev 1997;6:775–8.

66. Michnovicz JJ, Hershcopf RJ, Naganuma H, et al. Increased 2-hydroxylation of estradiol as a possible mechanism for the anti-estrogenic effect of cigarette smoking. N Engl J Med 1986;315:1305–9.

67. Austin H, Drews C, Partridge EE. A case-control study of endometrial cancer in relation to cigarette smoking, serum estrogen levels, and alcohol use. Am J Obstet Gynecol 1993;169:1086–91.

68. Brinton LA, Barrett RJ, Berman ML, et al. Cigarette smoking and the risk of endometrial cancer. Am J Epidemiol 1993;137:281–91.

69. Weir HK, Sloan M, Kreiger N. The relationship between cigarette smoking and the risk of endometrial neoplasms. Int J Epidmiol 1994;23:261–6.

70. Lucero J, Harlow BL, Barbieri RL, et al. Early follicular phase hormone levels in relation to patterns of alcohol, tobacco, and coffee use. Fertil Steril 2001;76:723–9.

71. Terry P, Vainio H, Wolk A, Welderpass E. Dietary factors in relation to endometrial cancer: a nationwide case-control study in Sweden. Nutrition & Cancer 2002;42:25–32.

72. Petridou E, Koukoulomatis P, Dessypris N, et al. Why is endometrial cancer less common in Greece than in other European Union countries? European J Cancer Prevention 2002;11:427–32.

73. Parazzini F, La Vecchia C, Moroni S, et al. Family history and the risk of endometrial cancer. Int J Cancer 1994;59: 460–2.

74. Gruber SB, Thompson WD. A population based study of endometrial cancer and familial risk in younger women. Cancer and Steroid Hormone Study Group. Cancer Epidemiol Biomarkers Prev 1996;5:411–7.

2

Molecular Pathogenesis of Endometrial Cancer

GEORGE L. MUTTER, MD

TAN A. INCE, MD, PhD

Genetic changes that cause endometrial cancer may be discovered by simple comparison of tumor with normal tissues and correlating clinicopathologic features with genotypic features. More difficult is the specific elaboration of those interacting events that may transpire in a particular sequence during a protracted interval of carcinogenesis. A small burden of premalignant cells makes them elusive targets for study, and their histopathologic plasticity complicates achieving diagnostic consensus and reproducibility among laboratories. Despite these formidable obstacles, the last decade has seen an explosion of new data regarding endometrial carcinogenesis. Cancer subtypes have been clearly divided along genetic and clinical lines, and a flood of information about genetic changes that cause endometrial cancer has been forthcoming from many sources, including nongynecologic tumor systems. The diagnosis of premalignant endometrial lesions, historically a confusing and contentious issue among pathologists, has achieved objectivity from biomarker studies and histomorphometric analysis. These data have yielded a scientific basis for standardization and revision of endometrial precancer diagnosis in a routine diagnostic setting. Lastly, experimental access to preclinical stages of premalignant endometrial disease, a phase of tumorigenesis that is the probable target of endocrine-associated risk factors, affords an opportunity for designing and evaluating cancer chemoprevention strategies.

GENETIC SUBGROUPS OF ENDOMETRIAL CANCER

Sporadic endometrial adenocarcinoma may be classified into dichotomous genotypic classes defined by polarized frequencies of inactivation of specific genes (Table 2–1). These genetic pathways of endometrial carcinogenesis are generally paralleled by endometrioid (type 1) and nonendometrioid (type 2) subtypes that comprise distinct clinicopathologic entities.[1–3] Approximately 70 to 80% of newly diagnosed cases of endometrial cancer in the United States are of endometrioid histology. Type 1 cancers have been associated with unopposed estrogen exposure and are often preceded by premalignant disease. Progression to carcinoma is highly inefficient, involving complex interactions between multiple genetic events (*PTEN*, K-*ras*, microsatellite instability) and ambient hormonal selection factors. In contrast, type 2 endometrial cancers have papillary serous or clear cell histology with a very aggressive clinical course. Hormonal risk factors have not been identified, nor have other nonhormonal factors become evident; there is no readily observed premalignant phase. Type 2 tumors characteristically present as fully developed malignancies and have *P53* tumor-suppressor gene defects. For purposes of discussion, type 1 and type 2 sporadic endometrial adenocarcinoma might just as well be considered separate diseases.

Table 2–1. ALTERED GENE FUNCTION IN SPORADIC ENDOMETRIOID AND NONENDOMETRIOID ENDOMETRIAL ADENOCARCINOMA				
Gene	Alteration	Endometrioid (%)	Nonendometrioid (%)	Refs
P53	Mutation	5–10	80–90	90,91
PTEN	Loss of function	55–83	11	5,25
K-ras	Mutational activation	13–26	0–10	15,63,90
β-Catenin	Mutation (immunoreactive)	25–38	Rare	63
MLH1	Microsatellite instability (epigenetic silencing)	17	5	33,35
P27	Loss of function	68–81	76	20
Cyclin D1	Increased expression	41–56	19	20
P16	Loss of function	20–34	10	20
RB	Loss of function	3–4	10	20
BCL2	Loss of function	65	67	15
BAX	Loss of function	48	43	15
Estrogen and progesterone receptors	Positive immunoreactivity	70–73	19–24	15

A third group are those rare endometrial adenocarcinomas that present as a manifestation of multi-cancer heritable syndromes (Table 2–2) (see Chapter 3).[4] The low frequency with which these are encountered in clinical practice belies their high level of scientific interest, as familial presentation affords unique opportunities to dissect those causal genetic events that may also be effective in a sporadic setting. The *PTEN* inactivation seen in Cowden disease and DNA mismatch repair defects of hereditary nonpolyposis colon cancer are frequent accompaniments to sporadic endometrial carcinogenesis.[5–11]

An overview of the most prevalent genetic changes in endometrial carcinoma can be obtained by detailed review of a relatively small number of individual genetic changes.

P53

P53 is a tumor-suppressor gene that is inactivated in half of all malignant human tumors.[12] As a multifunctional transcription factor, *P53* plays a central role in cell cycle regulation and apoptosis pathways. Despite substantial effort, it has not always been possible to link *P53* mutations with a particular histologic pattern or clinical outcome in many tumor types. Endometrial cancer is one of the exceptions, in which *P53* mutations are almost exclusively associated with a specific histologic subtype and not distributed stochastically among half the cases. Type 2 tumors, particularly serous papillary or clear cell histology, frequently (> 90%) harbor *P53* mutations.[13] A much lower *P53* mutational rate in type 1 tumors (< 10%) makes *P53* a useful molecular marker that distinguishes type 1 from type 2 endometrial cancers.[14–17]

In most studies, *P53* mutations have been detected by immunohistochemical staining of paraffin sections from endometrial cancers. Because wild-type *P53* is below detection levels and most mutations stabilize the protein causing its accumulation to a detectable level, positive staining has been used as an indication of a *P53* mutation. However, this interpretation is complicated by a few biologic factors. Whereas most *P53* mutations are missense mutations that lead to the accumulation of the mutant protein, a distinct subset are nonsense mutations or deletions that will be missed by this approach. In addition, wild-type *P53* can be induced to a detectable level in the absence of a mutation. For

Table 2–2. HERITABLE CONDITIONS ASSOCIATED WITH ENDOMETRIAL CANCER			
Condition	Gene(s)	Phenotype	Refs
Cowden disease	PTEN	Endometrial, endocrine, breast cancer	5
Hereditary nonpolyposis colon cancer	Mismatch repair MLH1, MSH2, MSH6	Colon, endometrial cancer	33,91,92

Adapted from Lynch HT et al.[6]

example, DNA damage in the case of radiation therapy can induce expression.[18,19] Altered expression of *MDM2* and *P15 ARF*, that regulate *P53* levels have been shown to cause detectable levels of *P53* in the absence of a mutation.[20,21]

Moreover, descriptive reporting of scattered positive P53 immunostaining has been misleading in that the clonal nature of the *P53* mutation is not considered in interpreting the results. Only diffuse and uniform (meaning an early mutation present in all tumor cells) or geographic focal clonal staining (meaning a second clonal event within the tumor) is biologically meaningful and useful in distinguishing the two endometrial cancer types (Figure 2–1). Therefore, a conventional descriptive scoring method used for most other immunostains in pathology (mild, moderate, severe, and so on) is inappropriate for *P53*.

For the above reasons, some of the earlier reports on *P53* found a less distinct difference between type 1 and type 2 endometrial carcinomas.[22] However, it is becoming evident now that this gene is almost exclusively mutated in type 2 endometrial cancers. In rare cases, when p53 protein is detected in type 1 cancers, it is generally not due to mutation.[20,21]

PTEN

Inactivation of the *PTEN* tumor-suppressor gene (formerly known as *MMAC1*) is the most common genetic defect in endometrial carcinoma. The PTEN

protein product is a dual specificity phosphatase, which acts to suppress cell division and enable apoptosis via an AKT-dependent pathway.[23,24] *PTEN* inactivation may be caused by a variety of mechanisms, including mutation or deletion.[5] Reported rates of *PTEN* inactivation in individual patient series are highly affected by the mix of tumor subtypes assembled and whether gene function is assessed by deletion (loss of heterozygosity) mutation or the presence of PTEN protein. Loss of *PTEN* function is most prevalent in the endometrioid subtype of endometrial cancers, reaching a peak rate of 83% in those tumors preceded by a histologically discrete premalignant phase.[25]

Additional support for *PTEN* inactivation in the genesis of endometrial cancers has been forthcoming from *PTEN* knockout mice and human syndromes caused by germline *PTEN* inactivation. Heterozygous *PTEN* inactivation produces an abnormal endometrial phenotype in mice, with 100% of mice developing hyperplastic lesions and 20% of animals progressing to endometrial carcinoma.[26] Humans with constitutive germline *PTEN* mutations may present with the heritable cancer syndrome of Cowden disease, which includes high rates of breast, thyroid, and other cancers in conjunction with hamartomas of multiple organs.[5,27] There appears to be an increased risk of endometrial cancer in women with Cowden disease, but only small numbers of these patients have been available for study, and the mag-

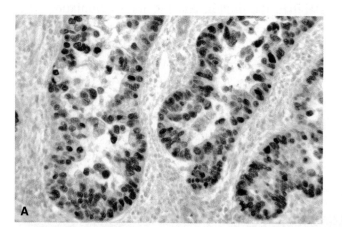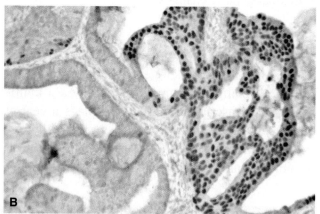

Figure 2–1.   P53 immunohistochemistry in endometrial adenocarcinomas. *A*, Mutant P53 protein in papillary serous type 2 endometrial adenocarcinoma presents as strong nuclear staining in a widespread distribution, indicating that *P53* mutation was present throughout tumor growth. In contrast, a geographic zone of *P53* staining (*B, right*) in a type 1 endometrioid carcinoma has emerged as a new subclone from a larger field of *P53*-negative (*B, left*) tumor. Accumulation of *P53* protein in endometrioid tumors is usually not due to mutation of the *P53* gene itself but rather changes in regulators of *P53* (P53 immunohistochemistry with monoclonal antibody [murine monoclonal *P53*-1801] diaminobenzidine detection and methyl green counterstain [×200 magnification]).

nitude of increased risk is modest. It is reasonable, therefore, to conclude that in humans, nongenetic factors combined with additional (non-*PTEN*) gene inactivation events are codeterminants of endometrial cancer risk.

Approximately a third of inactivated *PTEN* alleles in sporadic endometrial cancer are deletions involving chromosomal location 10q23. Detailed mapping of the long arm of chromosome 10 in endometrial cancers suggested the possibility that additional closely linked tumor suppressors might be deleted with *PTEN*.[28,29] The homeodomain containing the gene *EMX2* is a strong candidate for just such as gene.[30] Increased native *EMX2* expression is associated with diminished endometrial proliferative activity, a pattern that might be predicted for a tumor suppressor. Deletion of *EMX2*, with commensurate decline in expression, is seen in some endometrial adenocarcinomas.[30]

MICROSATELLITE INSTABILITY

Female carriers of the gene mutations associated with hereditary nonpolyposis colon cancer (HNPCC) syndrome have an extremely high cumulative incidence of endometrial cancer, estimated at 22 to 43%.[31] Patients with HNPCC have destabilization of small tandem repeats, referred to as microsatellite instability.[32] This is caused by structural defects in deoxyribonucleic acid (DNA) mismatch repair genes, such as *MLH1*, *MSH2*, and *MSH6*, which prevent replication repair of hairpin loops that form preferentially within palindromic or repetitive DNA sequences.[33] The microsatellite instability phenotype, manifest as a change in the number of repeat units within individual microsatellites, is seen in benign and malignant tissues, including the resultant endometrial cancers of HNPCC women.[9,33]

Microsatellite instability is not specific to familial forms of endometrial cancer but also accompanies 17 to 23% of sporadic endometrial carcinomas.[9–11,34,35] The cause of instability differs, however, as sporadic endometrial cancers with microsatellite instability infrequently contain mutations of mismatch repair genes that have been seen in hereditary (HNPCC) endometrial cancers.[36–38] Rather, sporadic endometrial cancers acquire microsatellite instability through epigenetic inactivation of the *MLH1* gene—a change not evident in the usual mutational screens initially used to query the functional integrity of *MLH1*.[33,37]

The manner in which microsatellite instability influences cellular function is complex. It is a widespread process that affects a large number of DNA motifs widely distributed throughout the genome. Secondary inactivation of specific genes may be accomplished by alteration of repeat sequences in coding regions, epigenetic inactivation of expanded microsatellites in regulatory domains, or a hypermutable state in nonrepeat areas.[39,40] The effects of microsatellite instability in endometrial carcinoma are not mediated by *P53*, K-*ras*, or *PTEN* inactivation, as changes in these genes are comparable in microsatellite unstable and stable cancers.[41,42]

Microsatellite instability is more common in endometrioid endometrial adenocarcinomas (17–19%) compared with nonendometrioid carcinomas (5–8%).[35,43] Population-specific or interstudy differences in the microsatellite instability rates of endometrial cancer are, thus, expected when the compared groups do not have the same mix of histologic types, confounding attempts to correlate this phenotype with overall survival.[43,44] In general, larger studies have not confirmed the survival predictive value of microsatellite instability.[43,45]

PREMALIGNANT PHASES OF (TYPE 1) ENDOMETRIOID ENDOMETRIAL CARCINOGENESIS

Current molecular techniques that have been informative in identifying precursor lesions to endometrial carcinoma include mutational and clonal analysis.[46] Comparison of precursor lesion genotype and clonal composition to that of matched carcinomas in individual patients enables establishment of lineage continuity between premalignant and malignant phases of endometrial carcinogenesis. Precursor lesions identified in this manner have acquired monoclonal genetic features (mutations, nonrandom X-chromosome inactivation, altered microsatellites) that differentiate them from neighboring normal tissues, but they have not acquired the full complement of changes necessary for the malignant phenotype

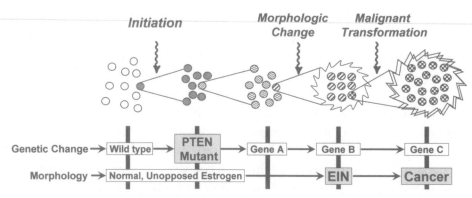

Figure 2–2. Clonal model of endometrial carcinogenesis. Endometrioid endometrial (type 1) adeno-carcinomas arise by successive genetic events that accumulate within nested hierarchical subclones of mutant cells. Starting from a polyclonal field of cells with a wild-type genotype (*left, open circles*), initiation by inactivation of the *PTEN* tumor-suppressor gene is not accompanied by any change in light microscopic histology. Patches of sparsely distributed PTEN-mutant glands are indistinguishable from those morphologically identical wild-type glands with which they are intermingled. This "latent," or subclinical, precancer phase converts to a clinically detectable stage when additional mutations produce a change in cytology and gland architecture diagnostic of endometrial intraepithelial neoplasia (EIN). Contiguous growth of closely packed glands in EIN lesions is due to an expansile localized geometry of mutant glands derived from a common progenitor (monoclonal). The number and specific identity of genetic changes necessary for progression to carcinoma are unknown, and are arbitrarily shown as "Genes A–C." Early events preceding morphologic change include microsatellite instability and *PTEN* inactivation. Less is known about subsequent events, which may include K-*ras* inactivation.

(Figure 2–2).[25,34,47–51] The monoclonal properties of histologically diagnosable precursors of a malignant phenotype (referred to as "precursor lesions") are a generalizable phenomenon, having been confirmed in premalignant tissues at a wide variety of tissue sites, including the vulva, cervix, oral mucosa, and esophagus.[52–55] The degree of elevated cancer risk conferred by a precursor lesion must be clinically defined at each specific site and probably changes dynamically with progression through a protracted and multistep premalignant phase. Changes in endometrial precursor lesion histopathology that accompany this process, which may be of practical use in stratifying cancer risk, are discussed below.

The high frequency and protracted course of premalignant disease that occur in endometrioid adeno-carcinomas are not seen in nonendometrioid endometrial cancers. More common in nonendometrioid tumors is the secondary surface spread of malignant cells (Figure 2–3), a condition that should not be construed as a premalignant state because it is not genetically different from the coexisting carcinomas and rarely occurs in the absence of a frank carcinoma elsewhere in the uterus.

Loss of *PTEN* function through mutation and/or deletion is the earliest known event in endometrial

carcinogenesis and is a biomarker for the detection of affected glands.[25,56] In the manner of a true "gatekeeper," *PTEN* expression is lost at the inception of clonal outgrowth in cells that are histologically indistinguishable from their normal companions and are dispersed in small patches within the polyclonal source field.[57] Immunohistochemical staining for PTEN protein in archival paraffin-embedded endometrial tissues is a highly sensitive method to identify these patches in routine pathologic materials.[58] A surprisingly high fraction, 43%, of endogenously cycling premenopausal women with a normal proliferative endometrium have acquired small numbers of PTEN-defective endometrial glands, which, on genetic analysis, bear sequence-confirmed *PTEN* mutations or deletions of 10q23 (Figure 2–4).[56] These PTEN-defective endometrial glands are incompletely shed during menses, growing out as morphologically unremarkable glands with each subsequent cycle. Exposure to estrogens unopposed by progestins produces a characteristic series of histologic changes in the endometrium, ranging from occasional glandular cystic dilatation to gland branching and thrombosis-induced foci of stromal breakdown. These endometria, which are variably diagnosed by pathologists as "anovulatory," "disor-

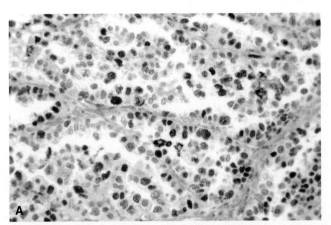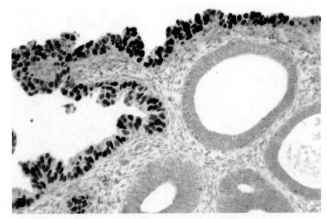

Figure 2–3. Surface spread of P53 mutant clear cell endometrial adenocarcinoma. *A,* Clear cell endometrial adenocarcinoma with nuclear P53 staining. *B,* Adjacent to invasive tumor, the uterine luminal surface has been overrun by malignant cells that stand out from subjacent benign glands. Surface spread is common in patients with invasive nonendometrioid endometrial carcinoma and does not necessarily represent an earlier stage of tumorigenesis. (P53 immunohistochemistry with monoclonal antibody [murine monoclonal P53-1801] diaminobenzidine detection and methyl green counterstain [×200 magnification].)

dered proliferative," or "simple nonatypical hyperplasias," have architectural changes uniformly distributed throughout in a nonlocalizing manner. Approximately half of these endometria have scattered, rare PTEN-null glands, presumably having been present prior to the onset of the hormonal imbalance.[56] PTEN-null glands of anovulatory endometria have a cytology and architecture that exactly matches that of their PTEN-expressing companion glands, including a similar extent of dilatation, branching, and tubal change. These preclinical phases of carcinogenesis are so frequent that they can be construed as a normal background event.

Progression of subclinical, or "latent," precursor lesions is highly inefficient and involves successive accumulation of additional genetic damage that culminates in an altered subclone with aberrant histomorphology and growth (see Figures 2–2 and 2–4). The point of origin of this subclone becomes the epicenter of an expanding localizing endometrial lesion that may be recognized by its altered cytology and crowded architecture. This is the stage at which pathologists are able to diagnose an atypical endometrial hyperplasia, and clonal analysis of physically contiguous glands confirms them to be derived from a common progenitor. Atypical endometrial hyperplasias have many of the genetic features seen in subsequent carcinomas including K-*ras* mutation, microsatellite instability, and β-catenin mutations.[34,47,49,59–64] Over half the atypical hyperplasias are

PTEN-null, and, in informative cases, the immunohistochemical staining pattern shows tight clusters of PTEN-null glands with an abnormal cytology.

CLINICAL IMPLICATIONS OF A REVISED CARCINOGENESIS MODEL

The current World Health Organization (WHO) endometrial hyperplasia diagnostic schema was developed at a time when the clonal origin of premalignant disease was unappreciated, and the only method to experimentally demonstrate a premalignant phenotype was to follow groups of patients and measure cancer incidence.[65] Histopathologic correlation with cancer outcome was a statistical process that failed to provide definitive classification of individual cases. With the advent of reliable markers for those features that characterize premalignant disease (presence of mutations, clonal pattern of growth), it became possible to resolve questions of classification in individual cases and assemble prototypical collections of genetically defined precancers.[66] These are valuable resources for de novo discovery of those histopathologic features that are pathognomonic of endometrial precursor lesions.

The selective growth advantage of monoclonal precursor lesions explains why the first histopathologic changes present in a localizing fashion. This contrasts with the global field effects of unopposed estrogens and the diffuse intermingling of patches of

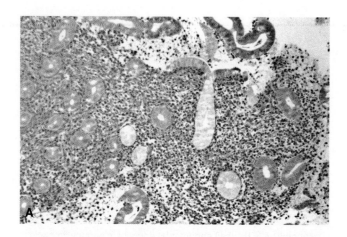

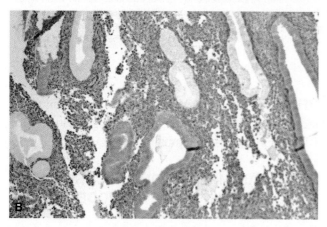

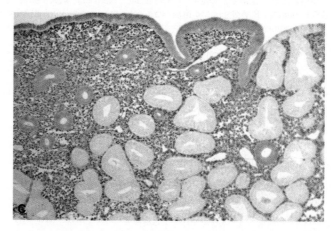

Figure 2–4. Emergent PTEN-null clones in endometrial carcinogenesis. PTEN-null glands (*pale*) are offset by PTEN-expressing glands (*brown*) in normal proliferative (*A*), anovulatory (*B*), and endometrial intraepithelial neoplasia (EIN) (*C*) endometria. The histology of PTEN-null glands is identical to that of PTEN-expressing glands in normal proliferative and anovulatory endometria. The PTEN-null glands of EIN lesions tend to be packed together in a focus (*C, center and right*) offset from the background of *PTEN*-expressing normal glands (*C, upper left*). Within the EIN area, gland area exceeds that of stroma, and cytology is altered. (PTEN immunohistochemistry with monoclonal antibody [murine monoclonal 6h2.1] diaminobenzidine detection and methyl green counterstain [×100 magnification]).

mutant cells with those normal tissues from which they are indistinguishable. Monoclonal putative endometrial precancers with acquired genetic changes that can be matched (in the same patient) to subsequent (type 1) endometrial cancers have undergone objective computerized morphometry to define their structural characteristics.[48] This morphometry disclosed that a very specific architectural change was highly associated with premalignant disease, namely, glandular crowding to the extent that the gland area exceeds that of the stroma. Cytology in the crowded focus always differs from that of the uncrowded background, suggesting that a relative internal comparison standard for judging cytologic "atypia" may be more reliable than a fixed or stereotypic cytologic standard. The idea that lesion architecture and cytology are codeterminants of premalignant behavior is quite contrary to the previous emphasis on cytology alone as the dominant predictor of endometrial cancer risk.[67]

A pitfall in using laboratory end points alone to define premalignant disease is that they may quickly become self-serving and fail to provide compelling evidence of increased cancer risk. There are established histomorphometric data of objectively measurable features of routine hematoxylin-eosin–stained endometrial histology that indicate an increase prospective clinical endometrial cancer risk.[68–70] Three features measured by computerized image analysis, when algorithmically reduced to a "D-score," are highly sensitive and specific in the prediction of future or concurrent endometrial cancer. Application of this objective image analysis procedure to a series of endometrial tissues of known clonal composition has confirmed that monoclonal precursor lesions have a histopathology identical to that known to increase endometrial cancer risk.[48] These lesions have been designated endometrial intraepithelial neoplasia or EIN, and criteria for their routine diagnosis by practicing pathologists are clearly specified (Table 2–3).[46,71–73] It has been proposed that EIN lesions should be treated with hormonal or surgical therapeutic ablation, which is currently applied to the diagnoses of atypical endometrial hyperplasia.

Table 2–3. ENDOMETRIAL INTRAEPITHELIAL NEOPLASIA: HISTOPATHOLOGIC PRESENTATION OF GENETICALLY DEFINED PREMALIGNANT ENDOMETRIAL LESIONS THAT CONFER INCREASED RISK OF CARCINOMA

EIN Diagnostic Criterion	Comments
1. Architecture	Area of glands exceeds that of stroma. Most often focal.
2. Cytologic change	Cytology is different in focus of crowded glands compared with background.
3. Size	Maximum dimension should exceed 1 mm. Smaller lesions have unknown clinical course.
4. Exclude benign mimics	Normal secretory, basalis, lower uterine segment, endometrial polyps, reparative changes, cystic atrophy, tangential sections, disruption artifact, etc.
5. Exclude cancer	Carcinoma if there are solid areas of epithelial growth, glands are mazelike and "rambling," or there is significant cribriforming

Genetically altered endometrial cells, which have not yet progressed to the point where they demonstrate the histopathologic features of EIN (see Table 2–3), have an undefined clinical outcome and, thus, no current basis to justify therapeutic intervention. Generally, this phase of disease is only discernible with specialized studies, such as PTEN immunohistochemistry, which, as stated previously, will disclose PTEN-null glands in almost half of normal women. Monitoring of this preclinical interval is of great interest in a research setting where protective effects of experimental therapies might be detected by changes in the prevalence or physical configuration of mutant cells.

ENDOCRINE MODIFIERS

Estrogens that are not opposed by the counterbalancing effects of progestins confer an increased risk of endometrioid (type 1) endometrial adenocarcinoma (also see Chapter 1).[74–77] Relevant exposures include hormone replacement therapy, excessive peripheral conversion in obesity, and endogenous production by estrogenic ovarian tumors or polycystic ovarian disease. The level of increased cancer risk is dependent on estrogen dose and duration, ranging from three- to 10-fold. Estrogen risks are obviated by the addition of progestins, such as medroxyprogesterone acetate, which protects against the development of endometrial hyperplasia and when administered in a combined low-dose oral contraceptive formulation may reduce endometrial cancer risk below that of the population background.[78–81]

Despite extensive epidemiologic data linking estrogens to increased endometrial cancer rates, there is surprisingly little evidence of those specific cellular mechanisms that are responsible. In some models, estrogens are thought to increase the rate of mutagenesis, but this is probably a very small effect.[82] Estrogens may indirectly elevate the endometrial mutational rate by increasing proliferative activity in general. The basal frequency with which new mutations arise through random mutagenesis is a combined function of field size and cell division rate.[83,84] Given a random mutagenesis rate of 10^{-7} per gene per cell division and an average menstrual cycle that regenerates over 10^9 cells (several grams at 10^9 cells/gram), each cycle produces hundreds of cells mutated for any selected gene.[83] Limiting conditions are those that define an advantage for a particular mutation, thereby allowing proliferation to a sufficient cell number so that a superimposed second hit can occur.[85,86] Estrogens may define just such an advantage for the *PTEN* gene, where physiologic expression in endometrial glands is high under estrogen-dominated conditions (Figure 2–5).[87] PTEN-null endometrial cells would be unable to exert the tumor-suppressor functions normally required in such a proliferative estrogenic state, thereby defining a growth advantage. In contrast, loss of PTEN function in a progesterone-rich environment may have few effects, as normal, genetically intact endometrial glands shut down expression of PTEN in that circumstance.

Large-scale expression profiling of endometrial tissue ribonucleic acids (RNAs) has enabled global comparisons of hormonal changes with those of malignant transformation.[88] Malignant (type 1 endometrioid) endometrial tissues most closely mimic the expression profile of estrogen-driven

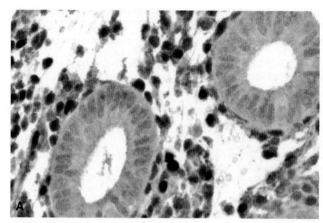
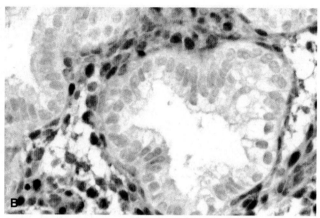

Figure 2–5. Hormonal regulation of endometrial glandular PTEN expression. *A,* PTEN protein (*brown*) is abundant under the dominant influence of estrogens in normal proliferative endometrial glands. *B,* After several days of progesterone exposure, midsecretory endometrial glands demonstrate a decline in PTEN abundance. (PTEN immunohistochemistry with monoclonal antibody [murine monoclonal 6h2.1] diaminobenzidine detection and methyl green counterstain [×200 magnification].)

normal proliferative endometrium and specifically fail to express most genes that increase in activity in normal secretory endometrium on progesterone exposure. Overall, loss of gene expression in cancers is the predominant alteration of neoplastic transformation, accounting for 8 of 10 discriminating changes in RNA abundance. Among the group of genes with reduced or lost expression in carcinoma are a small number of primarily inactivated tumor-supressor genes and a larger number of secondary effects not associated with primary mutation or deletion.[89]

Persistence of premalignant disease and its progression to carcinoma are heavily modified by endometrial tissue shedding and competitive remodeling. Precancers located within a noncycling endometrial compartment, such as the endometrial basalis or a hormonally nonresponsive endometrial polyp, are unlikely to be shed during a regular menstrual cycle. Correspondingly, unopposed estrogens prolong the interval between shedding episodes and do so under conditions that favor the outgrowth of precursor lesions. These considerations must be taken into account in devising a comprehensive picture of the evolution of what is an inherently unstable process. Although it is tempting to believe that the secrets of carcinogenesis will be discovered using high-resolution molecular tools, the regional context of complex tissue interactions should not be overlooked.

REFERENCES

1. Sherman ME, Sturgeon S, Brinton L, Kurman RJ. Endometrial cancer chemoprevention: implications of diverse pathways of carcinogenesis. J Cell Biochem 1995;59 Suppl 23:160–4.

2. Bokhman J. Two pathogenetic types of endometrial carcinoma. Gynecol Oncol 1983;15:10–7.

3. Deligdisch L, Holinka C. Endometrial carcinoma: two diseases? Cancer Detect Prev 1987;10:237–46.

4. Gruber S, Thompson W. A population based study of endometrial cancer and familial risk in younger women. Cancer Epidemiol Biomarkers Prev 1996;5:411–7.

5. Mutter GL. PTEN, a protean tumor suppressor. Am J Pathol 2001;158:1895–8.

6. Lynch HT, Casey MJ, Shaw TG, Lynch JF. Hereditary factors in gynecologic cancer. Oncologist 1998;3(5):319–38.

7. Risinger JI, Hayes AK, Berchuck A, Barrett JC. PTEN/MMAC1 mutations in endometrial cancers. Cancer Res 1997;57(21):4736–8.

8. Tashiro H, Blazes MS, Wu R, et al. Mutations in PTEN are frequent in endometrial carcinoma but rare in other common gynecological malignancies. Cancer Res 1997;57:3935–40.

9. Risinger JI, Berchuck A, Kohler MF, et al. Genetic instability of microsatellites in endometrial carcinoma. Cancer Res 1993;53:5100–3.

10. Burks RT, Kessis TD, Cho KR, Hedrick L. Microsatellite instability in endometrial carcinoma. Oncogene 1994;9:1163–6.

11. Duggan BD, Felix JC, Muderspach LI, et al. Microsatellite instability in sporadic endometrial carcinoma. J Natl Cancer Inst 1994;86:1216–21.

12. Soussil T, Berroud C. Assessing TP53 status in human tumours to evaluate clinical outcome. Nat Rev Cancer 2001;1:233–9.

13. Rose P. Endometrial carcinoma. N Engl J Med 1996;335:640–9.

14. Lax SF, Kendall B, Tashiro H, et al. The frequency of P53, K-ras mutations, and microsatellite instability differs in uterine endometrioid and serous carcinoma: evidence of distinct molecular genetic pathways. Cancer 2000;88(4):814–24.

15. Kounelis S, Kapranos N, Kouri E, et al. Immunohistochemical profile of endometrial adenocarcinoma: a study of 61 cases and review of the literature. Mod Pathol 2000;13(4):379–88.

16. Geisler JP, Geisler HE, Wiemann MC, et al. P53 expression as a prognostic indicator of 5-year survival in endometrial cancer. Gynecol Oncol 1999;74(3):468–71.

17. Kohlberger P, Gitsch G, Loesch A, et al. P53 protein overexpression in early stage endometrial cancer. Gynecol Oncol 1996;62(2):213–7.

18. MacCallum DE, Hupp TR. Induction of P53 protein as a marker for ionizing radiation exposure in vivo. Methods Mol Biol 1999;113:583–9.

19. Lu X, Lane DP. Differential induction of transcriptionally active P53 following UV or ionizing radiation: defects in chromosome instability syndromes? Cell 1993;75(4):765–78.

20. Schmitz MJ, Hendricks DT, Farley J, et al. p27 and cyclin D1 abnormalities in uterine papillary serous carcinoma. Gynecol Oncol 2000;77(3):439–45.

21. Soslow RA, Shen PU, Chung MH, Isacson C. Distinctive P53 and mdm2 immunohistochemical expression profiles suggest different pathogenetic pathways in poorly differentiated endometrial carcinoma. Int J Gynecol Pathol 1998;17(2):129–34.

22. Geisler JP, Wiemann MC, Zhou Z, et al. P53 as a prognostic indicator in endometrial cancer. Gynecol Oncol 1996;61(2):245–8.

23. Kurose K, Zhou X, Araki T, et al. Frequent loss of PTEN expression is linked to elevated phosphorylated Akt levels, but not associated with p27 and cyclin D1 expression, in primary epithelial ovarian carcinomas. Am J Pathol 2001;158:2097–106.

24. Zhu X, Kwon CH, Schlosshauer PW, et al. PTEN induces G1 cell cycle arrest and decreases cyclin D3 levels in endometrial carcinoma cells. Cancer Res 2001;61(11):4569–75.

25. Mutter GL, Lin MC, Fitzgerald JT, et al. Altered PTEN expression as a diagnostic marker for the earliest endometrial precancers. J Natl Cancer Inst 2000;92:924–30.

26. Stambolic V, Tsao MS, Macpherson D, et al. High incidence of breast and endometrial neoplasia resembling human Cowden syndrome in PTEN+/– mice. Cancer Res 2000;60(13):3605–11.

27. Eng C. Will the real Cowden syndrome please stand up: revised diagnostic criteria. J Med Genet 2000;37(11):828–30.

28. Simpkins SB, Peiffer-Schneider S, Mutch DG, et al. PTEN mutations in endometrial cancers with 10q LOH: additional evidence for the involvement of multiple tumor suppressors. Gynecol Oncol 1998;71(3):391–5.

29. Peiffer SL, Herzog TJ, Tribune DJ, et al. Allelic loss of sequences from the long arm of chromosome 10 and replication errors in endometrial cancers. Cancer Res 1995;55:1922–6.

30. Noonan FC, Mutch DG, Ann MM, Goodfellow PJ. Characterization of the homeodomain gene emx2: sequence con-

servation, expression analysis, and a search for mutations in endometrial cancers. Genomics 2001;76(1–3):37–44.

31. Millar AL, Pal T, Madlensky L, et al. Mismatch repair gene defects contribute to the genetic basis of double primary cancers of the colorectum and endometrium. Hum Mol Genet 1999;8(5):823–9.

32. Aaltonen LA, Peltomaki P, Mecklin JP, et al. Replication errors in benign and malignant tumors from hereditary nonpolyposis colorectal cancer patients. Cancer Res 1994;54:1645–8.

33. Esteller M, Levine R, Baylin SB, et al. MLH1 promoter hypermethylation is associated with the microsatellite instability phenotype in sporadic endometrial carcinomas. Oncogene 1998;17:2413–7.

34. Mutter GL, Boynton KA, Faquin WC, et al. Allelotype mapping of unstable microsatellites establishes direct lineage continuity between endometrial precancers and cancer. Cancer Res 1996;56:4483–6.

35. Faquin WC, Fitzgerald JT, Lin MC, et al. Sporadic microsatellite instability is specific to neoplastic and preneoplastic endometrial tissues. Am J Clin Pathol 2000;113(4):576–82.

36. Risinger J, Umar A, Boyd J, et al. Mutation of MSH3 in endometrial cancer and evidence for its functional role in heteroduplex repair. Nat Genet 1996;14:102–5.

37. Kowalski LD, Mutch DG, Herzog TJ, et al. Mutational analysis of MLH1 and MSH2 in 25 prospectively-acquired RER+ endometrial cancers. Genes Chromosomes Cancer 1997;18:219–27.

38. Katabuchi H, Van Rees B, Lambers AR, et al. Mutations in DNA mismatch repair genes are not responsible for microsatellite instability in most sporadic endometrial carcinomas. Cancer Res 1995;55:5556–60.

39. Parsons R, Li G, Longley M, et al. Hypermutability and mismatch repair deficiency in RER+ tumor cells. Cell 1993;75:1227–36.

40. Sutherland G, Haan E, Kremer E, et al. Hereditary unstable DNA: a new explanation for some old genetic questions? Lancet 1991;338:289–92.

41. Cohn DE, Basil JB, Venegoni AR, et al. Absence of PTEN repeat tract mutation in endometrial cancers with microsatellite instability. Gynecol Oncol 2000;79(1):101–6.

42. Swisher E, Peiffer-Schneider S, Mutch D, et al. Differences in patterns of TP53 and K-RAS2 mutations in a large series of endometrial carcinomas with or without microsatellite instability. Cancer 1999;85:119–26.

43. Basil JB, Goodfellow PJ, Rader JS, et al. Clinical significance of microsatellite instability in endometrial carcinoma. Cancer 2000;89(8):1758–64.

44. Maxwell GL, Risinger JI, Hayes KA, et al. Racial disparity in the frequency of PTEN mutations, but not microsatellite instability, in advanced endometrial cancers. Clin Cancer Res 2000;6(8):2999–3005.

45. MacDonald ND, Salvesen HB, Ryan A, et al. Frequency and prognostic impact of microsatellite instability in a large population-based study of endometrial carcinomas. Cancer Res 2000;60(6):1750–2.

46. Mutter GL. Histopathology of genetically defined endometrial precancers. Int J Gynecol Pathol 2000;19:301–9.

47. Mutter GL, Wada H, Faquin W, Enomoto T. K-ras mutations appear in the premalignant phase of both microsatellite

stable and unstable endometrial carcinogenesis. Mol Pathol 1999;52:257–62.

48. Mutter GL, Baak JPA, Crum CP, et al. Endometrial precancer diagnosis by histopathology, clonal analysis, and computerized morphometry. J Pathol 2000;190:462–9.

49. Jovanovic AS, Boynton KA, Mutter GL. Uteri of women with endometrial carcinoma contain a histopathologic spectrum of monoclonal putative precancers, some with microsatellite instability. Cancer Res 1996;56:1917–21.

50. Mutter GL, Chaponot M, Fletcher J. A PCR assay for nonrandom X chromosome inactivation identifies monoclonal endometrial cancers and precancers. Am J Pathol 1995;146:501–8.

51. Esteller M, Garcia A, Martinez-Palones JM, et al. Detection of clonality and genetic alterations in endometrial pipelle biopsy and its surgical specimen counterpart. Lab Invest 1997;76:109–16.

52. Tate JE, Mutter GL, Boynton KA, Crum CP. Monoclonal origin of vulvar intraepithelial neoplasia and some vulvar hyperplasias. Am J Pathol 1997;150:315–22.

53. Enomoto T, Haba T, Fujita M, et al. Clonal analysis of high-grade squamous intra-epithelial lesions of the uterine cervix. Int J Cancer 1997;73(3):339–44.

54. Califano J, Van der Riet P, Westra W, et al. Genetic progression model for head and neck cancer: implications for field cancerization. Cancer Res 1996;56:2488–92.

55. Zhuang Z, Vortmeyer AO, Mark EJ, et al. Barrett's esophagus: metaplastic cells with loss of heterozygosity at the APC gene locus are clonal precursors to invasive adenocarcinoma. Cancer Res 1996;56:1961–4.

56. Mutter GL, Ince TA, Baak JPA, et al. Molecular identification of latent precancers in histologically normal endometrium. Cancer Res 2001;61:4311–4.

57. Ali IU. Gatekeeper for endometrium: the PTEN tumor suppressor gene. J Natl Cancer Inst 2000;92(11):861–3.

58. Perren A, Weng L, Boag A, et al. Immunocytochemical evidence of loss of PTEN expression in primary ductal adenocarcinomas of the breast. Am J Pathol 1999;155:1253–60.

59. Enomoto T, Inoue M, Perantoni A, et al. K-ras activation in premalignant and malignant epithelial lesions of the human uterus. Cancer Res 1991;51:5304–14.

60. Sasaki H, Nishii H, Takahashi H, et al. Mutation of the Ki-ras protooncogene in human endometrial hyperplasia and carcinoma. Cancer Res 1993;53:1906–10.

61. Duggan BD, Felix JC, Muderspach LI, et al. Early mutational activation of the c-Ki-ras oncogene in endometrial carcinoma. Cancer Res 1994;54:1604–7.

62. Shibata D, Navidi W, Salovaara R, et al. Somatic microsatellite mutations as molecular tumor clocks. Nat Med 1996;2:676–81.

63. Matias-Guiu X, Catasus L, Bussaglia E, et al. Molecular pathology of endometrial hyperplasia and carcinoma. Hum Pathol 2001;32(6):569–77.

64. Saegusa M, Hashimura M, Yoshida T, Okayasu I. beta-Catenin mutations and aberrant nuclear expression during endometrial tumorigenesis. Br J Cancer 2001;84(2):209–17.

65. Scully RE, Bonfiglio TA, Kurman RJ, et al. Uterine corpus. Histological typing of female genital tract tumors. New York: Springer-Verlag; 1994. p. 13–31.

66. Mutter GL. Endometrial precancer type collection [online]. Available at: http://www.endometrium.org 2000 (accessed May 12, 2003).

67. Kurman R, Kaminski P, Norris H. The behavior of endometrial hyperplasia: a long term study of "untreated" hyperplasia in 170 patients. Cancer 1985;56:403–12.

68. Baak JPA, Nauta J, Wisse-Brekelmans E, Bezemer P. Architectural and nuclear morphometrical features together are more important prognosticators in endometrial hyperplasias than nuclear morphometrical features alone. J Pathol 1988;154:335–41.

69. Dunton C, Baak J, Palazzo J, et al. Use of computerized morphometric analyses of endometrial hyperplasias in the prediction of coexistent cancer. Am J Obstet Gynecol 1996;174:1518–21.

70. Orbo A, Baak JP, Kleivan I, et al. Computerised morphometrical analysis in endometrial hyperplasia for the prediction of cancer development. A long-term retrospective study from northern Norway. J Clin Pathol 2000;53(9):697–703.

71. Mutter GL, The Endometrial Collaborative Group. Endometrial intraepithelial neoplasia (EIN): will it bring order to chaos? Gynecol Oncol 2000;76:287–90.

72. Mutter GL. EIN central [online]. Available at: http://www.endometrium.org 2001 (accessed May 12, 2003).

73. Mutter GL. Endometrial intraepithelial neoplasia: a new standard for precancer diagnosis. Contrib Gynecol Obstet 2001;46:92–8.

74. Hulka BS. Links between hormone replacement therapy and neoplasia. Fertil Steril 1994;62 Suppl 2:168S–75S.

75. Levi F, La Vecchia C, Gulie C, et al. Oestrogen replacement treatment and the risk of endometrial cancer: an assessment of the role of covariates. Eur J Cancer 1993;29A:1445–9.

76. Parazzini F, La Vecchia C, Bocciolone L, Franceschi S. The epidemiology of endometrial cancer. Gynecol Oncol 1991;41:1–16.

77. Schottenfeld D. Epidemiology of endometrial neoplasia. J Cell Biochem 1995;59 Suppl 23:151–9.

78. Writing Group for the PEPI Trial. Effects of hormone replacement therapy on endometrial histology in postmenopausal women. The Postmenopausal Estrogen/Progestin Interventions (PEPI) Trial. JAMA 1996;275:370–5.

79. Woodruff JD, Pickar JH. Incidence of endometrial hyperplasia in postmenopausal women taking conjugated estrogens (Premarin) with medroxyprogesterone acetate or conjugated estrogens alone. Am J Obstet Gynecol 1994;170:1213–23.

80. Stanford JL, Brinton LA, Berman ML, et al. Oral contraceptives and endometrial cancer: do other risk factors modify the association. Int J Cancer 1993;54:243–8.

81. Rossouw JE, Anderson GL, Prentice RL, et al. Risks and benefits of estrogen plus progestin in healthy postmenopausal women: principal results. From the Women's Health Initiative randomized controlled trial. JAMA 2002;288:321–33.

82. Burcham PC. Internal hazards: baseline DNA damage by endogenous products of normal metabolism. Mutat Res 1999;443(1–2):11–36.

83. Jackson AL, Loeb LA. The mutation rate and cancer. Genetics 1998;148(4):1483–90.

84. Tomlinson IP, Novelli MR, Bodmer WF. The mutation rate and cancer. Proc Natl Acad Sci U S A 1996;93(25):14800–3.

85. Cairns J. Mutation and cancer: the antecedents to our studies of adaptive mutation. Genetics 1998;148(4):1433–40.

86. Rubin H. Selected cell and selective microenvironment in neoplastic development. Cancer Res 2001;61(3):799–807.

87. Mutter GL, Lin MC, Fitzgerald JT, et al. Changes in endometrial PTEN expression throughout the human menstrual cycle. J Clin Endocrinol Metab 2000;85:2334–8.

88. Mutter GL, Baak JP, Fitzgerald JT, et al. Global expression changes of constitutive and hormonally regulated genes during endometrial neoplastic transformation. Gynecol Oncol 2001;83(2):177–85.

89. Coller HA, Grandori C, Tamayo P, et al. Expression analysis with oligonucleotide microarrays reveals that MYC regulates genes involved in growth, cell cycle, signaling, and adhesion. Proc Natl Acad Sci U S A 2000;97(7):3260–5.

90. Sherman ME, Bur ME, Kurman RJ. P53 in endometrial cancer and its putative precursors: evidence for diverse pathways of tumorigenesis. Hum Pathol 1995;26:1268–74.

91. Berchuck A, Boyd J. Molecular basis of endometrial cancer. Cancer 1995;76 Suppl:2034–40.

92. Peltomaki P. Deficient DNA mismatch repair: a common etiologic factor for colon cancer. Hum Mol Genet 2001;10(7):735–40.

93. Lu KH, Broaddus RR. Gynecological tumors in hereditary nonpolyposis colorectal cancer: we know they are common—now what? Gynecol Oncol 2001;82(2):221–2.

3

Familial Endometrial Cancer

KAREN A. GRONAU, MD, MSc
JOAN MURPHY, MD, FRCSC
BARRY ROSEN, MD, FRCSC

Endometrial cancer occurs in 2.7% of women by the age of 70 years, making it the most commonly occurring gynecologic malignancy. Over the last 10 years, a hereditary component has been identified for some endometrial cancers. Most hereditary endometrial cancer occurs in families with hereditary nonpolyposis colorectal cancer (HNPCC). Endometrial cancer is the second most common cancer in women with a mutation in HNPCC genes.[1]

Some authors have proposed that endometrial cancer should be divided into two pathogenetic subtypes, each with a different prognosis. Estrogen-related endometrial cancer presents with abnormal vaginal bleeding, tends to be well differentiated histopathologically, and has an excellent prognosis after total abdominal hysterectomy.[2] Nonestrogen-related endometrial cancer is more likely to be poorly differentiated and aggressive (more often of the papillary serous or clear cell type) and, as such, carries a worse prognosis compared with the more common estrogen-related cancer (see Chapter 2).[2,3] It has been suggested that endometrial cancer in women with a genetic predisposition to it should be classified as a third subtype, which is usually diagnosed at a younger age and may or may not be estrogen related.[2,3]

This chapter will discuss genetic risk factors for endometrial cancer, the extracolonic cancer risk of HNPCC gene carriers, and the feasibility of screening for endometrial cancer.

MODIFIABLE AND NONGENETIC RISK FACTORS

Risk factors for endometrial cancer are well known and clearly defined (reviewed in Chapter 1). The most common cause of endometrial cancer is exposure to estrogen unopposed by progesterone. This estrogen can be exogenous (hormone replacement therapy, tamoxifen) or endogenous (obesity, nulliparity, late menopause, early menarche, or polycystic ovarian disease). Increased cancer risk due to unopposed estrogen is directly related to the dose of estrogen and duration of exposure and does not decline after discontinuation. Endometrial cancer is increased in populations with both diabetes and hypertension, but it is difficult to ascertain if these are independent risk factors or are related to obesity. Women with a personal history of breast or ovarian cancer are at increased risk of endometrial cancer, and this likely relates to tamoxifen therapy (see Chapter 13) and genetic risk. Atypical endometrial hyperplasia is the precursor lesion of endometrial cancer in 25% of cases (if untreated), but the time period of progression from hyperplasia to cancer is not well established.[4]

HEREDITARY NONPOLYPOSIS COLORECTAL CANCER

HNPCC or Lynch syndrome is a genetic condition accounting for 1 to 6% of all colon cancers.[5] The lifetime risk of colorectal cancer in this group is estimated to be 100%, with approximately 70% of tumors occurring in the proximal colon.[6] There are established screening and prevention protocols for those affected, involving repeated colonoscopies and prophylactic polypectomies.[7] Total colectomy is performed once colon cancer has been diagnosed in a gene carrier, as the risk of metachronous colorectal cancer is approximately 90%. The second most common metachronous cancer is endometrial cancer, and there is a 75% risk of various other metachronous cancers.[1,8]

HNPCC AND EXTRACOLONIC CANCERS

HNPCC involves two different clinical classifications. The first, Amsterdam I, has only colorectal carcinomas whereas the second, Amsterdam II, includes endometrial cancer or other adenocarcinomas along with colorectal cancer. The most common of these extracolonic cancers in women is endometrial cancer.

The risk of endometrial cancer is estimated to be as high as 30% by age 70 years for gene mutation carriers.[9] A higher incidence of 60% has been reported in a study showing a greater risk of endometrial cancer than of colon cancer (54%) in female gene carriers.[10] The age of onset of endometrial cancer in these patients is approximately 10 years younger than in the general population. The annual risk is on average, 1% between ages 40 and 60 years, and the median age at diagnosis is 49 years.[9] Therefore, the diagnosis of HNPCC should be considered in young endometrial cancer patients, and a careful family history should be obtained.[11]

A recent population-based cohort study has concluded that first-degree relatives of patients with double primary cancers of the colon and endometrium diagnosed at age < 50 years have a significantly increased risk of colon cancer or other HNPCC-associated cancers.[12] In a large Swedish database of second cancers after colorectal cancer, 100% of familial endometrial cancers came from families fulfilling the diagnostic criteria for HNPCC.[13] Some authors believe that endometrial carcinoma should be included in the main diagnostic criteria of Amsterdam II because synchronous or double primary tumors of the endometrium and colon rarely occur in non-

HNPCC families.[8] Endometrial cancer patients likely meet HNPCC diagnostic criteria in about 1% of cases.[14] Approximate risk estimates for cancers in other sites in HNPCC families are: stomach cancer, 19%; biliary tract cancer, 18%; urinary tract cancer, 10%; ovarian cancer, 9%.[14]

DIAGNOSIS OF HNPCC

HNPCC has a dominant pattern of inheritance. Germline mutations in six genes have been identified in this population.[15–19] These are the DNA mismatch repair (MMR) genes *MSH2*, *MSH6*, *MLH1*, *MLH3*, *PMS1*, and *PMS2*. More than 200 mutations have been identified, the majority of which are in *MSH2* and *MLH1*, with 87% of HNPCC families mapping to these loci.[20–23] Defects in these repair genes generally result in the replication error (RER) phenotype and lead to microsatellite instability in the resultant tumors.

Notwithstanding this detailed genetic picture, the definition of the disease is still largely clinical, on the basis of the Amsterdam criteria.[20] The criteria are: three relatives, one being a first-degree relative of the other two, with histologically verified colorectal cancer; at least two successive generations affected; at least one case diagnosed before age 50 years; and familial adenomatous polyposis excluded. Common clinical features among families meeting these criteria are an average age at diagnosis of 44 years (approximately 20 years younger than sporadic or nonhereditary colorectal cancer), tumors more commonly occurring in the proximal colon (approximately 70%) and multiple tumors in up to 40% of patients.

There is interest in molecular screening for this disease, in order to identify gene carriers and family members who may be at risk. When 509 consecutive colorectal tumors were analyzed in a Finnish study, 12% were found to have replication errors, and these patients were then screened for germline mutations of *MLH1* or *MSH2*.[24] Ten patients (2%) were found to have one of the germline mutations and to have a personal or family history of colorectal cancer, thus giving them a diagnosis of HNPCC. When 184 kindreds of families with clustering of colorectal or other HNPCC-associated cancers were screened for germline *MSH2* and *MLH1* mutations, 26% were found to be carriers, and multivariate analysis showed that younger age at diagnosis, fulfillment of the Amsterdam criteria, and a personal history of endometrial cancer were all independent predictors of mutation positivity.[25]

FAMILIAL ENDOMETRIAL CANCER

Familial endometrial cancer generally refers to HNPCC family members, although there may be a second group in which endometrial cancer is the primary malignancy (Figure 3–1). Until a site-specific endometrial cancer syndrome is recognized, all these patients should be considered potential HNPCC carriers and should be screened accordingly for colorectal cancer and other related cancers. Some authors believe that there is no genetic contribution to endometrial cancer in the absence of a personal history of HNPCC or other cancers.[26] One population-based study of family histories of 455 endometrial cancer patients and 3,216 controls aged 20 to 54 years found that about 5% of endometrial cancers may be associated with a positive family history of endometrial cancer alone, whereas about 2% occur with familial colorectal cancer.[27] When pedigrees of 80 women diagnosed with primary cancers of both the colon and endometrium at age < 70 years were analyzed, the relative risk of colorectal cancer was 16.1, which was increased to 30.5 if both cancers had been diagnosed in the proband at age < 55 years.[28]

Little is known about the importance of precursor lesions in high-risk patients. Recently, endometrial hyperplasia in women from HNPCC families with and without a germline mutation was examined for loss of MLH1 and MSH2 protein expression, and this loss was found to correlate with the presence of germline mutations.[29] Endometrial tumors from patients with multiple primary cancers were compared with tumors from patients with primary endometrial cancer, and the former were found to have a higher incidence of loss of MLH1 and MSH2 expression. This was particularly true if the patient was < 55 years of age.[12]

Those women who are HNPCC gene carriers have the highest risk of subsequent endometrial cancer, and some believe that they should undergo prophylactic total hysterectomy after childbearing is com-

pleted. Screening of those women at risk of HNPCC-related or site-specific endometrial cancer is controversial. Recently, an Australian study found the cumulative incidence of gynecologic malignancies in women aged 25 to 40 years from HNPCC families to be substantially higher than that in the general population. The authors concluded that surveillance should be offered to those at risk, but no surveillance guidelines were postulated.[30] Another recent study has suggested that first-degree relatives of a proband diagnosed at age < 50 years with double primary cancers of the colon and endometrium have an increased risk of colorectal or other HNPCC-related cancers and should be offered genetic testing.[31]

GENETICS OF ENDOMETRIAL CANCER

The molecular events responsible for endometrial cancer remain poorly defined. The histopathologic events of progression from hyperplasia to adenocarcinoma have been well described, but an understanding of the genetic basis of endometrial cancer is still incomplete (see Chapter 2). In endometrial cancer that is unrelated to estrogen exposure, no precursor lesion has been described. Estrogen and progesterone receptors are more often found in endometrioid than in serous tumors and, in general, are associated with low-grade, early-stage tumors, but their value as tumor markers is unclear.[32] PTEN, a dual-function phosphatase, is frequently lost or underexpressed in early lesions of the endometrium, making it a candidate tumor suppressor gene (see Chapter 2).

Several oncogenes have been studied in endometrial cancer, including members of the RAS family, HER2/neu (also called ERBB2) and c-Myc. The Ras family encodes p21 proteins, and mutations are seen in a variety of cancers. K-ras mutations occur in 10 to 37% of endometrial cancers and more often in endometrioid tumors. It is controversial whether these mutations are associated with an improved or worse prognosis.[2] HER2/neu overexpression occurs in a variety of cancers and may be associated with a worse prognosis in endometrial carcinoma, although this has not been shown consistently.[2] c-Myc is activated in colon, lung, breast, and ovarian cancers in addition to endometrial cancer. HER2/neu and c-Myc are implicated in less than 15% of cases. The tumor

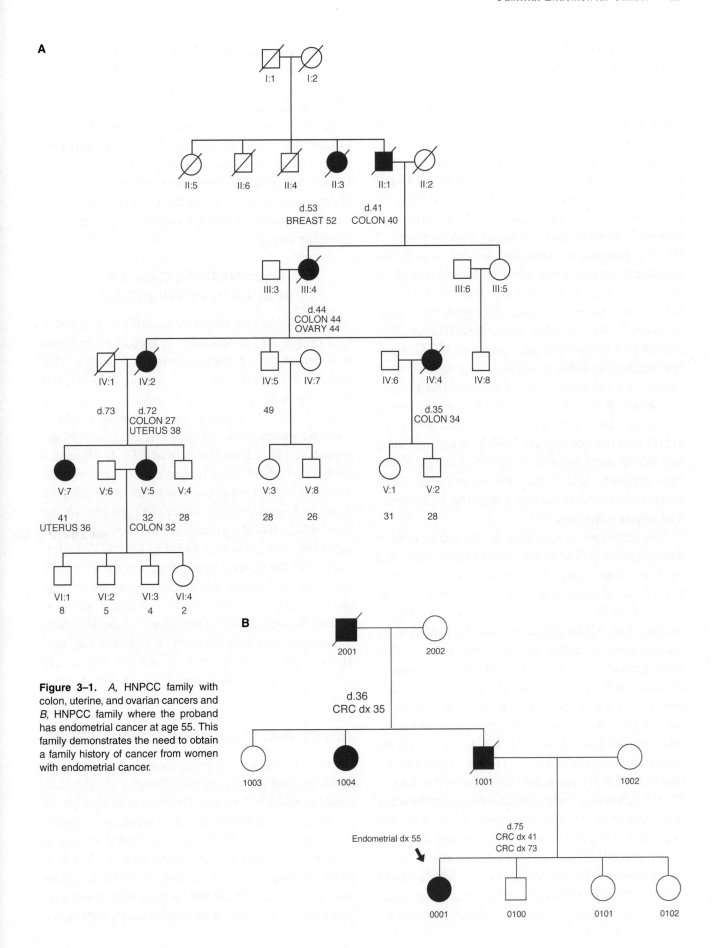

Figure 3–1. *A,* HNPCC family with colon, uterine, and ovarian cancers and *B,* HNPCC family where the proband has endometrial cancer at age 55. This family demonstrates the need to obtain a family history of cancer from women with endometrial cancer.

suppressor gene *P53* is mutated in up to 22% of endometrial cancers with rates of mutation lower in endometrial histology and higher in non-endometrioid histologies.[33] P53 overexpression is thought to be a late event in disease progression and occurs more often in papillary serous cancers.[32]

Microsatellite instability (MI) is a common feature in endometrial carcinomas, seen in 17 to 30% of both sporadic tumors and those related to HNPCC.[2,34] It seems to be more frequent with endometrioid tumors.[35] Normal and cancerous endometrium of HNPCC patients was analyzed for MI, and it was found only in cancerous cells.[36,37] Most MI-positive endometrial tumors have lost expression of MLH1 or MSH2, whereas those without MI express both gene products.[37] MI has also been identified in both endometrial hyperplasia and cancer of *MSH2* mutation carriers, possibly predicting more rapid disease progression and earlier onset of cancer in this group.[36] MI-positive tumors from women with a strong family history of cancer were shown to lack methylation of *MLH1* and did not express MSH2, again indicating that *MSH2* may contribute to inherited disease.[38] The most frequent *MSH2* mutation known (the Newfoundland mutation) confers a high risk of endometrial cancer to carriers.[39]

The technique of searching for MI can be used to distinguish tumors as synchronous or metastatic.[40] It has been shown that in endometrial tumors, immunohistochemical staining typically demonstrates correlation of *MLH1* or *MSH2* and evidence of an RER profile; thus, MMR deficiency may be predicted by immunohistochemistry, which is much faster than DNA analysis.[37] In one study of MI-positive sporadic endometrial tumors, no mutations of *MSH2* or *MLH2* were found, indicating that these genes do not play a role in the absence of hereditary risk.[41] However, other studies have shown that MI-positive sporadic endometrial tumors can have cytosine hypermethylation of the MLH1 promoter region, as well as loss of MLH1 expression, indicating that there may be some convergence in the molecular events of sporadic and familial endometrial cancers.[42–44] A recent study has shown that MLH1 carriers with endometrial cancer, but none with colorectal cancer, lacked MSH2 and/or MSH6 protein expression as well, suggesting selective *MSH2/MSH6* deficiency in those destined for

endometrial cancer only.[44] Mutations of *MSH6* were found in double primary colorectal and endometrial tumors, indicating that *MSH6* may actually contribute to the occurrence of these double primaries.[45] Only about one-third of tumors from MSH6 carriers exhibits MI.[36] A high prevalence of *MSH6* germline mutations has been found in atypical HNPCC families not fulfilling the Amsterdam criteria, and, in fact, endometrial cancer may be the most common clinical manifestation of HNPCC among MSH6 germline mutation carriers.[46]

ENDOMETRIAL CANCER IN BRCA1/2 POPULATIONS

The significance of *BRCA1/2* mutations in endometrial cancer, and specifically in hereditary endometrial cancer, is not well understood. The gene that encodes a BRCA1-associated protein, BARD1, has been shown to be mutated in sporadic endometrial cancer.[47] *BRCA1* probably does not play a role in sporadic endometrial carcinoma, as evidenced by the persistence of at least one normal *BRCA1* allele in a study in which 33 sporadic endometrial tumors were analyzed.[48] A retrospective cohort of 199 Ashkenazi Jews with endometrial cancer was genotyped for three *BRCA* founder mutations, and the incidence of germ-line mutations was found to be 1.5% (the frequency in the general population is 2%). This indicates that the lifetime risk of endometrial cancer may not be increased in individuals with *BRCA* germline mutations and that *BRCA* mutations are not increased in patients with endometrioid endometrial cancer.[49] However, there may be an increased risk of papillary serous carcioma of the endometrium in *BRCA* mutation carriers.[50]

SCREENING FOR ENDOMETRIAL CANCER

There is no role for screening for endometrial cancer in the general population (see Chapter 4). The incidence is just 2.7% by age 70 years in this group. In Japan, a mass endometrial cancer screening program was instituted in 1987, which included screening endometrial biopsy for all women 50 years of age or older, including those with abnormal uterine bleeding. In 1997, of the 29,808 women who underwent screening, 2.3% had suspicious biopsies, with only a

0.11% incidence of endometrial cancer.[44] With this low rate of detection, it is unlikely that this method of screening will prove to be cost effective. In a high-risk population, such as those with a genetic predisposition conferred by HNPCC, however, there may be a role for screening. An international HNPCC consortium has recommended endometrial cancer screening, but no protocol has been suggested.[41] Detection of premalignant, preclinical disease could be quite meaningful in terms of prevention and prognosis in this group. Of course, it remains to be seen if this screening would be cost effective and whether it would decrease the incidence and mortality from endometrial cancer.

There are no accepted strategies for dealing with women who are at increased genetic risk of endometrial cancer. At one extreme is hysterectomy after childbearing is complete, whereas the other option is to manage individuals on the basis of symptoms. The alternative would be to screen all at-risk women annually or semiannually using a method yet to be clearly established. Screening could be combined with hysterectomy at menopause, after symptoms or positive screening, or at the time of any abdominal surgery. It is unlikely that a randomized control trial would be possible, as it would require screening a large cohort of women for an extended period of time to establish whether any proposed screening strategy was effective at decreasing the mortality associated with endometrial cancer. Guidelines for surveillance and management of cancer risk in HNPCC carriers were established in 1996 at the International Collaborative Group-HNPCC annual meeting. Screening for colorectal cancer involves a colonoscopy every 2 years starting at age 25 years, or at 5 years younger than the youngest age of onset of colorectal cancer in that family. It has been proposed that screening for endometrial cancer should be done every 1 to 2 years starting at age 25 years and should include gynecologic examination, transvaginal ultrasonography, and serum cancer antigen (CA) 125 at age 30 to 35 years.[52] However, CA 125 is not a specific marker for endometrial cancer, and, in fact, there are no other known molecular or tumor markers that would be useful as screening tools.[53]

It is unlikely that these recommendations for endometrial cancer screening are followed world-wide in HNPCC centers. Furthermore, this method may not effectively pick up early endometrial cancers or premalignant changes. Certainly, a standardized protocol for screening these women is needed, and this must be tailored to target different groups of women (eg, women who are still menstruating may be more difficult to screen ultrasonographically than postmenopausal women in whom well-established endometrial thickness limits exist). In the absence of a markedly thickened endometrium, ultrasonography would not detect premalignant changes, such as complex hyperplasia, so these women may require tissue screening via periodic endometrial biopsy. This issue is something that the international HNPCC community should address so that consistency in clinical practice results, and these guidelines for endometrial cancer screening should be as standardized as the protocols in place for colon cancer screening.

CONCLUSION

Hereditary endometrial cancer seems to exclusively involve those women from families with Lynch syndrome II. Limited data suggest that alternative genetic abnormalities or genes that modify the *MMR* genes may predispose to a familial endometrial syndrome in which endometrial cancer is the only hereditary malignancy. This may be more important in certain circumstances, such as families in which multiple endometrial cancers have occurred with onset at a younger age. It seems likely, however, that the large majority of these cases will be from HNPCC families, albeit with atypical family history and clinical presentation. In any case, when a woman presents with endometrial cancer as a second primary, at age < 55 years or with a strong family history of endometrial and other cancers, consideration should be given to a diagnosis of HNPCC. Routine hysterectomy should be performed at the time of other abdominal surgeries in these women and may even be considered independently once childbearing is complete.

REFERENCES

1. Aarnio M, Mecklin JP, Aaltonen LA, et al. Lifetime risk of different cancers in hereditary non-polyposis colorectal cancer (HNPCC) syndrome. Int J Cancer 1995;64:430–3.
2. Bandera CA, Boyd J. The molecular genetics of endometrial carcinoma. Prog Clin Biol Res 1997;396:185–203.

3. Sandles LG, Shulman LP, Elias S et. al. Endometrial adeno-carcinoma: genetic analysis suggesting heritable site-specific uterine cancer. Gynecol Oncol 1992;47:167–71.

4. Kurman RJ, Norris HJ. The behaviour of endometrial hyperplasia: a long term study of untreated hyperplasia in 170 patients. CA Cancer J Clin 1985;56:403–12.

5. Ponz de Leon M. Prevalence of hereditary nonpolyposis colorectal carcinoma (HNPCC). Ann Med 1994;26(3):209–14.

6. Lynch HT, Lanspa SJ, Boman BM, et al. Hereditary nonpolyposis colorectal cancer—Lynch Syndromes I and II. Gastrointest Endosc Clin N Am 1988;17:679–712.

7. Jarvinen HJ, Mecklin JP, Sistonen P. Screening reduces colorectal cancer rate in hereditary nonpolyposis colorectal cancer (HNPCC) families. Gastroenterology 1995;108:1405–11.

8. Hakal T, Mecklin JP, Forss M, et al. Endometrial cancer in the cancer family syndrome. Cancer 1991;68:1656–9.

9. Watson P, Vasen HFA, Mecklin JP, et al. The risk of endometrial cancer in hereditary nonpolyposis colorectal cancer. Am J Med 1994;96:516–20.

10. Aarnio M, Sankila R, Pukkala E, et al. Cancer risk in mutation carriers of DNA-mismatch repair genes. Int J Cancer 1999;81:214–8.

11. Parc YR, Halling KC, Burgart LJ, et al. Microsatellite instability and hMLH1/hMSH2 expression in young endometrial carcinoma patients: associations with family history and histopathology. Int J Cancer 2000;86:60–6.

12. Maruyama A, Miyamoto S, Saito T, et al. Clinicopathologic and familial characteristics of endometrial cancer carcinoma with multiple primary carcinomas in relation to the loss of protein expression of MSH2 and MLH1. Cancer 2001;91:2056–64.

13. Hemminki K, Li X, Dong C. Second primary cancers after sporadic and familial colorectal cancer. Cancer Epidemiol Biomarkers Prev 2001;10:793–8.

14. Sagawa T, Yamada H, Yamamoto R, et al. Two cases of endometrial cancer meeting new clinical criteria for hereditary non-polyposis colon cancer. Gynecol Oncol 2000;79:327–31.

15. Fishel R, Lescoe MK, Rao MRS, et al. The human mutator gene homolog MSH2 and its association with hereditary nonpolyposis colon cancer. Cell 1993;75:1027–30.

16. Leach FS, Nicolaides NC, Papadopoulos N, et al. Mutations of mut-S homolog in hereditary nonpolyposis colorectal cancer. Cell 1993;74:1215–25.

17. Bronner CE, Baker SM, Morrison PT, et al. Mutation in the DNA mismatch repair gene homologue hMLH1 is associated with hereditary non-polyposis colon cancer. Nature 1994;368:258–61.

18. Papadopoulos N, Nicolaides NC, Wei Y-F, et al. Mutation of a mut-L homolog in hereditary colon cancer. Science 1994;371:75–80.

19. Nicolaides NC, Papadopoulos N, Liu B, et al. Mutations of two PMA homologues in hereditary colon cancer. Nature 1994;371:75–80.

20. Vasen HFA, Mecklin JP, Khan PM, Lynch HT. The International collaborative on hereditary nonpolyposis colorectal cancer (ICG-HNPCC). Dis Colon Rectum 1991;34(5):424–5.

21. Peltomaki P, Vasen HF. Mutations predisposing to hereditary nonpolyposis colorectal cancer: database and results of a collaborative study. Gastroenterology 1997;113:1146–58.

22. Lynch HT, Lynch J, Conway T, et al. Familial aggregation of carcinoma of the endometrium. Am J Obstet Gynecol 1994;171:24–7.

23. Sandkuijl L, Bishop T. Results of the joint analysis of the EUROFAP linkage data: summary. Copenhagen: EURO-FAP; 1993.

24. Aaltonen LA, Salovaara R, Kristo P, et al. Incidence of hereditary nonpolyposis colorectal cancer and the feasibility of molecular screening for the disease. N Engl J Med 1998;338:1481–7.

25. Wijnen JT, Vasen HF, Khan PM, et al. Clinical findings with implications for genetic testing in families with clustering of colorectal cancer. N Engl J Med 1998;339:511–8.

26. Olson JE, Sellers TA, Anderson KE, Folsom AR. Does a family history of cancer increase the risk for postmenopausal endometrial carcinoma? A prospective cohort study and a nested case-control family study of older women. Cancer 1999;85:2444–9.

27. Gruber SB, Thompson WD. A population-based study of endometrial cancer and familial risk in younger women. Cancer and Steroid Hormone Study Group. Cancer Epidemiol Biomarkers Prev 1996;5:411–7.

28. Pal T, Flanders T, Mitchell-Lehman M, et al. Genetic implications of double primary cancers of the colorectum and endometrium. J Med Gen 1998;35:978–84.

29. Berends MJW, Hollema H, Wu Y, et al. MLH1 and MSH2 protein expression as a pre-screening marker in hereditary and non-hereditary endometrial hyperplasia and cancer. Int J Cancer 2001;92:398–403.

30. Brown GJ, St John DJ, Macrae FA, Aittomaki K. Cancer risk in young women at risk of hereditary nonpolyposis colorectal cancer: implications for gynecologic surveillance. Gynecol Oncol 2001;80:346–9.

31. Cederquist K, Goolovleva I, Emanuelsson M, et al. A population based cohort study of patients with multiple colon and endometrial cancers: correlation of microsatellite instability, age at diagnosis and cancer risk. Int J Cancer 2001;91:486–91.

32. Kounelis S, Kapranos N, Kouri E, et al. Immunohistochemical profile of endometrial adenocarcinoma: a study of 61 cases and a review of the literature. Mod Pathol 2000;13:379–88.

33. Greenblatt MS, Bennett WP, Hollstein M, Harris CC. Mutations in the p53 tumor suppressor gene: clues to cancer etiology and molecular pathogenesis. Cancer Res 1994;54:4855–78.

34. Helland A, Borresen-Dale AL, Peltomak P, et al. Micorsatellite instability in cervical and endometrial carcinomas. Int J Cancer 1997;70:499–501.

35. Catasus L, Machin P, Matias-Guiu X, Prat J. Microsatellite instability in endometrial carcinomas: clinicopathologic correlations in a series of 42 cases. Hum Pathol 1998;29:1160–4.

36. Ichikawa Y, Lemon SJ, Wang S, et al. Microsatellite instability and expression of MLH1 and MSH2 in normal and malignant endometrial and ovarian epithelium in hereditary nonpolyposis colorectal cancer family members. Cancer Cytogenet 1999;112:2–8.

37. de Leeuw WJ, Dierssen J, Vasen HF, et al. Prediction of mismatch repair gene defect by microsatellite instability and immunohistochemical analysis in endometrial tumours from HNPCC patients. J Pathol 2000;192:328–35.

38. Chiaravalli AM, Furlan D, Facco C, et. al. Immunohistochemical pattern of hMSH2/hMLH1 in familial and sporadic colorectal, gastric, endometrial and ovarian carcinomas with instability in microsatellite sequences. Virchows Arch 2001;438:39–48.

39. Simpkins SB, Bocker T, Swisher EM, et al. MLH1 promoter of methylation and gene silencing is the primary cause of microsatellite instability in sporadic endometrial cancers. Hum Mol Genet 1999;8:661–6.

40. Batool T, Reginal PW, Hughes JH. Outpatient pipelle endometrial biopsy in the investigation of post-menopausal bleeding. Br J Obstet Gynaecol 1994;101:545–6.

41. Sato S, Matsunaga G, Konno R, Yajima A. Mass screening for cancer of the endometrium in Miyagi Prefecture, Japan. Acta Cytol 1998;42:295–8.

42. Lim PC, Tester D, Cliby W, et al. Absence of mutations in DNA mismatch repair genes in sporadic endometrial tumours with microsatellite instability. Clin Cancer Res 1996;2:1907–11.

43. Esteller M, Levine R, Baylin SB, et al. MLH1 promoter hypermethylation is associated with microsatellite instability phenotype in sporadic endometrial carcinomas. Oncogene 1998;17:2413–7.

44. Salvesen HB, MacDonald N, Ryan A, et al. Methylation of hMLH1 in a population-based series of endometrial carcinomas. Clin Cancer Res 2000;6:3607–13.

45. Schweizer P, Moisio AL, Kuismanen SA, et al. Lack of MSH2 and MSH6 characterizes endometrial but not colon carcinomas in hereditary non-polyposis colon cancer. Cancer Res 2001;61:2813–5.

46. Charmes GS, Millar AL, Pal T, et al. Do MSH6 mutations contribute to double primary cancers of the colon and endometrium? Hum Genet 2000;107:623–9.

47. Meijers-Heijboer H, Lindhout D, Menko F, et al. Familial endometrial cancer in female carriers of MSH6 germline mutations. Nat Genet 1999;23:142–4.

48. Thai TH, Du F, Tsan JT, et al. Mutations in the BRCA1-associated RING domain protein (BARD1) gene in primary breast, ovarian and uterine cancers. Hum Mol Genet 1998;7:195–202.

49. Liu FS, Ho ESC, Shih RTP, Shih A. Mutational analysis of the BRCA1 tumour suppressor gene in endometrial carcinoma. Gynecol Oncol 1997;66:449–53.

50. Levine DA, Lin O, Barakat RR, et al. Risk of endometrial carcinoma associated with BRCA mutation. Gynecol Oncol 2001;80:395–8.

51. Geisler JP, Sorosky JI, Duong HL, et al. Papillary serous carcinoma of the uterus: increased risk of subsequent or concurrent development of breast carcinoma. Gynecol Oncol 2001;83:501–3.

52. Burke W, Petersen G, Lynch P, et al. Recommendations for follow-up care of individuals with an inherited predisposition to cancer. I. Hereditary nonpolyposis colon cancer. Cancer Genetics Studies Consortium. JAMA 1997;277:915–9.

53. Consensus Statement. Recommendations for follow-up care of individuals with an inherited predisposition to cancer: I. hereditary nonpolyposis colon cancer. JAMA 1997;277:915–9.

4

Diagnosis, Screening, and Staging of Endometrial Carcinoma

ARLAN F. FULLER JR, MD

CLINICAL PRESENTATION

Abnormal uterine bleeding is, by far, the most common symptom of endometrial carcinoma and one that is generally considered as indicative of cancer by most patients. Despite this, in a number of patients, there may be a striking delay before seeking evaluation by a physician. For the majority of patients with low-grade tumors, this does not lead to decreased survival; however, among patients with high-grade lesions, there does appear to be a greater likelihood of advanced-stage disease at diagnosis.[1,2]

The development of abnormal uterine bleeding in premenopausal years can be a much more subtle symptom and one often attributed to what is termed dysfunctional uterine bleeding (DUB) in the absence of demonstrable endometrial pathology; this is even more common in the perimenopausal years, when it may be attributed to a luteal phase defect. The sine qua non in the management of *any* aberration in the menstrual cycle is endometrial biopsy or curettage. Although the usual approach to apparent dysfunctional uterine bleeding may be a therapeutic trial of progesterone, lack of prompt response customarily dictates the need for biopsy documentation of the endometrial histology. The prevalence of DUB in young women may be also attributed to intercurrent gynecologic problems, such as endometriosis and "infertility"; when the changes are temporally related to menopause, there may be a corresponding delay in diagnosis, both on the part of the patient and her physician.

Symptoms Associated with Premenopausal Endometrial Carcinoma

Abnormal Uterine Bleeding

In the nonpregnant premenopausal patient, abnormal uterine bleeding is most commonly a consequence of anovulation leading to DUB. Less common is heavy bleeding associated with menses, for example, the hypermenorrhea associated with fibroids or other benign intrauterine pathology. A third pattern of bleeding is the intermenstrual pattern, with irregular bleeding interspersed with "regular" menstrual cycles. Any one of these may be associated with endometrial hyperplasia and cancer. Typically, persistent estrogen stimulation unopposed by progesterone is the cause of anovulatory bleeding; some of these may ultimately develop into hyperplasia and carcinoma characteristic of type 1 endometrial carcinoma, which is most common among premenopausal women. The other two patterns may be more characteristic of type 2 endometrial carcinoma, developing in the absence of hyperplasia, which is relatively uncommon among premenopausal women (see Chapter 9).

In all these patterns of bleeding, the appropriate diagnostic intervention is an endometrial biopsy, demonstrating proliferative endometrium and confirming the clinical diagnosis of benign DUB. If the pattern of apparent DUB does not respond to progestin therapy, one must question the diagnosis and perform a dilatation and curettage (D&C), with or without hysteroscopy. The accuracy of endometrial biopsy with the various disposable sampling devices is related to the proportion of the endometrial surface involved by the disease process.[3] Diagnostic pelvic ultrasonography or hysteroscopy may be reserved for those patients who have an abnormal results from their pelvic examination or abnormal endometrial biopsy results or for those who do not respond to progestin therapy.

In the perimenopausal years, transient anovulatory bleeding may be common but as it is a manifestation of unopposed estrogen or diminished progestin response, as in the insufficient luteal phase, endometrial biopsy is necessary to exclude hyperplasia or to identify carcinoma. A high index of suspicion and a low threshold for endometrial biopsy may permit detection of hyperplasia that, although atypical, will reverse to normal with exogenous progestins. In both these time periods, lack of response to therapy of presumptive DUB should lead to prompt investigation with ultrasonography and/or hysteroscopy to identify associated benign conditions and exclude hyperplasia or carcinoma.

In a small series reported from Canada, 13 women with abnormal uterine bleeding (group 1) and 8 women with postmenopausal bleeding underwent hysteroscopy with the intention of endometrial ablation. All patients had inadequate or inconclusive preablation endometrial biopsies and were found to have cancer, either at the time (group 2) or subsequently (group 1). Among group 1 patients, 8 underwent complete resection and 5 had partial resection; in group 2 patients, malignancy was recognized, and resection was considered unwise. The tumor was found to be of microscopic extent in 2 patients in group 1. All 21 patients were alive and well following primary treatment for the disease at intervals ranging from 6 months to 9 years. Despite concerns about the potential role of hysteroscopy in intraperitoneal dissemination of disease, there was no evidence of intraperitoneal recurrence (see discussion on staging, below).[4]

Abnormal Cervical Cytology

As noted below in greater detail, Pap smear evidence of atypical glandular cells of uncertain significance (AGUS) may be indicative of underlying endometrial pathology, particularly if these cells appear to be atypical endometrial cells. In young women whose cervical evaluation does not demonstrate any endocervical pathology, endometrial biopsy should be performed. As described below, high-risk subtypes of endometrial carcinoma are more commonly associated with the finding of malignant cells in cytologic specimens, whereas low-grade lesions are associated with the AGUS smear.[5]

Symptoms Associated with Postmenopausal Endometrial Carcinoma

Uterine Bleeding

In the postmenopausal woman with vaginal bleeding who is not on hormonal replacement therapy (HRT), the diagnostic algorithms that have been proposed are described below.

For patients with an intact uterus who are on sequential HRT, withdrawal bleeding is not uncommon, and the diagnostic choices would be to discontinue HRT, carry out an endometrial biopsy, or both. With a continuous HRT regimen, bleeding is not unusual when the patient is immediately postmenopausal or converting from a sequential regimen. Nonetheless, persistent bleeding, heavy bleeding, an abnormal pelvic examination, or the presence of risk factors for hyperplasia or carcinoma should lead to biopsy and/or ultrasonographic evaluation, if the patient chooses to continue on HRT.

When tamoxifen is used in the management of breast cancer, with or without cytotoxic chemotherapy, there is a small but real increase in the risk of development of endometrial carcinoma. In these patients, postmenopausal bleeding should prompt evaluation with endometrial biopsy and ultrasonography. A thickened endometrium associated with benign subendometrial changes versus hyperplasia or carcinoma represents the usual differential diagnosis following diagnostic ultrasonography (see Chapter 13).

Abnormal Cervical Cytology

The presence of an atypical Pap smear or even a smear suspicious for or diagnostic of endometrial carcinoma is a relatively uncommon presentation of endometrial neoplasia, but one that can arise in a patient of any age. Eddy and colleagues reviewed the cervical cytology obtained prior to diagnosis in 112 patients with endometrial carcinoma or carcinosarcoma. Seventeen patients had a cytologic diagnosis of malignancy, 33 had AGUS smears, and the remainder were normal. Patients ranged in age from 35 to 89 years. The Pap smears were obtained within 3 months of diagnosis in 89 (79%) patients and within 6 months in an additional 16 (14%). Among patients with endometrioid tumors, grade 1 lesions were more commonly associated with AGUS smears, whereas high-grade lesions were commonly characterized by overt malignant cytology. Similarly, papillary serous and mixed mesodermal tumors were significantly more likely to be associated with malignant cytology.[5]

As one might expect, abnormal cervical cytology is more commonly associated with occult or gross cervical extension of an endometrioid neoplasm but is also associated with nonendometrioid histology and high tumor grade.[6] The latter phenomenon may be explained by decreased tumor adhesion and increased shedding of cells by these tumors. As described in Chapter 6, a positive cervical cytology is also associated with a higher risk of extrauterine spread of disease.[5,7]

Intra-abdominal Disease

Identification of a pelvic mass and ascites typically suggests the diagnosis of ovarian carcinoma. This may also be the clinical presentation in a minority of patients with endometrial carcinoma. In the experience published from our division of gynecologic oncology at the Massachusetts General Hospital, among more than 1,100 patients with endometrial carcinoma, 47 were found to have pathologic stage IV disease, and another 86 had stage III disease (51 with stage IIIA/IIIB and 35 patients with stage IIIC).[8,9] Among these patients, there was a preponderance of nonendometrioid histology and clinical symptoms indicative of advanced disease. Among the majority of stage IV patients, preoperative computed tomography (CT) was diagnostic of upper abdominal disease and multiple sites of spread of disease, including lung, liver, and bone. Given the preponderance of nonendometrioid or poorly differ-

entiated tumors in this group (only 3 patients had grade 1 tumors), the indication for preoperative CT becomes fairly well defined.

An important aspect of the evaluation of these patients with advanced disease, particularly those with isolated ovarian involvement, is the distinction between patients with ovarian metastasis from endometrial cancer and those with two separate and distinct primary neoplasms. In many cases, the final diagnosis is not determined until an exhaustive review of the pathology. The survival in these patients greatly exceeds that of either stage II ovarian cancer or stage III endometrial cancer, and treatment may vary greatly. In our series of 48 patients with surgical stage IIIA disease, we excluded an additional 4 patients with separate primaries on subsequent review. All 4 of these patients survived in excess of 10 years.[9] This problem in differential diagnosis continues to be one commonly seen in consultation in an academic referral center.

In a similar manner, identification of disseminated serous papillary carcinoma in the abdominal cavity in the absence of obvious primary ovarian disease leads one to the diagnosis of primary peritoneal neoplasia. Such a diagnosis cannot be conclusively reached in the absence of evaluation of a potential uterine primary source, either by excision of the uterus or prior curettage. In light of the benefit of cytoreductive surgery in this disease, identification of an occult bulky uterine primary is important.[10]

DIAGNOSTIC TECHNIQUES

Once the need for diagnostic evaluation is clear, the appropriate sequence for investigation may be initiated. Modalities for investigation include endometrial biopsy, D & C, pelvic, and transvaginal ultrasonography, sonohysterography, and hysteroscopy. The sequencing of these modalities into a diagnostic algorithm remains somewhat controversial; biases in favor of one or another modality may relate, in part, to the expertise and focus of the investigator with that diagnostic modality.

Many proposals have been made to evaluate the efficacy with which one can evaluate the patient with postmenopausal bleeding. As the vast majority of patients presenting with bleeding have atrophic endometrial changes and only about 10 to 20% of them have cancer or an atypical hyperplasia, the focus has been placed on a method of triage to identify those at high risk. Feldman and colleagues found that the patient who was age > 70 years, had diabetes, and was nulliparous had an 87% chance of having carcinoma or complex hyperplasia in contrast to the woman with no risk factors, who had a 3% chance of abnormal histology.[11]

Dilatation and Curettage

Dilatation of the cervix and endometrial curettage under general anesthesia in the operating room has traditionally been the definitive diagnostic procedure in patients suspected of having endometrial pathology. The inaccuracy of this procedure and the resources and costs involved have generally led to its replacement by any one of a number of office procedures carried out under paracervical anesthesia or, frequently, with no anesthesia, depending on the patient, the state of the cervix, and the nature of the underlying uterine pathology. In a recent study by Epstein and colleagues, 84 of 105 patients with postmenopausal bleeding and an endometrial stripe > 5 mm in double thickness were found to have significant pathology.[12] These patients underwent hysteroscopy followed by conventional D & C and then a repeat hysteroscopy to evaluate the adequacy of the D & C. Twenty-four patients underwent hysterectomy. The D & C, though suc-

cessful in identifying diffuse lesions within the uterus, missed 25 of 43 endometrial polyps, 5 of 10 hyperplasias, 3 of 5 complex atypical hyperplasias, and 2 of 19 (11%) carcinomas. Of patients with focal lesions, all or part of 87% of those lesions remained after curettage.

In addition to the "quantitative" aspects of endometrial curettage, Obermair and associates in the Austrian Gynecologic Oncology Study Group retrospectively reviewed the "qualitative" correlation between D&C and hysterectomy in 137 endometrial cancer patients with grade 1 disease at the time of initial curettage. Preoperative grade 1 correlated with the hysterectomy grade in 78% of cases; 20.4% were determined to be grade 2, and 1 patient had a grade 1 tumor in association with a carcinosarcoma (Figure 4–1).[13] Of patients with grade 2 histology and who had undergone hysterectomy, 38% had stage IC disease or more, in contrast to those with grade 1 final histology, 17% of whom had stage IC or more advanced disease.

These findings again raise the frequent concern that some patients treated conservatively with hormonal therapy may have more extensive or aggressive tumors and require close monitoring (see Chapter 9). Moreover, patients having limited surgery, such as a vaginal hysterectomy and bilateral salpingo-oophorectomy, may subsequently require laparoscopic node dissection because of increased tumor grade and the finding of deep myometrial invasion in the final hysterectomy specimen.

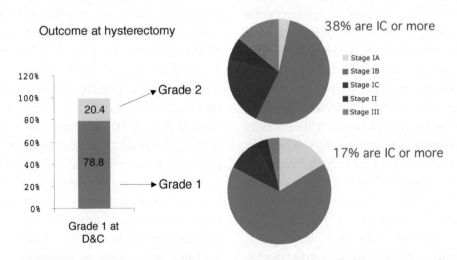

Figure 4–1.   Correlation of preoperative low-grade histology with the final hysterectomy grade and staging. Reproduced with permission from Obermair et al.[13]

Endometrial Biopsy

The instruments available for office procedures include both reusable devices, such as the Novak curette, and disposable instruments for one-time use, such as the Pipelle aspirator or Endocyte curette.[14] One clear point made by several investigators has been the lack of sensitivity of the Pipelle instrument in the detection of endometrial carcinoma and its precursors. In lesions that occupied < 5% of the endometrial surface, the Pipelle missed all 3 of 3 lesions; among those lesions that involved 5 to 25% of the endometrial surface, 4 of 12 were missed, and not until > 50% of the surface was involved was the disposable device 100% accurate (30 of 30).[3] Ferry and colleagues also evaluated the clinical significance of a "negative" Pipelle endometrial biopsy. They found that there was a 67% (25 of 37) agreement between biopsy and hysterectomy findings; of 12 described as "incorrect," there were 4 cases of atypical endometrium, 2 cases of atypical hyperplasia, 3 cases of necrotic hyalinized tissue, and 3 cases described as "nonspecific."[15] Indeed, all but the last three nonspecific findings would have prompted definitive surgical management. An additional study looked at the cost-effectiveness of the Pipelle biopsy alone as the definitive work-up prior to hysterectomy. In 56 patients with a preoperative biopsy only, all cancers were detected with 100% sensitivity; Pipelle biopsy was discordant with respect to tumor subtype in 6 of 56 (10.7%) cases and discordant with respect to grade in 3 of 41 cases.[16] The conclusion reached was that the Pipelle biopsy, if positive, was reliable in preoperative assessment of histology; the reservations that have remained are those related to a false-negative biopsy on the basis of limited endometrial disease, such as that arising in association with a polyp. These studies do indicate that when a lesion is missed, it is usually a manifestation of limited intrauterine disease, where close follow-up and reevaluation based on persistent symptoms will yield the correct diagnosis.

Dunn and colleagues defined an algorithm to determine the need for endometrial biopsy in 1,000 patients with abnormal uterine bleeding. The patients were separated into pre- and post-menopausal groups, with and without risk factors for carcinoma. Patients with a single risk factor for carcinoma (570 patients) underwent endometrial biopsy; among these, 5 were found to have endometrial carcinoma, with 3 additional cases of complex atypical hyperplasia.[17] In the other 430 patients not undergoing biopsy, none developed malignancy at short-term follow-up (2 years). The observations of this study suggest that one might limit the use of biopsies; however, the conclusion would have greater validity if one prospectively biopsied those without risk factors and could confirm the absence of significant pathology in those patients. Alternatively, a longer follow-up would be valuable, as would the knowledge that bleeding resolved in these patients without the need for histologic evaluation.

Pelvic Ultrasonography

A number of papers in the literature have addressed the initial evaluation with ultrasonography of patients with postmenopausal bleeding. These studies have shown that with an endometrial thickness of < 5 mm, the risk of endometrial carcinoma is less than 1%.[18,19] The controversy that exists relates to whether the initial approach of the clinician should involve an ultrasonographic study or an endometrial biopsy (see below).[20]

What is the fate of those patients whose endometrial thickness is < 5 mm at initial evaluation and who develop bleeding subsequent to investigation? This issue was addressed by Epstein and Valentin who followed up 97 patients with postmenopausal bleeding and an endometrial stripe < 5 mm in thickness. In this prospective study, 48 patients were allocated to primary evaluation by ultrasonography and 49 patients allocated to primary D & C. Over the course of the 1 year follow-up, 16 of 48 patients who had primary ultrasonographic evaluation developed recurrent bleeding compared with only 10 patients who underwent primary D & C. All of these patients had both ultrasonographic reevaluation and endometrial curettage. In the presence of increased thickening of the endometrium determined by ultrasonography, 33% were found to have significant pathology. In contrast, if there was no endometrial growth, only 4% of patients had significant endometrial lesions ($p = .008$).[21]

Tabor and colleagues have critically addressed the variability in the threshold of endometrial thickness at which the risk of neoplasia is negligible. They concluded that there was a significant variation in endometrial thickness among healthy women with abnormal uterine bleeding. Endometrial thickness was greater in premenopausal women and in postmenopausal women on HRT (Figure 4–2). Women using HRT who did not have endometrial neoplasia had a significantly thicker endometrium than those who did not use HRT (6.4 mm versus 2 mm, $p < .001$). There was a similar, and not unexpected, level of variation among symptomatic women with endometrial cancer and variation among centers as well (Figure 4–3). By comparing the median thickness of the endometrium among women with endometrial cancer to the median thickness of the endometrium in symptomatic women unaffected by endometrial cancer, they established a relationship of "multiples of the median (MoM)" that compensated for the variation among centers (Figure 4–4). At the same center, the median endometrial thickness for patients with endometrial cancer was 3.7 times the

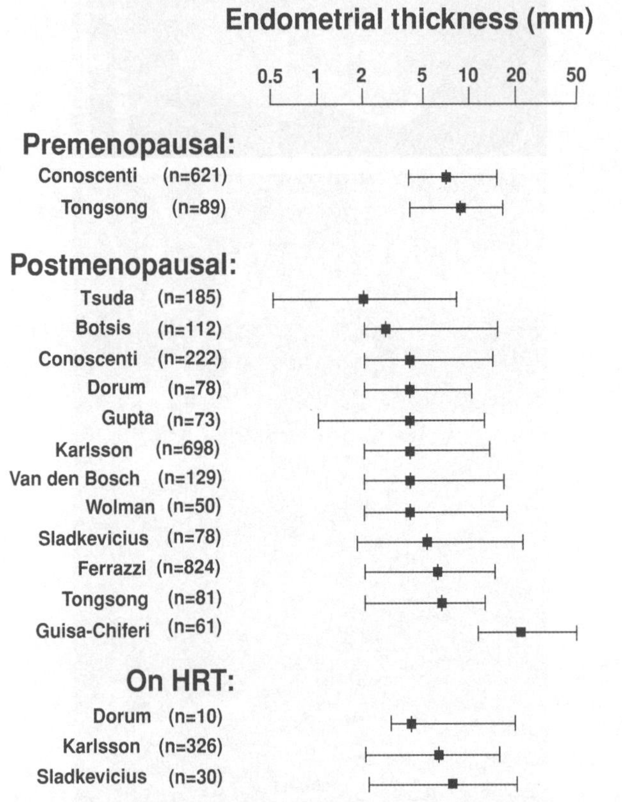

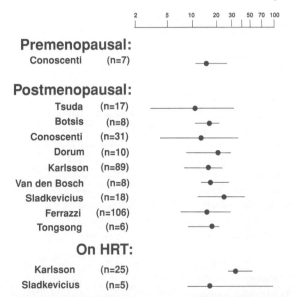

Figure 4–3. Measurements of endometrial thickness in a meta-analysis of published studies of 330 women with postmenopausal bleeding and determined to have endometrial cancer. HRT = hormone replacement therapy. Reproduced with permission from Tabor A et al.[22]

median thickness of unaffected women who had the same menopausal status and hormonal replacement status, with a range of 2.1 to 5.9 MoM. This meta-analysis confirmed the low, but "unacceptable" false-negative rate of 4% for a cutoff value of < 5 mm thickness of the endometrium. Their conclusion, as well as their recommendation, was that endometrial curettage should be performed on all postmenopausal patients with vaginal bleeding.[22] In an accompanying editorial, Runowicz disagreed, noting that the patient with a false-negative ultrasonogram, having an endometrial thickness below some arbitrary cutoff value will still be evaluated if symptoms persist.[23] Figure 4–5 demonstrates an example of a false-negative pelvic ultrasonogram in the presence of an isthmic endometrial cancer. The patient was asymptomatic, and the diagnosis was made incidental to an endometrial biopsy at the time of laparoscopic removal of a benign left ovarian neoplasm.

Pelvic and Transvaginal Ultrasonography versus Endometrial Biopsy

One controversial issue has been the choice of modality for initial screening of the patient with

Figure 4–2. Measurements of endometrial thickness in a meta-analysis of published studies of 3,483 women with postmenopausal bleeding and determined to be free of endometrial cancer. HRT = hormone replacement therapy. Reproduced with permission from Tabor A et al.[22]

Endometrial thickness (MOM)

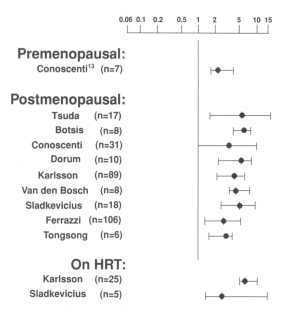

Figure 4–4. Symptomatic women (330) with endometrial cancer. Endometrial thickness presented as multiples of the median for unaffected women of the same menopausal status (stratified as well for use or nonuse of hormone replacement therapy [HRT]). Each study compares women in the same center. Reproduced with permission from Tabor A et al.[22]

postmenopausal bleeding. Goldstein and colleagues, in 1997, proposed an algorithm for ultrasonography-based triage of perimenopausal women with abnormal uterine bleeding. In this prospective study of 433 perimenopausal patients, transvaginal ultrasonography was used to determine endometrial thickness. If the endometrium was > 5 mm in double-layer thickness or not reliably visualized, saline infusion sonohysterography was performed. If this showed a single-layer endometrial thickness of < 3 mm, DUB was assumed to be the diagnosis. If focal lesions were noted, the patient went on to hysteroscopy and curettage; if the endometrium was globally thickened, then an endometrial biopsy was performed. Using this method of triage, 341 patients (79%) had no ultrasonographic abnormality, and DUB was diagnosed. Fifty-eight patients (13%) had focal lesions, which were removed hysteroscopically; 10 patients had globally thickened endometrium, and biopsy revealed hyperplasia in 5 and proliferative endometrium in the remaining 5. Two additional patients had unsatisfactory sonohysterography and also underwent hysteroscopy.[24]

Alternatively, given the prevalence of DUB in this group of perimenopausal patients described by Goldstein, it would seem reasonable to reserve evaluation for those patients who did not *immediately* respond to cyclic progestin therapy. This approach would eliminate the need for ultrasonography in as many as three-quarters of the patients in his study.

Weber and colleagues have proposed a cost-effectiveness analysis of office endometrial biopsy

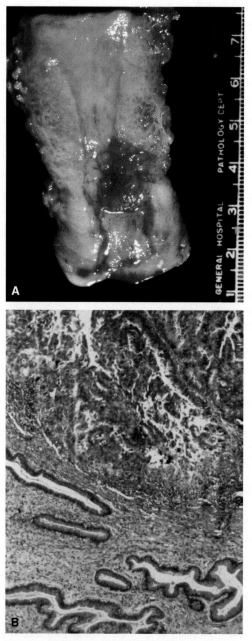

Figure 4–5. *A*, Ultrasound evaluation of postmenopausal bleeding in a 49-year-old patient who demonstrated a 4 mm endometrial stripe, and missed this superficially invasive grade 1 isthmic lesion shown microscopically (*B*).

versus transvaginal ultrasonography in the initial evaluation of the symptomatic postmenopausal patient.[25] Their conclusion that ultrasonography was more cost-effective than curettage was based on the inclusive cost for endometrial biopsy of $200 (US) and a corresponding cost of only $72 for the transvaginal ultrasonography (Figure 4–6). As these values are highly variable, one can easily imagine that in some locales, the costs-benefit would be reversed and the proper procedure would be the endometrial curettage first and the ultrasonography second. The curettage in this series is considered to be only a random endometrial biopsy with a rate of nondiagnosis of 28%. The efficacy would improve substantially if the curettage was performed with a Novak curet with the patient under local anesthesia. Most of the nondiagnostic studies included cases of endometrial polyps.

Medverd and colleagues used a similar approach of cost minimization in the evaluation of patients with postmenopausal bleeding.[26] Using standard Medicare reimbursement levels, they sought to identify the level of disease prevalence at which endometrial biopsy would be more cost effective, as histologic documentation of suspected endometrial abnormality is necessary. They determined that below the prevalence of atypical endometrial hyperplasia and carcinoma at 31%, transvaginal ultrasonography is more cost effective. Above the prevalence rate of 31% for a significant lesion,

endometrial biopsy as the initial part of the diagnostic work-up for postmenopausal bleeding is more cost effective.

Hysteroscopy in Diagnosis and Management

The use of diagnostic hysteroscopy in addition to endometrial biopsy has been evaluated in an incremental manner by Clark and colleagues; they showed that for patients having an endometrial biopsy as part of the diagnostic work-up of postmenopausal bleeding, the subsequent addition of hysteroscopy, but not ultrasonography, was associated with a significant increase in the diagnostic accuracy of "serious conditions."[27] Marchetti and associates evaluated hysteroscopy followed by endometrial biopsy and, in their experience, found a sensitivity of 93.10%, a specificity of 99.96%, a positive predictive value of 98.18%, and a negative predictive value of 99.85%. When endometrial biopsy was added to hysteroscopy, the sensitivity increased to 96.55% and specificity to 100%. In this case, the biopsy was directed by hysteroscopy.[28]

Hysteroscopy can certainly be carried out in either the outpatient operating suite or the office environment. The use of a small-caliber (4 mm OD) flexible hysteroscope provides a rapid diagnosis for the patient with postmenopausal bleeding with minimal discomfort. Unless there is a significant degree of cervical stenosis, the hysteroscope can be passed under direct vision with little difficulty. In the patient with stenosis of the cervix, dilatation under paracervical block is generally well tolerated and will facilitate introduction of the flexible hysteroscope. It is important to use minimal fluid pressure in distending the uterus in order to avoid uterine cramping.

Potential roles for office hysteroscopy include (1) the diagnosis of endometrial lesions, either benign or malignant; (2) determination of origin of a uterine lesion in the cervix versus the endometrium; and (3) identification of possible extension of an endometrial lesion to the cervix or vice versa. As far as the staging of endometrial carcinoma is concerned, hysteroscopy will identify occult stage II lesions, particularly in the upper endocervix (see "Surgical Staging of Endometrial Cancer").

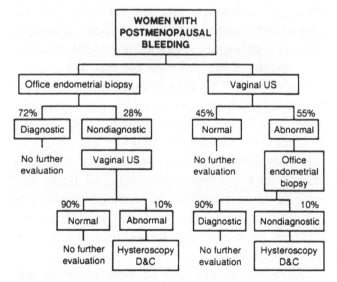

Figure 4–6. Alternative algorithms for evaluation of women with postmenopausal bleeding. D&C = dilatation and curretage; US = ultrasound. Reproduced with permission from Eddy GL et al.[5]

SCREENING FOR ENDOMETRIAL CARCINOMA

Principles of Screening

Development of a useful program of screening for endometrial cancer requires the identification of disease at a time when it is more curable than it is when the patient presents with symptoms. To be successful, ideally, there should be a preinvasive phase, where intervention is uniformly successful in attaining cure. This process can be termed "secondary prevention" and is critical to the success of screening, in contrast to "primary prevention," where the circumstances are altered to prevent even the development of precursors of the disease.

Historical Experience

One can (and should) make distinctions among the circumstances of cancer identification:

- *Screening*—the identification of disease or its precursors in the asymptomatic population
- *Early detection*—determination of occult symptoms in a population without complaints
- *Diagnosis*—the identification of the presence and extent of disease in a symptomatic patient

Problems with successful screening of patients with endometrial carcinoma are a consequence of:

- The high level of curability of the disease in patients presenting with clinical symptoms—notably vaginal bleeding
- The relatively invasive nature of the conventional screening method—the endometrial biopsy curet
- The costly and cumbersome nature of alternative techniques for early diagnosis—the endovaginal ultrasonographic probe and "office" hysteroscopy
- The recognition that many endometrial cancers arise de novo in the endometrium, without the appearance of preexisting hyperplasia—in fact, those tend to be the more aggressive, poorly differentiated carcinomas, the nonendometrioid carcinomas, and the "type II" endometrial carcinoma associated with atrophy

- When progression of a precursor lesion can be identified, the rate of progression may be slow, such that waiting for symptoms to arise would be a reasonable alternative

Those tumors that do arise in association with endometrial hyperplasia tend to be well differentiated and have a good prognosis. The risk factors for the genesis of endometrial hyperplasia are described in Chapter 9. Endometrial hyperplasia represents a descriptive term for a very heterogeneous group of histologic findings with an equally variable risk of progression to carcinoma.[29] These changes may be described in both architectural and cytologic terms (See "Identification of Groups at High-Risk of Development of Carcinoma from Preexisting Hyperplasia" and Chapter 5).

Screening for Development of Endometrial Carcinoma

Surveillance of large populations for endometrial carcinoma is likely to identify many patients with low-risk, slow-growing, asymptomatic carcinomas and will ensure a good prognosis, whether the patients were diagnosed on screening or when they become symptomatic. A large series of patients screened by Nakagawa-Okamura and colleagues compared 126 cases diagnosed at mass screening with 1,069 symptomatic cases identified in the outpatient setting of 22 Japanese hospitals.[14] Eighty-eight percent of the screened patients had stage I disease in contrast to 65% of the symptomatic patients. Seventy-five percent of the screened patients had grade 1 disease versus 61% of the symptomatic population. In the screened (prevalent) cases, the 5-year survival was 94.0% compared with 84.3% in the symptomatic (incident) population. The results of this study do confirm the hypothesis that low-grade lesions have a substantial preclinical phase and may be more prevalent in screened populations (length-time bias), in contrast to high-grade lesions that may grow more rapidly and present at a more advanced stage.

A similar comparison between prevalent and incident cases was performed for transvaginal ultrasonography and reported in 1995.[30] Osmers and colleagues compared 22 asymptomatic patients with endometrial carcinoma detected by transvaginal ultrasonography with 61 patients whose diagnosis was established after investigation of postmenopausal bleeding. The screened patients had a mean depth of myometrial invasion of 4 mm, and 45% had well-differentiated tumors; the symptomatic patients had a mean depth of myometrial invasion of 10 mm, and only 18% had low-grade tumors. The conclusion reached was that "asymptomatic endometrial carcinomas screened by transvaginal ultrasonography were more likely to have a better prognosis than symptomatic cancers." One cannot reach the conclusion, however, that transvaginal ultrasonography improves the prognosis of endometrial cancer.

To this end, Gerber and colleagues compared 190 postmenopausal patients with symptomatic endometrial cancer with 123 asymptomatic patients with suspicious endometrium detected by transvaginal ultrasonography. In this retrospective study, they concluded that symptomatic patients were significantly older ($p < .05$), more frequently obese, and hypertensive. The duration of bleeding prior to diagnosis did correlate with the stage of the disease; however, there was no prognostic advantage for screened patients when compared with those with bleeding of < 8 weeks' duration. In their experience, patients at high risk of endometrial cancer tended to avoid screening with transvaginal ultrasonography; moreover, the use of the diagnostic modality for screening "often results in unnecessary operations and increased morbidity and costs."[31] Transvaginal ultrasonography does show evidence of a high negative predictive value but poor specificity with multiple false positives related to endometrial polyps, benign fluid accumulations in the uterus, and varying degrees of hyperplasia, which reduces its clinical utility. The consensus appears to be strongly in favor of only screening women at high risk of the disease, if that group can be adequately delineated.

In another study of 577 women in the Postmenopausal Estrogen/Progestin Interventions (PEPI) trial, 45% of women examined by transvaginal ultrasonography had atrophic (< 5 mm) endometria; of the 55% of women with an endometrial thickness of 5 mm or more, only 5% (11 patients) had any serious abnormality. There was a negative predictive value of 99% but only a 9% positive predictive value for detecting any abnormality above that threshold of 5 mm.[18] Little argument could be made for the routine use of transvaginal ultrasonography in the screening of asymptomatic women.

In 1995, Koss pursued a systematic search for the identification of occult endometrial carcinoma and carried out a series of endometrial biopsies at annual intervals for 2,586 peri- or postmenopausal women. Sixteen occult endometrial carcinomas were found by screening, and 2 additional cases were later identified, producing a prevalence of about 7/1,000 women in the screened population. Follow-up examination of 1,754 women then led to the estimated incidence rate of 1.7/1,000 woman-years.[32] The decrease in the number of women available in the subsequent year for follow-up was undoubtedly related to the discomfort of annual endometrial sampling experienced by asymptomatic women.

One observation that further addresses the issue of the value of early diagnosis in this group of patients comes from Menczer and colleagues in Tel Hashomer, Israel. They studied a group of 181 women, with a substantial delay in diagnosis or treatment, and found no significant difference in outcome when all prognostic factors were considered for patients with a delay in diagnosis of < 1 year or a delay from diagnosis to treatment of < 4 months.[2] There seems to be little justification under the circumstances for invasive or costly monitoring of a disease with what appears to be a dichotomous presentation—where one encounters either a hormonally responsive low-grade tumor that has a slow pattern of growth and early symptoms or a high-grade lesion with anaplastic growth and early spread to distant sites.

Identification of Groups at High-Risk of Development of Carcinoma from Preexisting Hyperplasia

Once hyperplasia has been identified at curettage, the risk of subsequent and concurrent carcinoma can be predicted by classification of the hyperplastic changes (Table 4–1): simple hyperplasia, complex hyperplasia, simple atypical hyperplasia, and complex atypical hyperplasia. In a series reported by Xie

Table 4–1. DEFINITIONS OF HYPERPLASIA

Simple hyperplasia	Increased number of glands with luminal dilatation, decreased stroma, lacking back-to-back crowding
Complex hyperplasia	Increased number of glands with irregular outline, structural complexity and back-to-back crowding without atypia
Simple atypical hyperplasia	Simple hyperplasia as above with cytologic atypia
Complex atypical hyperplasia	Complex hyperplasia as above with cytologic atypia

and colleagues, who retrospectively studied 150 patients with hyperplasia detected by curettage, all of whom had subsequent hysterectomy, the accuracy of endometrial curettage range from 77 to 92%, depending on the nature of the hyperplastic change. Atypical changes in either simple hyperplasia or, more frequently, complex hyperplasia were likely to coexist with occult carcinoma (Table 4–2).[33] Although endometrial hyperplasia does not invariably progress to carcinoma, the findings of cytologic and architectural atypia present the clearest association with carcinoma. Even so, identification of those few with a significant risk of neoplastic progression remains a problem—and one for which the presence of one or more molecular markers may be predictive (*PTEN*, K-*ras*, *P53*, as discussed in Chapter 2).[34,35]

These findings emphasize the importance of an adequate tissue diagnosis and close follow-up if one is considering conservative management with hormonal therapy or observation only in young patients or in patients with complex medical problems. The marginal benefit of additional radiographic studies or hysteroscopy is as yet unknown (see Chapter 9).

Distinguishing between Endometrial Hyperplasia and Carcinoma

Generally speaking, the finding of severely atypical endometrial hyperplasia will be an indication for hysterectomy. If conservative hormonal management might be considered, the ability to distinguish hyperplasia from overt carcinoma could be valuable. Emoto and associates used transvaginal color Doppler techniques in differentiating between hyperplasia and carcinoma.[36] In 71 patients evaluated for hyperplasia or carcinoma, transvaginal color Doppler ultrasonography (TV CDU) detected intratumoral blood flow in 38 of 53 patients with carcinoma (72%); abnormal blood flow was found in only 1 of 18 patients with hyperplasia (5.6%). This one false

positive appeared to be associated with a pyometrium. Abnormal intratumoral blood flow in the group of patients with carcinoma was positively associated with myometrial invasion, high-grade tumor, and lymph node metastases (see Chapter 6).

The success of surgical management in this group of patients with atypical hyperplasia can be seen in a study by Hunter and colleagues, where 54 patients with simple or complex endometrial hyperplasia *with atypia* underwent hysterectomy. Nineteen of 54 patients were found to have coexisting carcinoma, predominantly grade 1 and pathologic stage I; three patients had grade 2 disease (stage IB, stage IC, and stage IIIA). All patients survived without recurrence at a mean follow-up of 3 years.[37]

RISK FACTORS FOR THE DEVELOPMENT OF ENDOMETRIAL CARCINOMA

A number of epidemiologic factors have been identified with an increased risk of endometrial carcinoma, notably obesity, diabetes mellitus, and, to a lesser extent, hypertension (see Chapter 11). Most studies indicate that although there is an increased risk associated with hypertension, it is not an independent variable when corrections are made for other fac-

Table 4–2. RELATIONSHIP BETWEEN DIAGNOSIS WITH ENDOMETRIAL CURETTAGE AND FINAL DIAGNOSIS AT HYSTERECTOMY IN 150 CASES

Curettage	Surgical Findings (n)					
	SH	CH	SAH	CAH	EC	Total
SH	50	2	1	0	0	53
CH	6	3	0	1	1	11
SAH	7	2	13	1	3	26
CAH	2	0	1	27	30	60
Total	65	7	15	29	34	150

CAH = complex atypical hyperplasia; CH = complex hyperplasia; EC = endometrial carcinoma; SAH = simple atypical hyperplasia; SH = simple hyperplasia. Adapted from Xie X et al.[33]

tors.[38,39] Obviously, the use of estrogen replacement therapy is associated with an increased risk of developing a well-differentiated adenocarcinoma; however, most data suggest a very favorable survival. In one study from King County, Washington, the survival among patients with endometrial carcinoma acquired on exogenous estrogen therapy was more than 100% of age-matched controls. Conversely, cigarette smoking has a protective effect, in the postmenopausal, but not premenopausal, woman.[40,41] The effect appeared confined to those smoking more than 20 cigarettes per day and was not related to body mass index, which might be expected to be lower in smokers. The observation that the protective effect was largely in postmenopausal women suggests that it may be mediated by the inhibition of aromatase function in adipose tissue, hence the lack of association with high or low body mass index.

Race has been considered a risk factor for endometrial carcinoma. Many studies have observed that African Americans tend to have more poorly differentiated tumors, a higher prevalence of adverse histologic subtypes, more advanced-stage disease, less access to adequate health care, and a correspondingly poorer prognosis.[42] In data from the National Cancer Database, the decrease in survival has been estimated at 25% compared with non-Hispanic Whites and Hispanics.[43] A subsequent study suggested that the excess mortality among Blacks could be predominantly attributed to the lower use of estrogen therapy.[44] The latest data suggest a racial disparity in ribosomal deoxyribonucleic acid (DNA) methylation and a poorer survival, stage for stage, in patients with low levels of rDNA methylation. How these differences might translate into lower survival in African American women with endometrial cancer is unclear (see Chapter 6).[45]

As far as genetic risk is concerned, the most substantial association is with hereditary nonpolyposis colorectal cancer (HNPCC) (see Chapter 3). This is an autosomal dominant disease with high penetrance. The disease is caused by defects in mismatch repair genes, such as *hMLH1* on chromosome 3p, *hMSH2* on chromosome 2p, or less common genes involved in mismatch repair.[46] Although some authors have recommended "screening" for endometrial carcinoma in populations known to be affected by the

genes, Lynch and colleagues have observed 1,018 women from 86 families and has determined the cumulative incidence of endometrial cancer to be 20% by age 70 years (versus 3% in the general population) although other investigators have suggested a higher cumulative incidence (reviewed in Chapter 3).[47] In the highest-risk group most likely to carry the HPNCC gene, the average annual risk from 40 to 60 years of age was more than 1% per year.[48] Prophylactic transabdominal hysterectomy with bilateral salpingo-oophorecotomy (TAH/BSO), not screening, was recommended for this very-high-risk group.

Further support for either expectant management or prophylactic surgery for this disease comes from a prospective study of women at risk of HNPCC and familial colorectal carcinoma, in which 269 women were followed up with screening pelvic ultrasonography for a period up to 13 years. Two cases of endometrial carcinoma were reported; neither was diagnosed at surveillance, but both presented with symptomatic early-stage disease. Both patients were long-term survivors. No evidence of a role for surveillance by ultrasonography could be identified.[49] The American Cancer Society (ACS) recommends that annual screening for endometrial biopsy should be offered for women by the age of 35 who have, or are at risk of HNPCC. Women in this high-risk group should be informed of the risks and symptoms of endometrial cancer, and should be informed of potential benefits, risks, and limitations of testing for early endometrial cancer detection.

At present, there are no data indicating that annual screening of women with HNPCC does or does not detect endometrial cancers at a sufficiently early stage to improve survival compared to diagnosis when symptoms are present.[50]

SURGICAL STAGING OF ENDOMETRIAL CANCER

Endometrial carcinoma is unusual among malignant neoplasms in that the formal staging system (Table 4–3) is not uniformly applied to all patients. A discussion of surgical staging, therefore, addresses not only the staging system itself but also the rationale for the selective application of this staging system to endometrial neoplasms with widely varying risks of

Table 4–3. SURGICAL STAGING OF ENDOMETRIAL CANCER	
Stage	**Extent of Disease**
IA	Endometrial only
IB	Less than half myometrial invasion
IC	Greater than half myometrial invasion
IIA	Mucosal involvement of cervix
IIB	Stromal invasion of cervix
IIIA	Involvement of uterine serosa, adnexa, or cytologically positive peritoneal washings
IIIB	Metastatic disease to the vagina
IIIC	Retroperitoneal extension to pelvic or para-aortic nodes
IVA	Extension to bladder mucosa or bowel mucosa
IVB	Distant metastasis including spread to the abdominal contents and inguinal nodes

Adapted from International Federation of Gynecology and Obstetrics, 1988. Classification and staging of gynecologic malignancies. ACOG Technical Bulletin Number 155—May 1991 (replaces No. 47, June 1977). Int J Gynaecol Obstet 1992;38(4):319–23.

disease extension beyond the uterine corpus.

Given the relatively low risk of extrauterine disease in some patients with low-grade lesions associated with endometrial hyperplasia, some patients may not be staged at all. As noted in Chapter 9, some patients may be treated with hormonal therapy, a treatment that is considered "conservative" only in the sense that it conserves the uterus; this eliminates any consideration of staging when even the primary tumor is not removed (see Chapter 6). Other patients may be treated by vaginal TAH/BSO, not affording the opportunity for even clinical assessment of pelvic nodes. Development of a consistent and widely applicable algorithm for the selective application of this staging system is essential to compare treatment plans and outcomes between institutions. The first prerequisite of this development is an understanding of the appropriate preoperative assessment on which such an algorithm can be based.

A number of prognostic variables are available preoperatively to assist in the determination of risk of nodal metastasis as well as other extrauterine spread of disease. Given the large proportion of women with limited disease and a good prognosis, it is appropriate that even this low morbidity of staging not exceed the potential benefit of early delineation and treatment of extrauterine disease. This is also particularly true for patients with early disease, on clinical grounds, who have complicating medical ill-

nesses that may make staging more risky, and an anticipated lifespan correspondingly shorter.

Challenges To Be Addressed by a Preoperative Staging Algorithm

Preoperative evaluation of the patient should include sufficient information to identify patients with low-grade histology and disease anticipated to be confined to the uterus who will not require node dissection. The presence of gross cervical disease requires the exclusion of a primary cervical cancer; if the lesion is determined to be secondary to cervical stromal invasion by endometrial carcinoma, then primary therapy will be modified accordingly.

Of concern as well is the use of routine *fractional* D&C to identify occult cervical stromal invasion. This is not routinely carried out in the absence of clinical suspicion of cervical involvement. An enlarged cervix, a Pap smear positive for adenocarcinoma, or fragments of tissue extruding through a normal cervix might suggest this. The question is whether the preoperative identification of cervical stromal involvement will modify therapy in a meaningful manner in order to justify fractional curettage. An ongoing problem that remains is the histologic distinction between tumor in endocervical curettings and tumor actually invading the endocervical glandular epithelium. It should also be noted, of course, that endocervical curettage will not preoperatively identify those patients with tumor extension exclusively into the endocervical stroma without mucosal involvement.

Similarly, preoperative identification of an adnexal mass may facilitate the intraoperative discrimination between metastatic disease to the ovary and primary ovarian cancer. Other than influencing the choice of a vertical incision to gain adequate access to the upper abdomen, the preoperative identification of an adnexal mass will have no other impact on treatment. The suggestion of either a simultaneous primary ovarian neoplasm or stage III endometrial carcinoma may indicate the need for a referral by the obstetrician/gynecologist to a subspecialist in gynecologic oncology.

The value of preoperative ultrasonography in patients with endometrial cancer may lie not only in the identification of adnexal masses but also in the assessment of myometrial invasion and extension to the cervical stroma. Szantho and colleagues identified 7 of 10 patients with occult cervical stromal invasion in their series of 52 patients; myometrial invasion was "accurately identified" in 46 of those 52 patients.[51] In a similar study, Alcazar evaluated 50 patients prospectively by ultrasonography and cancer antigen (CA) 125; 35 (70%) had < 50% myometrial invasion and 15 (30%) had > 50% invasion. Transvaginal ultrasonography revealed that deeply invasive lesions were associated with a thicker endometrial epithelium (18.7 mm) than those with superficially invasive lesions (13.4 mm). Similarly, the CA 125 level in deeply invasive lesions was 30 IU/mL compared with a value of 16.9 IU/mL with superficial invasion. Transvaginal ultrasonography was more sensitive than CA 125 in the detection of myometrial invasion.[52]

The Preoperative Evaluation Should Assess the Relevant Variables

Once the patient with endometrial cancer has been identified, the initial evaluation includes precise clinical examination of the uterus with attention to both gross and occult cervical or endocervical extension of disease. If the exocervix is normal to speculum examination, does bimanual examination reveal any bulbous contour to the cervix or uterine isthmus? Paracervical and uterosacral ligaments should be normal without induration or shortening. The uterine corpus itself should be of a size comparable with the age and menopausal status of the patient in the absence of uterine fibroids.

The adequacy of clinical examination varies greatly with respect to body habitus and the degree of abdominal and pelvic muscular relaxation. If the examination is not determined to be adequate, then the addition of pelvic ultrasonography (if not already performed) may aid in the assessment of the extent of intrauterine disease and the risk of extrauterine disease as well. The use of pelvic ultrasonography may be particularly valuable to exclude occult adnexal disease in patients with grade 1 lesions who are considered for vaginal surgery.

If an adnexal mass is identified, abdominal exploration should be preceded by an appropriate bowel

preparation so that complete surgical excision may be performed. There should be no reservation about the appropriateness of cytoreduction surgery irrespective of the diagnosis in the medically fit patient, as this is appropriate for either diagnosis.[8,10,53]

In all patients, radiographic evaluation should include chest radiography. For patients with an abnormal uterus, poorly differentiated endometrioid tumors, or nonendometrioid histology, abdominopelvic computed tomography (CT) will visualize gross extrauterine metastatic disease. Evidence of gross cervical invasion will also increase the likelihood of retroperitoneal nodal metastases (Table 4–4).

The value of endocervical curettage as part of a fractional D & C is limited by the absence of demonstrable therapeutic benefit to radical hysterectomy over total extrafascial hysterectomy in the management of patients with stage II disease that is clinically occult. It should easily be recognized that there are two types of stage II disease: (1) that which is clinically evident and treated by radical hysterectomy or preoperative radiation therapy, and (2) that which is identified histologically by the pathologist as occult invasion. The majority of cases are the latter. Several retrospective studies have shown no benefit to radical hysterectomy in patients with clinically occult disease when compared with treatment with total extrafascial hysterectomy and postoperative pelvic radiation therapy.[54–58] Recognition that clinically occult endometrial carcinoma involving the cervix will be managed differently from that which is clinically identifiable has led to the recommendation that these two lesions be separated, with the former to be described as "stage II occult"; this observation is further supported by the improved survival in patients with clinically occult disease.[55] Data suggesting an advantage for radical hysterectomy are necessarily predicated on the clinical identification of gross cervical disease and have not been prospectively randomized. Nonethe-

Table 4–4. PREOPERATIVELY AVAILABLE FACTORS ASSOCIATED WITH AN INCREASED RISK OF EXTRAUTERINE DISEASE

Elevated CA 125
Positive cervical cytology or gross cervical disease
Nonendometrioid histology
Adnexal mass

CA = cancer antigen.

less, in order to avoid cutting through gross tumor, either preoperative radiation followed by total hysterectomy or radical hysterectomy appears to be appropriate local therapy. In a large clinical study by Sartori and colleagues, radical hysterectomy improved the rate of local control with a local failure rate of 35% after simple hysterectomy but no local vaginal recurrences after radical hysterectomy.[58]

Boente and colleagues confirmed these observations, noting also that 27 of 84 patients (32%) with clinical evidence of gross cervical involvement had extrauterine disease and that radical hysterectomy in this group of patients was associated with an improved survival. In patients with gross cervical disease having radical hysterectomy, the 5-year actuarial survival was 75%; in contrast, the survival among patients with total hysterectomy and preoperative radiation therapy was 48% and only 33% with postoperative radiation therapy. Although patient selection had some influence within this group, the outcome was even more marked for those patients with gross cervical disease of > 3 cm. The actuarial 5-year survival was 74% for radical hysterectomy patients with or without postoperative radiation therapy but only 18% for those with preoperative radiation therapy followed by total hysterectomy. This group were of the opinion "that gross cervical involvement should be considered by the FIGO staging committee as a separate entity."[59] This recommendation is certainly supported by the available data and is based on a logical separation of clinical entities.

Use of Hysteroscopy in the Delineation of the Extent of Intrauterine Disease

Hysteroscopy can identify the extent of disease within the endometrial cavity as well as the potential for extension to the cervix. Although a number of different techniques have been used to identify early stage II disease, direct physical inspection of the endocervix seems to be a logical and cost-effective approach, particularly as it can be carried out in an office setting with a flexible hysteroscope. The disadvantage, of course, is that this technique identifies only patients with mucosal or mucosal plus stromal involvement by tumor; it cannot detect tumor that spreads directly to the cervical stroma without mucosal involvement.

Garuti and colleagues prospectively evaluated with hysteroscopy 60 women who were to undergo laparotomy and staging for endometrial cancer. In a group of patients with predominantly grade 1 and grade 2 tumors (53 of 60), although there was no correlation of stage or survival with the *morphology* of the tumor, the extent of spread within the endometrial cavity was significantly related to stage, grade, and survival. Involvement of less than 50% of the endometrial cavity was associated with predominantly low-grade, stage I disease and 100% survival.[60] In their experience, hysteroscopy detected all 4 tumors that had metastasized to the cervix, 2 of which had invaded the cervical stroma. They did note, however, that 8 patients were "overdiagnosed" with endocervical extension not documented by histology. Also, 3 patients with gross cervical disease underwent modified radical hysterectomy, suggesting that hysteroscopy detected 1 additional case with a substantial false-positive rate.

A retrospective study from Hong Kong evaluating the benefit of preoperative hysteroscopic assessment of cervical invasion in 200 consecutive patients revealed that hysteroscopy identified 28 of 41 patients with cervical invasion; however, gross examination was equally accurate. More than 20% of their unselected patients had extension of cancer to the cervix; this large proportion of patients with gross cervical disease is uncommon in our experience and may reflect regional variations in care.[56] Hysteroscopy missed all 8 patients with stromal invasion only, as one might expect. However, 50% of patients with stage IIA disease were also missed. Three of 4 patients with mucosal involvement only that were not detected had been examined by CO_2 hysteroscopy, which was determined to be inferior to normal saline that was used in this study as well. Of patients with both mucosal and stromal involvement, 25 of 29 (86.2%) were correctly identified with both modalities. This study does raise the question of the additional, incremental benefit to preoperative assessment of the cervix beyond meticulous clinical evaluation. No comment was made as to the extent of surgical management or how that changed with identification of cervical invasion.[61]

In an anatomic situation where there is continuity between the vaginal vault and peritoneal cavity through patent fallopian tubes, it is no surprise that cells in the endometrial cavity are desquamated both into the vagina and the pelvic peritoneal cavity. Multiple studies have documented an increased prevalence of positive peritoneal cytology following diagnostic hysteroscopy, raising the question as to whether there is an increased risk of recurrence.[62–65] No such determination has been made following sonohysterography, but certainly the same reservation can be made. In fact, in two studies from the Czech Republic, there was an increase in the prevalence of positive pelvic washes from the cul-de-sac after dilatation and curettage alone.[66,67] At this point, there is reassuring evidence that an increased prevalence of positive peritoneal cytology does not result in a decreased survival among patients with clinical stage I disease undergoing hysteroscopy prior to definitive laparotomy.[64,68]

Alternative approaches have included endocervical curettage and various radiographic studies, ranging from endocervical ultrasonography to magnetic resonance imaging (MRI). In a study of preoperative uterine ultrasonography in the evaluation of occult cervical disease, of 30 patients with endometrial carcinoma assessed by both transvaginal and endocervical ultrasonography, both modalities identified 3 of 4 patients with cervical stromal invasion, although endocervical ultrasonography had greater specificity. Endocervical ultrasonography identified all three patients with stage IIA disease with an additional 3 false positives. Transvaginal ultrasonography was less sensitive, with an equal number of false positives, and tended to overstage mucosal disease as stromal invasion. False positives were associated with protrusion of the polypoid endometrial lesion into the endocervical canal.[69] In this study, although recognition of occult cervical involvement was described as important in determining the extent of hysterectomy, there was no description of modification in surgical technique of hysterectomy nor outcome.

The Value of a CA 125 Level in Determining the Need for Staging Procedures

The association of an elevated CA 125 level with occult extrauterine disease in patients with clinically apparent disease limited to the uterus has been long

recognized but does not appear to be generally integrated into clinical practice.[70,71] Recent studies have looked at a cutoff value in CA 125 either as an upper limit for vaginal hysterectomy or as a lower limit for pelvic and para-aortic lymphadenectomy. The generally accepted cutoff value described by Sood and colleagues was 20 U/mL for grade 1 lesions suitable for vaginal hysterectomy.[72] They found that values > 35 U/mL were significantly associated with a greater risk of myometrial invasion, positive cytology, and nodal metastases. Values > 65 U/mL were 6.5 times more likely to have metastatic disease as those below this value. The optimal cutoff value of CA 125 above which most nodal metastases are identified remains controversial and potentially could reflect regional variation.

Dotters identified a cutoff value of 20 U/mL; grade 3 histology, a value > 20, or both predicted 87% of patients requiring staging. Among patients whose tumors had grade 1 or 2 histology, 9 of 12 patients with nodal metastases were identified at a cutoff level of > 20 U/mL but only 6 of 12 if the cutoff value was > 35 U/mL.[73] This observation was consistent with a prior choice of a cutoff value of > 15 U/mL, as Koper and colleagues identified 32 of 60 patients with positive nodes at this level but only 10 of 60 if the value was > 35 U/mL. In this retrospective study, the addition of grade 3 histology permitted identification of 39 of 60 patients at the > 20 U/mL level but only 22 of 60 at the > 35 U/mL level.[74]

In multivariate analysis, Hsieh and colleagues determined that lymph node metastases had the most significant effect on CA 125 elevation. They employed receiver operating curve (ROC) analysis to determine that, in their population, a cutoff value at 40 U/mL produced the best sensitivity (77.8%) with a higher specificity (81.0%) than a cutoff value at 35 U/mL.[75] Kurihara and colleagues extended these observations to premenopausal women as did Ebina and colleagues; both groups looked at a higher level of CA 125 as a cutoff value in premenopausal patients and confirmed the validity of the value of > 20 U/mL for postmenopausal women[76,77] The lower cutoff values chosen were > 20 U/mL for postmenopausal patients and > 70 U/mL for premenopausal patients. On the basis of ROC analysis and logistic regression analysis, they identified nuclear

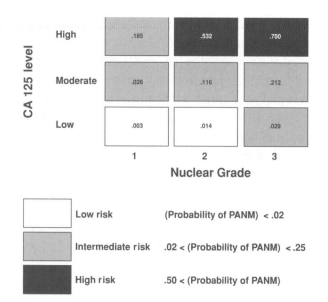

Low risk   (Probability of PANM) < .02

Intermediate risk   .02 < (Probability of PANM) < .25

High risk   .50 < (Probability of PANM)

Figure 4–7. Prediction of para-aortic nodal metastases (PANM) based on cancer antigen (CA) 125 level and histologic grade. Reproduced with permission from Ebina Y et al.[74]

grade and CA 125 level as the significant variables predicting para-aortic nodal metastasis (Figure 4–7).

Value of Gross Intraoperative Examination of the Uterus

No patient undergoing hysterectomy should undergo that surgery without intraoperative evaluation of the opened uterus (see below). This simple procedure can eliminate the surprise postoperative finding of endometrial carcinoma, which was preoperatively unsuspected. In a patient with known endometrial carcinoma, visualization of the interface between tumor and myometrium may aid in predicting risk of extrauterine metastases, particularly to the pelvic lymph nodes. The accuracy described in visual examination alone has varied widely; Doering and colleagues reported this evaluation as sensitive in identifying the extent of myometrial invasion, but others have suggested that it is less accurate.[78] Noumoff and colleagues noted that the gross examination was in accord with the histologic specimens only two-thirds of the time and that the error was usually one of underestimation of depth of invasion.[79] Goff and Rice clarified this issue by correlating the accuracy of gross inspection with the tumor grade. Evaluation of grade 2 tumors did not correlate with final

histology in 35.1% of cases; with grade 3 tumors an error was present, usually underestimation of invasion, in 69.2%.[80] This latter error has diminished significance in light of the fact that patients with grade 3 tumors, irrespective of depth of myometrial invasion, have sufficient risk of nodal metastases to warrant routine pelvic node dissection. It is the grade 2 tumor with limited intrauterine disease for which frozen section evaluation might be beneficial. It is our experience, however, that bilateral pelvic lymph node dissection can be completed by the time that frozen section information is available. This author's personal view is that in patients with gross residual intrauterine grade 2 disease, on inspection of the sectioned uterus, bilateral pelvic node dissection should be performed in the absence of medical contraindications.

Bilateral pelvic node dissection is also probably indicated in patients with visual evidence of less than one-third myometrial invasion and grade 1 disease. In those patients with grade 1 lesions who are to be considered for vaginal hysterectomy, there may be a role for preoperative evaluation of CA 125 in order to identify an increased risk of extrauterine disease.[73] Alternatively, laparoscopic bilateral pelvic lymph node dissection may be carried out at an interval after the final histologic evaluation of the uterus is complete. Para-aortic node dissection is reserved for those patients with palpable nodes at that level, or those with positive pelvic nodes, either by clinical examination or by frozen section evaluation. It should be noted that the size of pelvic lymph nodes does not necessarily indicate the presence or absence of metastatic disease and strongly suggests a role for routine lymphadenectomy in high-risk patients.[81] Reich and colleagues compared the size of positive and negative lymph nodes in 32 patients with node-positive endometrial cancer, with 143 negative nodes recovered from 5 patients with node-negative endometrial cancer. As expected, there was a correlation between the overall size of a positive node and the size of the metastasis within it. Nonetheless, 68 of 125 (54%) were positive nodes or < 10 mm in overall diameter. Conversely, 46 of 160 (29%) negative nodes in the node-positive patients were > 10 mm in diameter.[82] This study emphasizes the importance of frozen section examination of pelvic nodes if one is to base the decision to carry out para-aortic lymph node dissection on the status of pelvic nodes.

The decision to perform pelvic and para-aortic lymphadenectomy does not appear to affect the overall morbidity and mortality associated with the primary treatment of endometrial carcinoma in most clinical series.[83–85] The only exception to these observations has been that of Franchi and colleagues, from Varese, Italy, who studied 206 patients with endometrial carcinoma, of whom 133 underwent pelvic node dissection. The complication rate in this entire group of 206 was 26.7%; patients who underwent node dissection were more likely to have had complications. The removal of 14 nodes or more was significantly associated with the development of one complication. The removal of 19 nodes or more was significantly associated with development of two complications.[86] In contrast, Giannice and colleagues examined 36 elderly (> 70 years) patients undergoing either pelvic (28 patients) or pelvic and para-aortic (8 patients.) node dissection and compared them with age-matched controls having similar complicating medical conditions and extent of underlying malignancy. There was no difference in morbidity or mortality for those patients having complete surgical staging.[87]

Laparoscopic Surgical Staging as an Adjunct to Hysterectomy

Laparoscopy may be employed both as part of the planned primary therapy of endometrial carcinoma along with vaginal hysterectomy and bilateral salpingo-oophorectomy. It may also be an appropriate course of evaluation in patients who are found incidentally to have endometrial carcinoma after their primary surgical procedure for presumed benign disease. In the hands of experienced laparoscopists, this is a safe, efficient, and effective means of carrying out a complete pelvic node dissection, with the potential for lower morbidity and, in particular, an earlier return to functional status.[88–94] The increased cost associated with a longer operative time appears to be offset by a shorter hospital stay, with a little apparent

difference in overall cost.[93,95,96] Although there was an increased risk of positive peritoneal cytology with laparoscopic surgery, this did not appear to result in a corresponding increase in intraperitoneal recurrence.[97,98] Laparoscopy appeared to have advantages in reduced morbidity that extended to patients of moderate obesity as well as advanced age.[89,91,99,100] The use of laparoscopy for para-aortic node dissection in endometrial carcinoma may have a more limited role and can usually be reserved for patients with positive pelvic nodes, as may be the case with corresponding open surgery. One distinction to be made with respect to para-aortic node dissection for ovarian cancer is that less emphasis can be placed on dissecting those highest para-aortic nodes at the renal hilus.

CONCLUSION AND RECOMMENDATIONS

As described in this chapter and in Chapter 6 on prognosis, one can identify a number of factors that can predict the identification of extrauterine disease at staging laparotomy. Other than grade, CA 125 level, and radiographic identification of extrauterine disease, there may be little practical benefit at this time to extensive molecular characterization of the tumor identified as endometrial cancer at D & C. It is important to separate out low-risk patients who can be treated either medically or by vaginal hysterectomy from those who will require staging according to the International Federation of Gynecology and Obstetrics (FIGO) criteria.[102,103] The additional prognostic information relating to tumor size and depth of myometrial invasion gleaned from evaluation of the excised uterus may provide further confirmation of the preoperative risk assessment in patients to be managed conservatively (Table 4–5).[104] The presence of a positive Pap smear should alert the physician to a greater likelihood of cervical involvement as well as a poorer prognosis. AGUS smears are more likely to be associated with low-grade lesions; overt malignant smears are more likely to be associated with high-grade lesions or nonendometrioid histology.

Preoperative identification of occult cervical stromal involvement appears to have limited benefit; in the absence of extrauterine disease, the choice of surgical therapy does not appear to affect survival

Table 4–5.   A SCHEME FOR DEFINITIVE STAGING, BASED ON APPROPRIATE RISK AND BENEFIT

		Anovulatory	Ovulation induction*
Grade 1 tumor, clinically confined to the uterus	Desire for preserving fertility (see Chapter 9)	Obese	Progestin therapy*
	No indication for childbearing	Uterine descent	Vaginal hysterectomy and BSO*
		No uterine descent	Abdominal hysterectomy and BSO; node dissection determined by extent of intrauterine disease
		Medical contraindications to surgery	Progestin therapy
Grade 2 or 3 tumor clinically confined to the uterus	Uterine descent and indications for vaginal surgery		Vaginal hysterectomy, BSO and laparoscopic node dissection, as indicated
	No indications for vaginal surgery		Abdominal hysterectomy, BSO and node dissection
Cervical invasion	Gross cervical involvement	Medically fit for radical surgery	Radical hysterectomy, BSO and pelvic node dissection
		Not fit for radical surgery	Preoperative brachytherapy followed by total abdominal hysterectomy, BSO and node dissection
	Occult cervical involvement		Postoperative pelvic radiation therapy + possible Brachytherapy ± brachytherapy
Adnexal involvement	Isolated disease in one ovary at laparotomy	Benign by frozen section	Treat as stage 1 with variation by grade
		CA 125, question second primary at laparotomy	Abdominal hysterectomy, BSO, omentectomy, node dissection, including para-aortics
		Probable metastasis at laparotomy	Abdominal hysterectomy, BSO, omentectomy, node dissection, including para-aortics
	Other foci of disease in the pelvis and/or abdomen		Complete cytoreductive surgery, if technically feasible and medically tolerated

*CA 125 < 20 U/mL.
BSO = bilateral salpingo-oophorectomy.

for stage II (occult) disease. Stage II gross disease is best treated with preoperative radiation therapy or radical hysterectomy, if appropriate, being mindful of a high risk of extrauterine disease.

As better therapies are developed for the treatment of metastatic disease, in particular for those tumors of nonendometrioid histology, surgical staging of endometrial carcinoma will have a more powerful role. Its greater value in the diagnosis of metastatic disease will be validated with better therapy and improved overall outcome.

REFERENCES

1. Obermair A, Hanzal E, Schreiner-Frech I, et al. Influence of delayed diagnosis on established prognostic factors in endometrial cancer. Anticancer Res 1996;16(2):947–9.

2. Menczer J, Krissi H, Chetrit A, et al. The effect of diagnosis and treatment delay on prognostic factors and survival in endometrial carcinoma. Am J Obstet Gynecol 1995;173(3 Pt 1):774–8.

3. Guido RS, Kanbour-Shakir A, Rulin MC, Christopherson WA. Pipelle endometrial sampling. Sensitivity in the detection of endometrial cancer. J Reprod Med 1995;40(8):553–5.

4. Vilos GA, Harding PG, Silcox JA, et al. Endometrial adenocarcinoma encountered at the time of hysteroscopic endometrial ablation. J Am Assoc Gynecol Laparosc 2002;9(1):40–8.

5. Eddy GL, Wojtowycz MA, Piraino PS, Mazur MT. Papanicolaou smears by the Bethesda system in endometrial malignancy: utility and prognostic importance. Obstet Gynecol 1997;90(6):999–1003.

6. Fukuda K, Mori M, Uchiyama M, et al. Preoperative cervical cytology in endometrial carcinoma and its clinicopathologic relevance. Gynecol Oncol 1999;72(3):273–7.

7. Larson DM, Johnson KK, Reyes CN Jr, Broste SK. Prognostic significance of malignant cervical cytology in patients with endometrial cancer. Obstet Gynecol 1994;84(3):399–403.

8. Goff BA, Goodman A, Muntz HG, et al. Surgical stage IV endometrial carcinoma: a study of 47 cases. Gynecol Oncol 1994;52(2):237–40.

9. Schorge JO, Molpus KL, Goodman A, et al. The effect of postsurgical therapy on stage III endometrial carcinoma. Gynecol Oncol 1996;63(1):34–9.

10. Chi DS, Welshinger M, Venkatraman ES, Barakat RR. The role of surgical cytoreduction in stage IV endometrial carcinoma. Gynecol Oncol 1997;67(1):56–60.

11. Feldman S, Cook EF, Harlow BL, Berkowitz RS. Predicting endometrial cancer among older women who present with abnormal vaginal bleeding. Gynecol Oncol 1995;56(3):376–81.

12. Epstein E, Ramirez A, Skoog L, Valentin L. Dilatation and curettage fails to detect most focal lesions in the uterine cavity in women with postmenopausal bleeding. Acta Obstet Gynecol Scand 2001;80(12):1131–6.

13. Obermair A, Geramou M, Gucer F, et al. Endometrial cancer: accuracy of the finding of a well-differentiated tumor at dilatation and curettage compared to the findings at subsequent hysterectomy. Int J Gynecol Cancer 1999;9(5):383–6.

14. Nakagawa-Okamura C, Sato S, Tsuji I, et al. Effectiveness of mass screening for endometrial cancer. Acta Cytol 2002;46(2):277–83.

15. Ferry J, Farnsworth A, Webster M, Wren B. The efficacy of the pipelle endometrial biopsy in detecting endometrial carcinoma. Aust N Z J Obstet Gynaecol 1993;33(1):76–8.

16. Schneider J, Centeno MM, Ausin J. Use of the Cornier pipelle as the only means of presurgical histologic diagnosis in endometrial carcinoma: agreement between initial and final histology. Eur J Gynaecol Oncol 2000;21(1):74–5.

17. Dunn TS, Stamm CA, Delorit M, Goldberg G. Clinical pathway for evaluating women with abnormal uterine bleeding. J Reprod Med 2001;46(9):831–4.

18. Langer RD, Pierce JJ, O'Hanlan KA, et al. Transvaginal ultrasonography compared with endometrial biopsy for detection of endometrial disease. N Engl J Med 1997;337(25):1792–8.

19. Smith-Bindman R, Kerlikowske K, Feldstein VA, et al. Endovaginal ultrasound to exclude endometrial cancer and other endometrial abnormalities. JAMA 1998;280:1510–7.

20. Goldstein RB, Bree RL, Benson CB, et al. Evaluation of the woman with postmenopausal bleeding: Society of Radiologists in Ultrasound-Sponsored Consensus Conference statement. J Ultrasound Med 2001;20(10):1025–36.

21. Epstein E, Valentin L. Rebleeding and endometrial growth in women with postmenopausal bleeding and endometrial thickness < 5 mm managed by dilatation and curettage or ultrasound follow-up: a randomized controlled study. Ultrasound Obstet Gynecol 2001;18(5):499–504.

22. Tabor A, Watt HC, Wald NJ. Endometrial thickness as a test for endometrial cancer in women with postmenopausal vaginal bleeding. Obstet Gynecol 2002;99(4):663–70.

23. Runowicz C. Can radiological procedures replace histologic examination in the evaluation of abnormal vaginal bleeding? Obstet Gynecol 2002;99(4):529–30.

24. Goldstein SR, Zeltser I, Horan CK, et al. Ultrasonography-based triage for perimenopausal patients with abnormal uterine bleeding. Am J Obstet Gynecol 1997;177(1):102–8.

25. Weber AM, Belinson JL, Bradley LD, Piemonte MR. Vaginal ultrasound versus endometrial biopsy in women with postmenopausal bleeding. Am J Obstet Gynecol 1997;177:924–9.

26. Medverd JR, Dubinsky TJ. Cost analysis model: US versus endometrial biopsy in evaluation of peri- and post-menopausal abnormal vaginal bleeding. Radiology 2002;222(3):619–27.

27. Clark TJ, Bakour SH, Gupta JK, Khan KS. Evaluation of outpatient hysteroscopy and ultrasonography in the diagnosis of endometrial disease. Obstet Gynecol 2002;99(6):1001–7.

28. Marchetti M, Litta P, Lanza P, et al. The role of hysteroscopy in early diagnosis of endometrial cancer. Eur J Gynaecol Oncol 2002;23(2):151–3.

29. Tabata T, Yamawaki T, Yabana T, et al. Natural history of endometrial hyperplasia. Study of 77 patients. Arch Gynecol Obstet 2001;265(2):85–8.

30. Osmers RG, Osmers M, Kuhn W. Prognostic value of transvaginal sonography in asymptomatic endometrial cancers. Ultrasound Obstet Gynecol 1995;6(2):103–7.

31. Gerber B, Krause A, Muller H, et al. Ultrasonographic detection of asymptomatic endometrial cancer in postmenopausal patients offers no prognostic advantage over symptomatic disease discovered by uterine bleeding. Eur J Cancer 2001;37(1):64–71.

32. Koss LG. Detection of occult endometrial carcinoma. J Cell Biochem 1995;23 Suppl:165–73.

33. Xie X, Lu WG, Ye DF, et al. The value of curettage in diagnosis of endometrial hyperplasia. Gynecol Oncol 2002;84(1):135–9.

34. Konopka B, Paszko Z, Janiec-Jankowska A, Goluda M. Assessment of the quality and frequency of mutations occurrence in PTEN gene in endometrial carcinomas and hyperplasias. Cancer Lett 2002;178(1):43–51.

35. Lemon SL, Teneriello M, Norris HJ, Birrer MJ. Molecular characterization of premalignant and malignant endometrial curettings for the early detection of endometrial carcinoma [meeting abstract]. Proc Ann Meet Am Assoc Cancer Res 1995;36:A3769.

36. Emoto M, Tamura R, Shirota K, et al. Clinical usefulness of color Doppler ultrasound in patients with endometrial hyperplasia and carcinoma. Cancer 2002;94(3):700–6.

37. Hunter JE, Tritz DE, Howell MG, et al. The prognostic and therapeutic implications of cytologic atypia in patients with endometrial hyperplasia. Gynecol Oncol 1994;55(1):66–71.

38. Cohen CJ, Rahaman J. Endometrial cancer. Management of high risk and recurrence including the tamoxifen controversy. Cancer 1995;76 10 Suppl:2044–52.

39. Maatela J, Aromaa A, Salmi T, et al. The risk of endometrial cancer in diabetic and hypertensive patients: a nationwide record-linkage study in Finland. Ann Chir Gynaecol 1994;208 Suppl:20–4.

40. Terry PD, Miller AB, Rohan TE. A prospective cohort study of cigarette smoking and the risk of endometrial cancer. Br J Cancer 2002;86(9):1430–5.

41. Weiderpass E, Baron JA. Cigarette smoking, alcohol consumption, and endometrial cancer risk: a population-based study in Sweden. Cancer Causes Control 2001;12(3):239–47.

42. Barrett RJ, Harlan LC, Wesley MN, et al. Endometrial cancer: stage at diagnosis and associated factors in black and white patients. Am J Obstet Gynecol 1995;173(2):414–22.

43. Partridge EE, Shingleton HM, Menck HR. The National Cancer Data Base report on endometrial cancer. J Surg Oncol 1996;61(2):111–23.

44. Hill HA, Coates RJ, Austin H, et al. Racial differences in tumor grade among women with endometrial cancer. Gynecol Oncol 1995;56(2):154–63.

45. Powell MA, Mutch DG, Rader JS, et al. Ribosomal DNA methylation in patients with endometrial carcinoma. Cancer 2002;94(11):2941–52.

46. Tannergard P, Wahlberg S, Kolodner R, et al. Characterization of genetical changes in families with HNPCC [meeting abstract]. Proc Ann Meet Am Assoc Cancer Res 1995; 36:A3737.

47. Burke W, Petersen G, Lynch P, et al. Recommendations for follow-up care of individuals with an inherited predisposition to cancer. I. Hereditary nonpolyposis colon cancer. Cancer Genetics Studies Consortium. JAMA 1997;277(11):915–9.

48. Lin KM, Shashidharan M, Thorson AG, et al. Cumulative incidence of colorectal and extracolonic cancers in MLH1 and MSH2 mutation carriers of hereditary nonpolyposis colorectal cancer. J Gastrointest Surg 1998;2(1):67–71.

49. Dove-Edwin I, Boks D, Goff S, et al. The outcome of endometrial carcinoma surveillance by ultrasound scan in women at risk of hereditary nonpolyposis colorectal carcinoma and familial colorectal carcinoma. Cancer 2002; 94(6):1708–12.

50. Szantho A, Szabo I, Csapo ZS, et al. Assessment of myometrial and cervical invasion of endometrial cancer by transvaginal sonography. Eur J Gynaecol Oncol 2001;22(3):209–12.

51. Smith RA, von Eschenbach AC, Wender R, et al. American Cancer Society guidelines for the early detection of cancer: update of early detection guidelines for prostate, colorectal, and endometrial cancers. CA Cancer J Clin;51(1):38–75

52. Alcazar JL, Jurado M, Lopez-Garcia G. Comparative study of transvaginal ultrasonography and CA 125 in the preoperative evaluation of myometrial invasion in indometrial carcinoma. Ultrasound Obstet Gynecol 1999;14(3):210–4.

53. Munkarah A. Is there a role for surgical cytoreduction in stage IV endometrial cancer? Gynecol Oncol 2000;78(2):83–4.

54. Leminen A, Forss M, Lehtovirta P. Endometrial adenocarcinoma with clinical evidence of cervical involvement: accuracy of diagnostic procedures, clinical course, and prognostic factors. Acta Obstet Gynecol Scand 1995;74(1):61–6.

55. Eltabbakh GH, Moore AD. Survival of women with surgical stage II endometrial cancer. Gynecol Oncol 1999;74(1): 80–5.

56. Feltmate CM, Duska LR, Chang Y, et al. Predictors of recurrence in surgical stage II endometrial adenocarcinoma. Gynecol Oncol 1999;73(3):407–11.

57. Ng TY, Nicklin JL, Perrin LC, et al. Postoperative vaginal vault brachytherapy for node-negative stage II (occult) endometrial carcinoma. Gynecol Oncol 2001;81(2):193–5.

58. Sartori E, Gadducci A, Landoni F, et al. Clinical behavior of 203 stage II endometrial cancer cases: the impact of primary surgical approach and of adjuvant radiation therapy. Int J Gynecol Cancer 2001;11(6):430–7.

59. Boente MP, Yordan EL Jr, McIntosh DG, et al. Prognostic factors and long-term survival in endometrial adenocarcinoma with cervical involvement. Gynecol Oncol 1993; 51(3):316–22.

60. Garuti G, De Giorgi O, Sambruni I, et al. Prognostic significance of hysteroscopic imaging in endometrioid endometrial adenocarcinoma. Gynecol Oncol 2001;81(3):408–13.

61. Lo KW, Cheung TH, Yim SF, Chung TK. Hysteroscopic dissemination of endometrial carcinoma using carbon dioxide and normal saline: a retrospective study. Gynecol Oncol 2002;84(3):394–8.

62. Lo KW, Cheung TH, Yim SF, Chung TK. Preoperative hysteroscopic assessment of cervical invasion by endometrial carcinoma: a retrospective study. Gynecol Oncol 2001; 82(2):279–82.

63. Arikan G, Reich O, Weiss U, et al. Are endometrial carcinoma cells disseminated at hysteroscopy functionally viable? Gynecol Oncol 2001;83(2):221–6.

64. Obermair A, Geramou M, Gucer F, et al. Does hysteroscopy facilitate tumor cell dissemination? Incidence of peritoneal cytology from patients with early stage endometrial carcinoma following dilatation and curettage (D & C) versus hysteroscopy and D & C. Cancer 2000;88(1):139–43.

65. Egarter C, Krestan C, Kurz C. Abdominal dissemination of malignant cells with hysteroscopy. Gynecol Oncol 1996; 63(1):143–4.

66. Kudela M, Pilka R. Is there a real risk in patients with endometrial carcinoma undergoing diagnostic hysteroscopy (HSC)? Eur J Gynaecol Oncol 2001;22(5):342–4.

67. Kuzel D, Toth D, Kobilkova J, Dohnalova A. Peritoneal washing cytology on fluid hysteroscopy and after curettage in women with endometrial carcinoma. Acta Cytol 2001; 45(6):931–5.

68. Gucer F, Tamussino K, Reich O, et al. Two-year follow-up of patients with endometrial carcinoma after preoperative fluid hysteroscopy. Int J Gynecol Cancer 1998;8(6):476–80.

69. Kikuchi A, Sultana J, Okai T, et al. Intrauterine sonography for preoperative assessment of cervical invasion in endometrial carcinoma. Gynecol Oncol 1997;65:415–20.

70. Patsner B, Mann WJ, Cohen H, Loesch M. Predictive value of preoperative serum CA-125 levels in clinically localized and advanced endometrial carcinoma. Am J Obstet Gynecol 1988;158:399–402.

71. Duk JM, Aalders JG, Fleurin GJ, de Bruijn HWA. CA-125: a useful marker in endometrial carcinoma. Am J Obstet Gynecol 1986;155:1097–102.

72. Sood AK, Buller RE, Burger RA, et al. Value of preoperative CA 125 level in the management of uterine cancer and prediction of clinical outcome. Obstet Gynecol 1997; 90(3):441–7.

73. Dotters DJ. Preoperative CA 125 in endometrial cancer: is it useful? Am J Obstet Gynecol 2000;182(6):1328–34.

74. Koper NP, Massuger LF, Thomas CM, et al. Serum CA 125 measurements to identify patients with endometrial cancer who require lymphadenectomy. Anticancer Res 1998;18(3B):1897–902.

75. Hsieh C-H, Chang Chien C-C, Lin H, et al. Can a preoperative CA 125 level be a criterion for full pelvic lymphadenectomy in surgical staging of endometrial cancer? Gynecol Oncol 2002;86:28–33.

76. Ebina Y, Sakuragi N, Hareyama H, et al. Para-aortic lymph node metastasis in relation to serum CA 125 levels and nuclear grade in endometrial carcinoma. Acta Obstet Gynecol Scand 2002;81(5):458–65.

77. Kurihara T, Mizunuma H, Obara M, et al. Determination of a normal level of serum CA125 in postmenopausal women as a tool for preoperative evaluation and postoperative surveillance of endometrial carcinoma. Gynecol Oncol 1998;69(3):192–6.

78. Doering DL, Barnhill DR, Weiser EB, et al. Intraoperative evaluation of depth of myometrial invasion and stage I endometrial adenocarcinoma. Obstet Gynecol 1989;74:930–3.

79. Noumoff J, Menzin A, Mikuta JJ, et al. The ability to evaluate prognostic variables on frozen section in hysterectomies performed for endometrial carcinoma. Gynecol Oncol 1991;42:202–8.

80. Goff BA, Rice LW. Assessment of depth of myometrial invasion in endometrial adenocarcinoma. Gynecol Oncol 1990; 38:46–8.

81. Larson DM, Johnson KK. Pelvic and para-aortic lymphadenectomy for surgical staging of high-risk endometrioid adenocarcinoma of the endometrium. Gynecol Oncol 1993;51(3):345–8.

82. Reich O, Winter R, Pickel H, et al. Does the size of pelvic lymph nodes predict metastatic involvement in patients with endometrial cancer? Int J Gynecol Cancer 1996;6: 445–7.

83. Larson DM, Johnson K, Olson KA. Pelvic and para-aortic lymphadenectomy for surgical staging of endometrial cancer: morbidity and mortality. Obstet Gynecol 1992; 79(6):998–1001.

84. Homesley HD, Kadar N, Barrett RJ, Lentz SS. Selective pelvic and periaortic lymphadenectomy does not increase morbidity in surgical staging of endometrial carcinoma. Am J Obstet Gynecol 1992;167(5):1225–30.

85. Fanning J, Firestein S. Prospective evaluation of the morbidity of complete lymphadenectomy in endometrial cancer. Int J Gynecol Cancer 1998;8(4):270–3.

86. Franchi M, Ghezzi F, Riva C, et al. Postoperative complications after pelvic lymphadenectomy for the surgical staging of endometrial cancer. J Surg Oncol 2001;78(4): 232–7.

87. Giannice R, Susini T, Ferrandina G, et al. Systematic pelvic and aortic lymphadenectomy in elderly gynecologic oncologic patients. Cancer 2001;92(10):2562–8.

88. Fram KM. Laparoscopically assisted vaginal hysterectomy versus abdominal hysterectomy in stage I endometrial cancer. Int J Gynecol Cancer 2002;12(1):57–61.

89. Manolitsas TP, McCartney AJ. Total laparoscopic hysterectomy in the management of endometrial carcinoma. J Am Assoc Gynecol Laparosc 2002;9(1):54–62.

90. Langebrekke A, Istre O, Hallqvist AC, et al. Comparison of laparoscopy and laparotomy in patients with endometrial cancer. J Am Assoc Gynecol Laparosc 2002;9(2):152–7.

91. Scribner DR Jr, Walker JL, Johnson GA, et al. Surgical management of early-stage endometrial cancer in the elderly: is laparoscopy feasible? Gynecol Oncol 2001;83(3):563–8.

92. Eltabbakh GH, Shamonki MI, Moody JM, Garafano LL. Laparoscopy as the primary modality for the treatment of women with endometrial carcinoma. Cancer 2001; 91(2):378–87.

93. Malur S, Possover M, Michels W, Schneider A. Laparoscopic-assisted vaginal versus abdominal surgery in patients with endometrial cancer—a prospective randomized trial. Gynecol Oncol 2001;80(2):239–44.

94. Magrina JF, Mutone NF, Weaver AL, et al. Laparoscopic lymphadenectomy and vaginal or laparoscopic hysterectomy with bilateral salpingo-oophorectomy for endometrial cancer: morbidity and survival. Am J Obstet Gynecol 1999;181(2):376–81.

95. Fram KM. Laparoscopically assisted vaginal hysterectomy versus abdominal hysterectomy in stage I endometrial cancer. Int J Gynecol Cancer 2002;12(1):57–61.

96. Scribner DR Jr, Mannel RS, Walker JL, Johnson GA. Cost analysis of laparoscopy versus laparotomy for early endometrial cancer. Gynecol Oncol 1999;75(3):460–3.

97. Vergote I, De Smet I, Amant F. Incidence of positive peritoneal cytology in low-risk endometrial cancer treated by laparoscopically assisted vaginal hysterectomy. Gynecol Oncol 2002;84(3):537–8.

98. Sonoda Y, Zerbe M, Smith A, et al. High incidence of positive peritoneal cytology in low-risk endometrial cancer treated by laparoscopically assisted vaginal hysterectomy. Gynecol Oncol 2001;80(3):378–82.

99. Scribner DR Jr, Walker JL, Johnson GA, et al. Laparoscopic pelvic and paraaortic lymph node dissection in the obese. Gynecol Oncol 2002;84(3):426–30.

100. Eltabbakh GH, Shamonki MI, Moody JM, Garafano LL. Hysterectomy for obese women with endometrial cancer: laparoscopy or laparotomy? Gynecol Oncol 2000;78 (3 Pt 1):329–35.

101. Scribner DR Jr, Walker JL, Johnson GA, et al. Laparoscopic pelvic and paraaortic lymph node dissection: analysis of the first 100 cases. Gynecol Oncol 2001;82(3):498–503.

102. Kamura T, Yahata H, Shigematsu T, et al. Predicting pelvic lymph node metastasis in endometrial carcinoma. Gynecol Oncol 1999;72(3):387–91.

103. van Doorn HC, Van Der Zee AG, Peeters PH, et al. Preoperative selection of patients with low-stage endometrial cancer at high risk of pelvic lymph node metastases. Int J Gynecol Cancer 2002;12(2):144–8.

104. Mariani A, Webb MJ, Keeney GL, et al. Low-risk corpus cancer: is lymphadenectomy or radiotherapy necessary? Am J Obstet Gynecol 2000;182(6):1506–19.

5

Pathology of Endometrial Carcinoma

ROBERT H. YOUNG, MD, FRCPath
PHILIP B. CLEMENT, MD

In this chapter, we use, with some modification, the classification of endometrial carcinomas based on cell type formulated by the International Society of Gynecological Pathologists (ISGYP) under the auspices of the World Health Organization (WHO) (Table 5–1).[1] Tumors with two or more cell types are placed in the category of a carcinoma of mixed cell type, provided the minor component(s) accounts for at least 10% of the tumor. Even smaller components of second cell types that may have prognostic significance (eg, serous) should be recorded in the pathology report.

These various subtypes will be discussed in turn. Their gross features do not differ for the most part and will be considered together as will certain general microscopic features.

GROSS AND GENERAL MICROSCOPIC FEATURES OF ENDOMETRIAL CARCINOMA

There is a great variation in the gross characteristics of endometrial carcinoma. Examination of the hysterectomy specimen in the usual case will show an appearance typical of one or more of the gross morphologic appearances of carcinoma in other hollow viscera. The endometrium may be lined in part or totally by irregular shaggy granular tissue (Figure 5–1). In some cases, striking polypoid masses project into and sometimes fill the cavity (Figure 5–2). The tumor tissue is typically pale tan to white and fleshy but occasionally is firm to gritty. Foci of hemorrhage and necrosis may be apparent. Gross inspection may show no or or varying degrees of myometrial invasion but is not always reliable, even in high-grade tumors, in determining the extent of myometrial invasion (see Chapter 6 for further illustrations on this issue). In some cases, visual inspection of the specimen may be indistinguishable from normal tissue, but carcinoma is detected on microscopic examination. Particularly in the case of high-grade tumors, there may be diffuse, or almost diffuse, myometrial invasion that is grossly obvious (Figure 5–3). It should be noted that a lush normal secretory endometrium may be grossly misinterpreted as neoplastic.

Table 5–1. CLASSIFICATION OF ENDOMETRIAL CARCINOMA
Endometrioid adenocarcinoma
Serous adenocarcinoma
Clear cell adenocarcinoma
Mucinous adenocarcinoma
Squamous cell carcinoma
Transitional cell carcinoma
Undifferentiated carcinoma
Carcinoma of mixed cell type

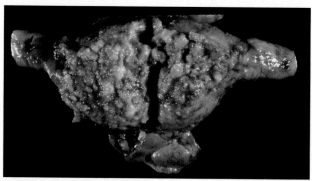

Figure 5–1. Endometrioid carcinoma. The endometrial cavity is completely lined with irregular friable neoplastic tissue.

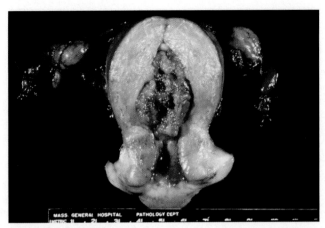

Figure 5–2. Endometrioid carcinoma. A polypoid tumor fills the endometrial cavity.

Careful gross evaluation of a hysterectomy specimen is important in leading to judicious sampling. In cases with extensive disease of the uterus and adjacent tissues, including adnexa, or in cases in which the anatomy is distorted by extensive leiomyomas or adhesions, meticulous sectioning and recording of the site of origin of particular blocks may be crucial in determining such issues as the extent of local or regional spread and even the site of origin of the tumor, given the frequent multicentricity of mullerian neoplasia of the female genital tract. Any variant of endometrial carcinoma may be associated with a histologically similar tumor involving one or both

ovaries. When this is seen with tumors in the endometrioid category (Figure 5–4), the uterine and ovarian tumors are most often independent primary tumors.[2] When the tumors are higher-grade neoplasms, particularly those in the serous group, the tumors are metastatic from one site to the other in a greater number of the cases. Criteria for determining the primary site in endometrioid tumors are presented in Tables 5–2, 5–3, and 5–4, and many of the principles apply to the evaluation of other cell types.[3] In the endometrioid group, particularly in the case of low-grade tumors, the relation between the two tumors can usually be resolved with confidence, but for higher grade endometrioid tumors and tumors of other cell types, it may be impossible to resolve the issue with certainty.

Gross evaluation is also important in judging whether a tumor may be primarily in the lower uterine segment.[4-6] Some recent evidence suggests that

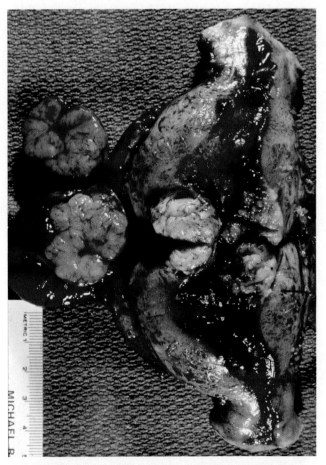

Figure 5–4. Synchronous endometrioid carcinoma of the uterine corpus and ovaries. One ovary (*left*) contains a well-delineated solid mass and the corpus (*right*) an independent primary.

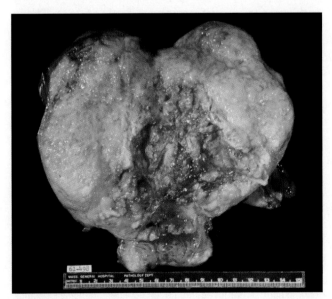

Figure 5–3. Endometrioid carcinoma. There is extensive tumor lining the endometrium and an abnormal-appearing myometrium due to extensive myometrial invasion.

Table 5–2.   ENDOMETRIOID TUMORS OF OVARY AND ENDOMETRIUM: INDEPENDENT PRIMARY TUMORS

1. Histologic dissimilarity of tumors
2. No or only superficial myometrial invasion of endometrial tumor
3. No vascular space invasion of endometrial tumor
4. Atypical endometrial hyperplasia present
5. Absence of other evidence of spread of endometrial tumor
6. Ovarian tumor unilateral (80 to 90% of cases)
7. Ovarian tumor located in parenchyma
8. No vascular space invasion, surface implants, or predominant hilar location in ovary
9. Absence of other evidence of spread of ovarian tumor
10. Ovarian endometriosis or adenofibroma present

Table 5–4.   ENDOMETRIOID TUMORS OF OVARY AND ENDOMETRIUM: OVARIAN PRIMARY; ENDOMETRIAL SECONDARY

1. Histologic similarity of tumors
2. Large ovarian tumor—small endometrial tumor
3. Ovarian endometriosis or adenofibroma present
4. Location in ovarian parenchyma
5. Direct extension from ovary predominantly into outer wall of uterus
6. Spread elsewhere in typical pattern of ovarian carcinoma
7. Ovarian tumor unilateral (80 to 90% of cases) and forming single mass
8. No atypical hyperplasia in endometrium

such tumors, which account for 3 to 6% of all uterine corpus carcinomas, are disproportionately common in young women (under 50 years) and are often high grade and more deeply invasive than tumors elsewhere in the corpus. Endometrial carcinomas in young women, which include rare cases in teenagers,[7] are usually low-grade endometrioid carcinomas (see Chapter 9). Most high-grade endometrioid tumors or high-risk variants, such as serous or clear cell carcinoma, occur in postmenopausal patients. However, a subset of patients under 40 years old with a low body mass index in a recent study had tumors with unfavorable histology; that is, serous or clear cell carcinoma.[8]

The general microscopic features of endometrial carcinoma are as varied as their gross appearances, which are exemplified by the amount and distribution of tumor in a hysterectomy specimen. Most of the endometrium may be lined by tumor, or the tumor may have striking focality and an abrupt interface with adjacent endometrium (Figure 5–5). Sometimes, the tumor, usually of the endometrioid type, is multifocal within a background of endometrial hyperplasia (Figure 5–6), but others occur on a background of atrophy (Figure 5–7). There may be striking polypoid intracavitary growth of tumor without any myometrial invasion or, conversely, striking myometrial invasion may be seen in cases with minimal endometrial tumor or none at all if the surface tumor has been removed by a prior curettage.

ENDOMETRIOID CARCINOMA

Our classification of endometrioid carcinoma and its subtypes again follows that of the ISGYP/WHO with minor modifications (Table 5–5). These tumors account for about 80% of all endometrial carcinomas.

Table 5–4.   ENDOMETRIOID TUMORS OF OVARY AND ENDOMETRIUM: ENDOMETRIAL PRIMARY; OVARIAN SECONDARY

1. Histologic similarity of tumors
2. Large endometrial tumor—small ovarian tumor(s)
3. Atypical endometrial hyperplasia present
4. Deep myometrial invasion
   a. Direct extension into adnexa
   b. Vascular space invasion in myometrium
5. Spread elsewhere in typical pattern of endometrial carcinoma
6. Ovarian tumors bilateral and/or multinodular
7. Hilar location, vascular space invasion, surface implants, or combination in ovary
8. Ovarian endometriosis or adenofibroma absent

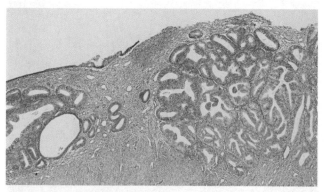

Figure 5–5. Endometrioid carcinoma, low grade, confined to the endometrium. A large aggregate of confluent neoplastic glands forms a rounded aggregate within the endometrium and occupies most of the right half of the illustration. It is separated from a smaller focus of tumor (*left*) by essentially normal endometrium.

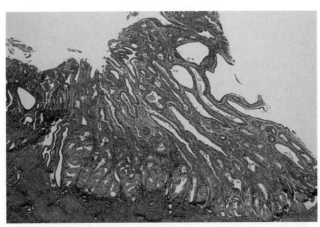

Figure 5–6. Endometrioid carcinoma, low grade. The tumor is occurring on the background of hyperplasia. The superficial half of the field shows only hyperplasia whereas the lower half, particularly to the *left*, shows a cribriform pattern of grade 1 endometrioid carcinoma.

Typical Endometrioid Carcinoma

The typical endometrioid carcinoma is composed of tubular glands that are mostly medium sized but may range from small to cystically dilated (Figure 5–8). They are lined by stratified or pseudostratified columnar cells that may have cilia (Figure 5–9). Mucin is usually absent or confined to luminal tips of the cells, but minor foci of mucinous differentiation (cells with intracellular mucin) are present in almost half the tumors (Figure 5–10). If more than 10% of the cells are mucinous, the tumor should be classified as a tumor of mixed cell type with a notation on the approximate extent of each component. Luminal mucin may be prominent in an endometrioid carcinoma and does not warrant categorization

Table 5–5. ENDOMETRIOID CARCINOMA OF THE UTERINE CORPUS
Variants
With squamous differentiation
Secretory
Villoglandular
With small nonvillous papillae
Other

of the tumor as a mucinous carcinoma. The cells of endometrioid carcinoma typically have an unimpressive amount of pale to eosinophilic cytoplasm (see Figure 5–9), although occasionally it is more abundant and strikingly eosinophilic.[9] Nuclear pleomorphism is most often only mild to moderate (Figure 5–11) but occasionally is severe. Stromal foamy histiocytes (Figure 5–12) occur in approximately 15% of tumors, usually those that are well differentiated, and this finding in a curettage specimen should suggest the possibility of endometrial carcinoma. About one-third of endometrioid adenocarcinomas are associated with endometrial hyperplasia, a finding less commonly seen in tumors arising in the lower uterine segment. The epithelial component of a malignant mixed mullerian tumor (MMMT) (see Chapter 15) often has the microscopic appearance of endometrioid carcinoma, but a tumor is placed in the latter category only when a sarcomatous stromal component is also present. In some endometrioid carcinomas, there are spindled epithelial cells (Figure 5–13), which may lead to a misdiagnosis of MMMT. The spindle cells in the pure carcinomas are less atypical than those of an MMMT, merge

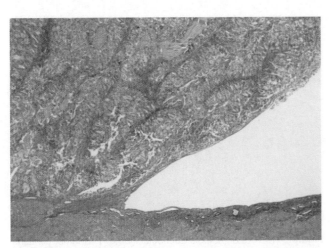

Figure 5–7. Endometrioid adenocarcinoma. This grade 2/3 tumor (*left*) is arising on the background of an atrophic endometrium (*right*).

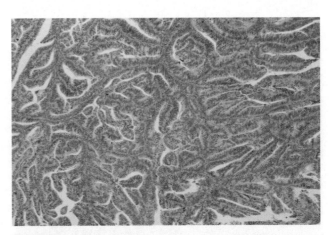

Figure 5–8. Endometrioid carcinoma. Typical low-power appearance of tubular glands of varying sizes and shapes, most being of moderate size.

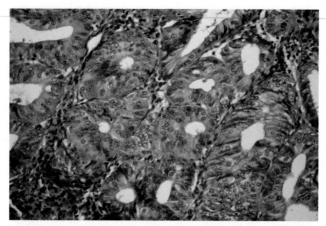

Figure 5–9. Endometrioid adenocarcinoma. Typical cytologic features of a low-grade neoplasm showing lightly eosinophilic cytoplasm and pseudostratified epithelial cells with mild atypia. Reproduced with permission from Clement PB, Young RH.[10]

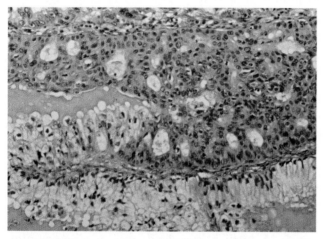

Figure 5–10. Endometrioid adenocarcinoma. This tumor is associated with a minor component of mucinous cells that have basally located nuclei and pale mucin-rich cytoplasm.

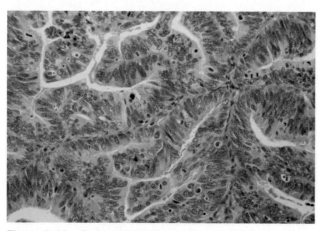

Figure 5–11. Endometrioid adenocarcinoma. This tumor shows brisk mitotic activity and modest cytologic atypia.

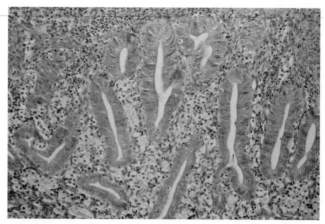

Figure 5–12. Endometrioid adenocarcinoma. The neoplastic glands are separated by stroma containing numerous foam cells.

more imperceptibly with the glandular epithelial cells, and often show focal small whorls indicative of abortive squamous differentiation.[10] Some equate MMMT with sarcomatoid carcinoma, an approach that the authors do not agree with. MMMT is of epithelial cell origin, but tumors should be categorized on their morphologic features, not just their histogenesis; otherwise, many tumors with differing appearances and behavior would be grouped together.

Tumors with a small glandular pattern often cause diagnostic problems in biopsy or curettage material, especially when an associated neutrophilic infiltrate and luminal mucin are present (Figure 5–14), which result in a superficial resemblance to microglandular hyperplasia of the cervix.[11,12] Careful attention to cytologic features and, in some cases,

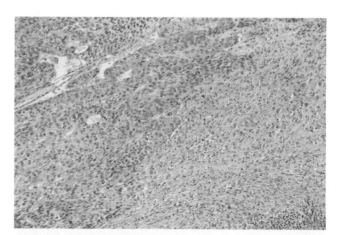

Figure 5–13. Endometrioid adenocarcinoma. This tumor contains a component of spindled epithelial cells occupying the *right* portion of the illustration (sarcomatoid carcinoma).

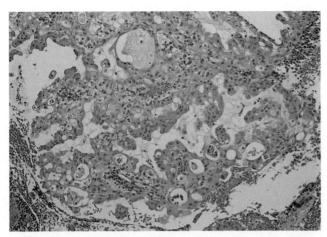

Figure 5–14. Endometrioid adenocarcinoma. This tumor has a microglandular pattern, focal mucin, and a neutrophilic infiltrate. The appearance superficially resembles that of microglandular hyperplasia.

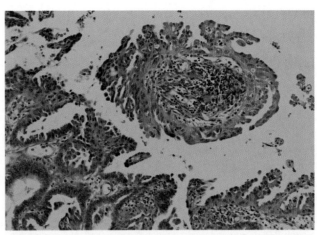

Figure 5–15. Endometrioid adenocarcinoma. The surface of this neoplasm shows a syncytial growth of cells and micropapillae simulating the benign process of syncytial papillary metaplasia.

the presence of a minor component of more typical endometrioid carcinoma will resolve this problem. Certain knowledge that the problematic tissue is from the endometrial cavity is also important, and uncertainty should be resolved by hysteroscopic evaluation. When a hysterectomy is performed in these cases, the microglandular pattern is usually superficial, with typical endometrioid neoplasia beneath it. Tumors in this general category are typically low grade. In other endometrioid carcinomas, surface changes may resemble syncytial papillary metaplasia (Figure 5–15), and this finding alone in a scanty curettage specimen may require additional sampling to exclude an associated carcinoma.[13]

Occasionally endometrioid carcinomas (and for that matter other cell types, most notably serous carcinoma) arise within an endometrial polyp (Figure 5–16) or rarely even in an adenomyoma.[10] In many cases, there is also tumor outside the polyp or adenomyoma, and deciding where it actually arose from is often impossible. Otherwise, carcinomas associated with endometrial polyps have no special features. A similar comment pertains to carcinomas found in pregnant patients.[14]

Endometrioid Carcinoma with Squamous Differentiation

About one-quarter of endometrioid carcinomas contain focal to extensive squamous elements ranging from intraluminal rounded aggregates (morules) (Fig-

ure 5–17) of immature squamous cells with bland nuclear features (adenoacanthoma) to foci that, viewed in isolation, would be considered squamous cell carcinoma (adenosquamous carcinoma).[15–18] This old subdivision into adenoacanthoma and adenosquamous carcinoma is no longer advocated. Diverse patterns of squamous differentiation are seen ranging from individual cell keratinization to the formation of large masses of keratin. Necrosis may be seen within rounded foci of the morular type. The immature squamous cells that constitute the classic morule may become confluent (see Figure 5–17) and impart a solid appearance. Appreciation by the pathologist that the cells are immature squamous cells is important so that

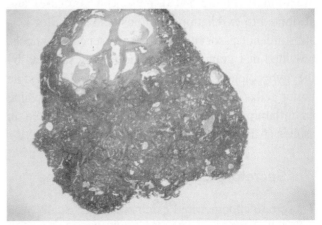

Figure 5–16. Endometrioid adenocarcinoma. This tumor arose in a polyp, remnants of which are seen at the top in the form of cystically dilated glands separated by a cellular fibrous stroma (senile cystic polyp). Most of the picture shows overgrowth of the polyp by carcinoma.

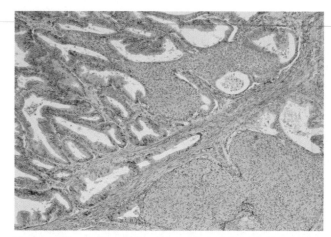

Figure 5–17. Endometrioid adenocarcinoma. Rounded intraluminal aggregates of bland epithelial cells (morules) just above the center of the field represent abortive squamous differentiation. At the *bottom right*, the morules have become confluent with a solid pattern, but the immature squamous features and bland cytologic features distinguish them from the solid pattern of a high-grade carcinoma.

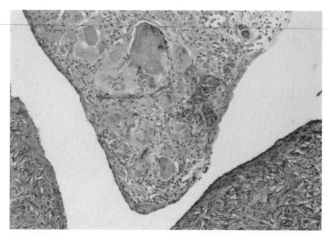

Figure 5–18. Peritoneal keratin granuloma. A small focus of keratin and associated foreign-body giant cells are closely apposed to the surface of the ovary from this patient who had uterine endometrioid carcinoma with squamous differentiation. Keratin has exfoliated from the tumor and implanted on the ovary, a finding not associated with adverse prognostic consequences.

the tumor is not given a higher grade than it should. Their uniform, bland cytology and, in some cases, association with focal overt squamous differentiation are helpful diagnostically. The behavior of tumors with squamous differentiation is dependent on the grade of the glandular component and is similar to that of typical endometrioid carcinomas when matched for grade and depth of myometrial invasion. Rare features of these tumors include those in which the squamous cells are spindled or have clear glycogen-rich cytoplasm. The latter should be carefully distinguished from clear cell carcinoma on the basis of their lack of distinctive patterns of that tumor. Peritoneal keratin granulomas (Figure 5–18), present in rare cases and attributed to exfoliation and transtubal spread of keratin, are not associated with a worsened prognosis, provided that granulomas are thoroughly sampled by the gynecologist and pathologist to exclude viable tumor cells.[19] The authors know of one case in which an inflammatory reaction to the keratin resulted in ascites (A.F. Fuller, personal communication)

Secretory Endometrioid Carcinoma

These rare endometrioid carcinomas are usually well differentiated and contain cells with subnuclear and/or supranuclear glycogen vacuoles (Figure 5–19).[20–22] The appearance is attributed to an endogenous or exogenous progestational stimulus in some cases, but

in most cases there is no obvious cause. This appearance has no therapeutic or prognostic implications. It is important that the clarity of the cell cytoplasm does not lead to a misdiagnosis of clear cell adenocarcinoma. The latter has distinctive patterns of its own (which will be presented later) that do not include secretory features.

Villoglandular Endometrioid Carcinoma

About 10% of endometrioid carcinomas contain an appreciable component characterized by villouslike papillae with thin fibrovascular cores (Figure

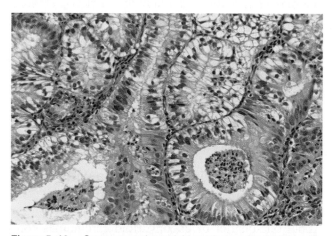

Figure 5–19. Secretory endometrioid carcinoma. Most of the cells have striking subnuclear vacuoles and many also have supranuclear vacuoles.

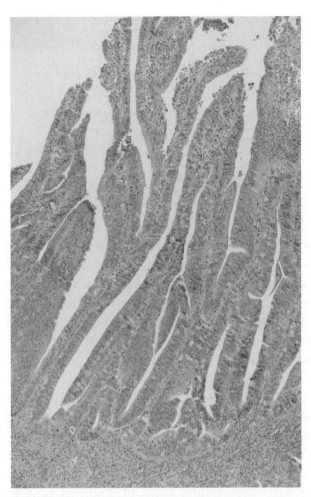

Figure 5–20. Endometrioid adenocarcinoma with villoglandular papillary pattern. The papillae are tall and fingerlike and lack the budding typically seen in serous carcinoma.

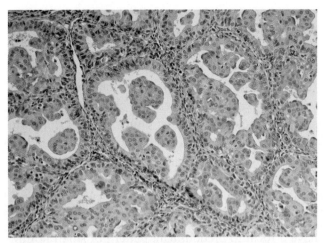

Figure 5–21. Endometrioid adenocarcinoma with small nonvillous papillae. The papillae lack the high-grade cytologic features usually seen in serous carcinoma. Reproduced with permission from Clement PB, Young RH.[10]

Endometrioid Carcinoma with Small Nonvillous Papillae

This pattern of endometrioid carcinoma (Figure 5–21), which is particularly apt to be confused with serous papillary carcinoma, has only recently been described and is seen at least focally in about 8% of endometrioid carcinomas.[25] The mean age of patients was intermediate between that of patients with endometrioid carcinoma of the usual type and that of patients with serous papillary carcinoma. Patients had an overall 5-year survival of 84%, which is similar to that of patients with typical endometrioid carcinoma and more than double that of patients with serous papillary carcinoma. These tumors are characterized by small papillae occurring within glands of otherwise typical endometrioid carcinoma or on the villous projections of villoglandular endometrioid carcinoma. Most of the papillae are in the form of buds of cells with ample eosinophilic cytoplasm, perhaps in some tumors reflecting abortive squamous differentiation, and a low nuclear-cytoplasmic ratio. Some papillae may have a more complex pattern in which they anastomose with the formation of slitlike spaces enhancing the confusion with serous carcinoma. A combination of a more complex papillary pattern, greater degree of cellular budding, more conspicuous slit-like spaces, and greater cytologic atypia generally point to the diagnosis of serous carcinoma.

5–20).[23,24] Approximately 40% of tumors, which are almost always grade 1 or 2, are pure, whereas the rest are mixed with typical endometrioid carcinoma or occasionally another histologic type. The villous pattern tends to be most striking in superficial foci of tumor but may also be seen in tumor invasive of the myometrium. The behavior is similar to that of typical endometrioid carcinoma of similar grade in most studies. Ambros and colleagues, however, found that myoinvasive tumors in this group had a higher frequency of vascular invasion and nodal involvement and a worse outcome than myoinvasive endometrioid carcinoma of usual type.[23] The two types, however, had a similar behavior when confined to the endometrium. The generally tall papillae, lack of conspicuous cellular budding, and usually lower grade distinguish these tumors from serous carcinoma.

Rare Variants of Endometrioid Carcinoma and Miscellaneous Rare Findings

Hendrickson and Kempson described an unusual type of tumor they designated "ciliated carcinoma," which consisted of sheets of cells punctured by small extracellular lumina imparting a cribriform appearance.[26] The tumor cells have grade 1 nuclear features and cilia that project into extracellular and intracellular lumina. The behavior is similar to that of typical endometrioid carcinoma. This same comment pertains to rare endometrioid carcinomas that have a focal to predominant pattern of small hollow or solid tubules lined by columnar cells with apical, occasionally clear, cytoplasm, as well as short slender cords.[27] In other rare cases, stromal hyalinization can entrap the epithelial cells of endometrioid carcinoma with the formation of sex cord-like structures.

Psammoma bodies can occur rarely in otherwise typical endometrioid carcinomas as may benign heterologous elements in the stroma (fat, osteoid).[28,29] The presence of the former should not lead to the misdiagnosis of serous carcinoma nor should the latter result in a misdiagnosis of MMMT.

Two rare subtypes of endometrioid carcinoma with a poor prognosis are those that show focal trophoblastic differentiation and those with a giant cell component.[30,31] The former may feature isolated syncytiotrophoblastic cells or foci of typical choriocarcinoma. The trophoblastic elements are immunoreactive for human chorionic gonadotropin (hCG). Tumors are typically associated with elevated serum levels of hCG that decline after hysterectomy. In tumors with a malignant giant cell component, poorly cohesive sheets and nests of bizarre multinucleated giant cells are present. There is a marked inflammatory infiltrate in half the cases. Pure or almost pure giant cell tumors should be considered a variant of undifferentiated carcinoma (see below).

DIFFERENTIAL DIAGNOSIS OF ENDOMETRIOID CARCINOMA

Various benign processes may be misinterpreted as endometrioid adenocarcinoma, particularly in curettage or biopsy material when the diagnosis of endometrioid carcinoma is usually first established.

Table 5–6. BENIGN MIMICS OF ENDOMETRIOID CARCINOMA

1. Artifactual (curettage-induced)
   Pseudopapillarity of atrophic endometrium
   Compaction of normal endometrial glands
   Telescoping
2. Menstrual-associated collapse with glandular crowding and regeneration
3. Intravascular menstrual endometrium
4. Adenomyosis with atrophic stroma
5. Intravascular adenomyosis
6. Florid squamous metaplasia
7. Polyps with epithelial proliferations or atypia

A list of these benign processes is presented in Table 5–6. The first category in the table includes appearances that are induced, in large part, by the curettage procedure, and mere familiarity with the entity and lack of cytologic atypia of the epithelial cells should facilitate the correct interpretation. The second category includes the glandular crowding and regeneration that is typical of menstrual collapse. The menstrual background in these cases is a clue to the correct diagnosis. In some cases, menstrual endometrium may extend into vascular channels within the myometrium; we have seen this misinterpreted as extensive vascular invasion by endometrioid carcinoma. Intravascular plugs of epithelial cells are associated with stromal cells, which one would not expect if it were carcinoma. Adenomyosis may also involve vascular channels, and the presence of endometrial stroma is again a clue to the diagnosis, as is the presence of associated conventional adenomyosis. In postmenopausal patients, adenomyosis typically has an atrophic stroma, and when there is extensive adenomyosis with limited stroma, the dispersed glands may be misinterpreted as invasive endometrioid carcinoma. However, there is no stromal reaction to the glands, which have a somewhat even distribution and lack cytologic atypia. Problems caused by florid squamous metaplasia are mentioned elsewhere in the text. Polyps may have varying degrees of epithelial proliferation within them, which, when florid, can be problematic. The association with atrophic cystic glands of a senile cystic polyp and other evidence of an associated polyp are clues to the diagnosis. Polyps of an adenomyomatous type, particularly when associated with epithelial atypia (so-called atypical polypoid adenomyoma), can be particularly challenging in a curettage specimen when the well-circumscribed gross nature of the lesion evident in a hysterectomy is generally not appreciable. The background smooth muscle that is present is a clue to the diagnosis, as is the fact that the smooth muscle resembles cellular leiomyomatous smooth muscle, rather than the normal smooth muscle of the myometrium.

GRADING OF ENDOMETRIOID CARCINOMA WITH COMMENTS ON PROGNOSTIC FACTORS TO BE NOTED IN PATHOLOGY REPORT

The 1988 International Federation of Gynecology and Obstetrics (FIGO)/ISGYP grading for endometrioid adenocarcinomas, with modifications suggested by Zaino and colleagues in 1995, considers both pattern and nuclear features.[1,32] Tumors that are < 5% solid are grade 1; 5 to 50% solid are grade 2; and > 50% solid are grade 3. Solid foci due to the presence of a squamous component are discounted. The presence of grade 3 nuclear features (marked nuclear pleomorphism, coarse chromatin, and prominent nucleoli) in the majority of neoplastic cells in architecturally grade 1 or 2 tumors increases their grade by 1 (see Figure 5–11). More recently, Takeshima and colleagues found that architectural grade 1 or 2 tumors with > 25% of grade 3 nuclei had a similar behavior to those with > 50% grade 3 nuclei.[33] Taylor and colleagues have proposed a two-tier grading system based on the FIGO system, in which low-grade tumors have 20% or less nonsquamous solid areas, whereas high-grade tumors had > 20% non-squamous solid areas.[34] They found that this system was less cumbersome, had less interobserver variation, and had the same or better prognostic significance as the three-grade system.

Recently, Lax and colleagues have also proposed a binary architectural grading system for endometrioid carcinomas, which they found to be more reproducible than the FIGO system and identified subsets of advanced-stage tumors with favorable and unfavorable prognosis.[35] In this system, a tumor was classified as high grade if at least two of the following three criteria were present: (1) > 50% solid growth (without distinction of squamous from nonsquamous

epithelium); (2) a diffusely infiltrative, rather than expansile, growth pattern; and (3) tumor cell necrosis. For tumors confined to the endometrium, only criteria 1 and 3 are evaluated, and if both are present, the tumors are considered high grade. This system stratified patients into three prognostic groups based on grade and surgical staging: (1) patients with stage IA or IB low-grade tumors had a 100% 5-year survival; (2) patients with higher-stage (IC, II–IV), low-grade tumors and those with high-grade tumors confined to the myometrium (IB and IC) had a 5-year survival of 67 to 76%; and (3) patients with advanced-stage, high-grade tumors had a 26% 5-year survival rate.

Factors to mention in the pathology report, in addition to the histologic type, include the grade, depth of myometrial invasion, special features (if any) of invasive tumor, and the presence or absence of involvement of lymphovascular spaces, the cervix (see below), the serosa, the parametrium, the adnexa, and other tissues submitted, such as lymph nodes.

PATTERNS OF INVASION BY ENDOMETRIOID CARCINOMA

A confluent arrangement of neoplastic glands within the endometrium or a disorderly distribution of clearly malignant glands generally makes recognition of endometrial stromal invasion obvious (see Figure 5–5). It is sometimes erroneously thought that carcinomas that do not invade the myometrium lack a metastatic potential, but such is not always the case. Transtubal spread to the peritoneum and implantation at the vaginal apex are the two most obvious examples, the former being particularly common in cases of serous carcinoma and other poor-prognosis subtypes. Endometrioid carcinomas and other tumors that are typically low grade may implant at the vaginal apex as may high-grade tumors.

Endometrioid carcinoma commonly extends into adenomyosis, and care should be taken not to misinterpret this as myometrial invasion. Adjacent uninvolved adenomyosis should prompt the pathologist to consider carcinomatous involvement of adenomyosis. Such foci typically have smooth contours at their periphery (Figure 5–22) without the disorderly distribution of invasive glands that characterize many, but

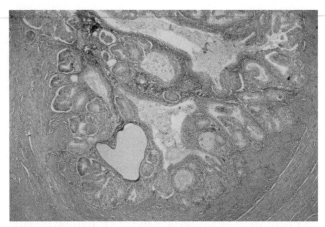

Figure 5–22. Endometrioid adenocarcinoma involving adenomyosis. The cystic gland with flattened epithelium (*lower left*) is a clue that this focus of carcinoma involves adenomyosis. The relatively well-circumscribed margin of the glandular proliferation also favors involvement of adenomyosis.

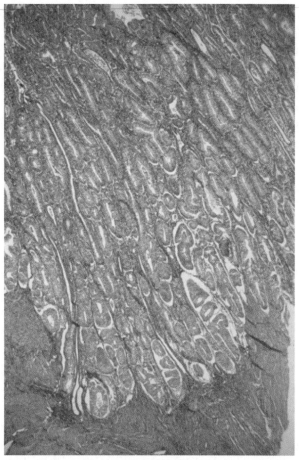

Figure 5–23. Endometrioid adenocarcinoma. The bulbous pushing base of this lesion does not represent invasion, the latter requiring a more conspicuous confluent growth of carcinomatous glands or irregular infiltration.

not all, invasive tumors. Traces of associated adenomyosis (either residual benign endometrioid glands or stroma) at the edge of the foci of tumor or within it (see Figure 5–22), should be sought to substantiate the diagnosis of carcinoma involving adenomyosis. When the tumor in the myometrium is confined to adenomyotic foci, the prognosis is not adversely affected.[36,37]

Most myoinvasive tumors show an irregular penetration of the myometrium. It should be noted that at the base of many tumors confined to the endometrium, there is a bulbous contour that is not considered invasion of the myometrium (Figure 5–23). In most cases of early myometrial invasion, the infiltrating glands have a random disorderly arrangement (Figure 5–24). In some cases, however, tumor invades in smoothly contoured, sometimes rounded, aggregates (Figure 5–25), but low-power microscopy that demonstrates a confluent proliferation and effacement of the underlying myometrium generally readily distinguishes this pattern of early invasion from the bulbous irregularity of tumor confined to the endometrium noted above (see Figure 5–23). Some tumors have a distinctive pattern of myoinvasion, in which individual glands are widely spaced in the myometrium ("diffusely infiltrating" pattern) (Figure 5–26).[38] The prognostic significance of this pattern, on the basis of the largest study of the phenomenon, does not differ from that of typical invasion. When glands in such cases are deceptively benign appearing, the term "adenoma malignum" pattern has been

used, but the authors do not recommend it.[38] Carcinoma invasive of the myometrium is usually at least focally gland forming, but sheets, nests, or small clusters of tumor cells or single cells may be seen. A desmoplastic reaction or a lymphocytic response may be seen and sometimes the stromal response is myxoid. Occasionally, myoinvasive endometrioid glands undergo a peculiar but distinctive change characterized by microcystic or slitlike glands with a lining of flattened epithelial cells (Figure 5–27).[10]

EFFECTS OF TREATMENT ON THE HISTOLOGIC APPEARANCE OF ENDOMETRIAL CARCINOMA

Radiation-induced changes include the disappearance of tumor; necrosis of tumor; tumor cell cytoplasm that is increased in the amount and degree of

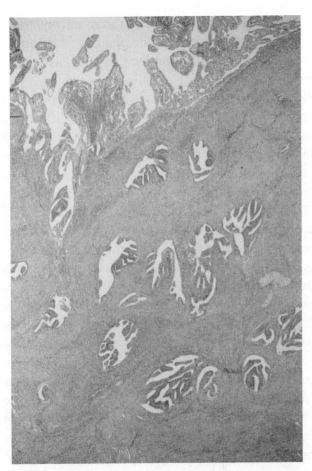

Figure 5–24. Endometrioid adenocarcinoma with superficial myometrial invasion. In contrast to the prior figure, there are irregularly dispersed and abnormally branching glands in the superficial myometrium.

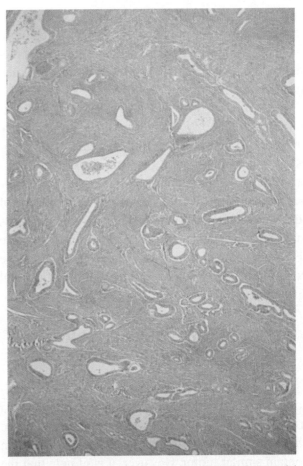

Figure 5–26. Endometrioid adenocarcinoma with myometrial invasion. The glands are widely separated with little or no stromal reaction, an appearance that represents the so-called diffusely infiltrating or adenoma malignum pattern of myometrial invasion, the latter term being used when cytologic features are relatively bland.

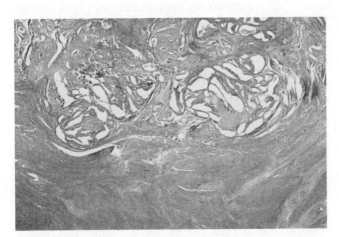

Figure 5–25. Endometrioid adenocarcinoma with superficial myometrial invasion. Although having a well-circumscribed boundary with the adjacent myometrium, the low-power confluence of the glands indicates the presence of myometrial invasion.

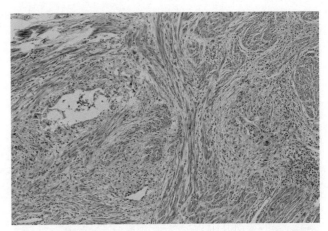

Figure 5–27. Endometrioid adenocarcinoma with myometrial invasion. There is a peculiar pattern of invasion characterized by small clusters of cells (*3 o'clock*) and a cystic gland lined by flattened epithelium (*9 o'clock*). There is also a desmoplastic stromal reaction.

vacuolation; nuclei that are bizarre, pyknotic, or karyorrhectic; and enlarged nucleoli.[39] The tumor may become more differentiated, and squamous elements that are absent in a pretreatment specimen may become prominent.

Progestins can also induce changes in endometrioid carcinomas. Well-differentiated tumors have been occasionally successfully treated with progestins, suggesting that at least some of them disappear entirely (see Chapter 9). Those that persist may become better differentiated, with the appearance of squamous metaplasia within the tumor. The glands may become smaller with an atrophic appearance (Figure 5–28), and there may be an increase in the ratio of stroma to tumor, with prominent decidual change of the stroma.

DISTINCTION BETWEEN ENDOMETRIAL AND ENDOCERVICAL CARCINOMAS

The distinction between an endometrial adenocarcinoma and an endocervical adenocarcinoma in a fractional dilatation and curettage specimen may be challenging when both components of the specimen contain similar tumor. However, it is of note that the typical endometrial carcinoma is endometrioid, and, in our experience, endometrioid carcinomas of the cervix are rare. The typical endocervical primary adenocarcinoma, that is, the so-called endocervical-type adenocarcinoma of the cervix, has a distinctly

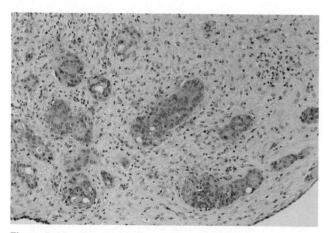

Figure 5–28. Endometrioid adenocarcinoma in patient on progesterone therapy. The picture differs from that of usual endometrioid adenocarcinoma due to the effect of the hormonal therapy. The stroma is prominent and somewhat decidualized. Glands are barely visible, and those present are very small.

different histologic appearance from endometrioid carcinoma of the corpus. The glands of the former are generally smaller, and their lining cells tend to have more intense amphophilic to eosinophilic cytoplasm, are more mitotically active, and show more apoptosis.[40] Despite these morphologic differences in the great majority of cases, there are other cases in which morphologic overlap is such that other findings may aid in the distinction. Colposcopic and hysteroscopic findings, as well as the presence of associated atypical endometrial hyperplasia or endocervical adenocarcinoma in situ, can be helpful. Much has been written about the role of immunohistochemistry in their distinction, in the authors' opinion, to a degree that is not matched by the aid obtained in routine practice.[41] Nonetheless, some brief comment on the topic is indicated. Endometrial adenocarcinomas are generally characterized by a vimentin (VIM)-positive, estrogen-receptor (ER)-positive, and carcinoembryonic antigen (CEA)-negative profile, whereas endocervical adenocarcinomas are characterized by the opposite findings.[42,43] The detection of human papillomavirus (HPV) by in situ hybridization also favors an endocervical origin, although it is by no means always present in such tumors.[44]

Other immunohistochemical studies have compared the immunoprofile of endometrial endometrioid adenocarcinomas with that of endometrial serous carcinomas. Kounelis and colleagues reported that endometrioid carcinomas have a much lower expression of P53 than do serous carcinomas (35% versus 76%).[45] Most of the P53-positive endometrioid carcinomas were high grade; similar findings have been reported in other studies. In the same study, ER and progesterone receptors (PRs) were much more commonly present (in 70% and 72.5%, respectively) in endometrioid carcinomas than in serous carcinomas (in 23.8% and 19%, respectively).

CERVICAL INVOLVEMENT BY ENDOMETRIAL CARCINOMA

Assessment of the cervix by a pathologist is an important facet of the staging of endometrial carcinoma. In stage IIA disease, tumor is confined to the endocervical epithelium (Figure 5–29), whereas in IIB disease, tumor is invasive of the endocervical

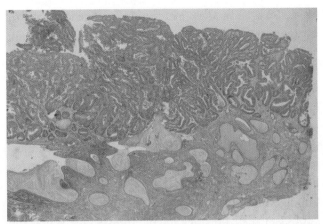

Figure 5–29. Endometrioid adenocarcinoma with spread to endo-cervical mucosa. There is no cervical stromal invasion (stage IIA endometrial cancer).

stroma (Figure 5–30). In most studies, stage IIB disease is associated with a worse prognosis in comparison to stage I, but stage IIA disease is not. The diagnosis of stage II disease in the 1988 FIGO staging system for endometrial carcinoma is based on examination of the hysterectomy specimen. In some institutions, however, preoperative radiation treatment is still given to patients in whom stage II disease is diagnosed by clinical examination in conjunction with an endocervical curettage (ECC). Histologic diagnosis of stage II disease on the basis of the findings within an ECC specimen can be difficult because these specimens are often artifactually contaminated by tumor from the endometrial cavity. Artifactual contamination most commonly takes the form of tumor fragments unattached to

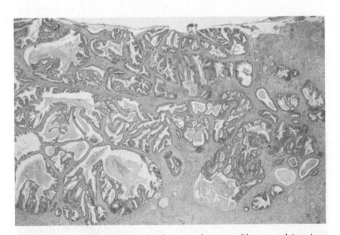

Figure 5–30. Endometrioid adenocarcinoma with spread to uterine cervix. There is stromal invasion (stage IIB endometrial carcinoma). The confluence of the glandular proliferation indicates stromal invasion.

stroma admixed with normal endocervical tissue. In such cases, the presence of detached fragments of adenocarcinoma, without definite cervical involvement should be noted. Failure to do so can result in the tumor being inappropriately considered stage IIB and potentially lead to overly extensive treatment. Abeler and Kjorstad for example, reviewed 278 ECC specimens initially considered positive for involvement by endometrial carcinoma and concluded that only 24% of them represented unequivocal stage IIB disease, as indicated by the presence of stromal invasion in tissue fragments that were covered by normal squamous or endocervical glandular epithelium.[46] The diagnosis of cervical involvement by an endometrial endometrioid carcinoma is usually more straightforward in a hysterectomy specimen, as is the distinction between stage IIA and stage IIB disease. However, some problems can arise. Although stromal invasion is usually manifested by an irregular penetration of individual glands that are obviously malignant, sometimes there are leisurely patterns of growth that can be somewhat deceptive. For example, as seen in Figure 5–30, glands are growing in a somewhat organized fashion without overt single gland infiltration of the stroma. However, the distribution of glands in the superficial stroma is too confluent for one to avoid the conclusion that there has been endocervical stromal invasion. Even more challenging are cases in which the glands are separated and small and unassociated with a stromal reaction (Figure 5–31). In some of these cases, it is possible to misinterpret the glands as benign endocervical glands mesonephric remnants. Careful high-power microscopic scrutiny is crucial, and comparison of the glands with differentiated glands of the endometrial primary should enable the conclusion that the cervical process represents extension from the corpus neoplasm.

SEROUS ADENOCARCINOMA

The frequency of this important subtype of endometrial carcinoma varies in the literature from 1 to 10% because of difficulties that may arise in its distinction from other papillary endometrial carcinomas, including the two papillary variants of endometrioid carcinoma already considered, as well as clear cell carci-

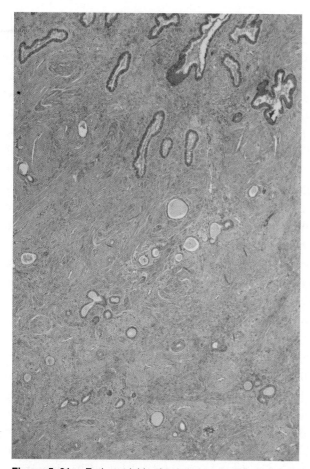

Figure 5–31. Endometrioid adenocarcinoma with spread to uterine cervix. This form of stromal invasion (stage IIB endometrial carcinoma) may be diagnostically challenging. The glands are widely separated, mostly small, and bland in appearance, with limited stromal reaction. These features may result in their being misinterpreted as a benign process, such as hyperplasia of mesonephric remnants. Normal endocervical glands are seen at the top.

noma (see "Clear Cell Adenocarcinoma").[47–63] Patterns of patient referral may also influence its prevalence in clinical series because recognition of the adverse prognosis associated with its diagnosis on curettage may lead to referral to specialized treatment centers. It is inappropriate for a pathologist to sign a case out as papillary adenocarcinoma because this descriptive term can refer to several different subtypes of endometrial carcinoma. Most patients with serous carcinoma present with postmenopausal bleeding, but some have a serous or serosanguineous vaginal discharge. Some tumors are discovered on examination of a Pap smear. Occasional patients have had the *BRCA1* germline mutation, indicating that some serous carcinomas are a component of the familial

breast–ovarian cancer syndrome.[57] A background of estrogen use is much less common in patients with serous carcinoma compared with patients with endometrioid carcinoma. Occasional patients have a history of pelvic radiation. Some patients with serous carcinoma of the endometrium present with an ovarian or peritoneal serous carcinoma with clinical evidence of ascites. In such cases, where there is unilateral or bilateral ovarian disease and extensive peritoneal implants, determining whether the uterine tumor is the primary or part of multifocal mullerian neoplasia may be difficult or impossible. When the endometrium is extensively involved and there is transmural spread with significant myometrial vascular permeation and only superficial involvement of one or both ovaries, classification of the tumor as an endometrial primary is appropriate. In some cases, endometrial involvement by serous carcinoma represents part of a massive pelvic neoplasia, and when the endometrial neoplasia is much less bulky than the extrauterine neoplasia, particularly that of the peritoneal surfaces, a peritoneal primary tumor is usually the correct interpretation.

On gross examination, serous carcinoma has no unique features (Figure 5–32). However, in our experience, the tumor is generally not as bulky within the uterus as is often the case with endometrioid carcinoma, presumably because the propensity of serous carcinoma to rapidly spread leads the patient to come to clinical attention before there is a massive bulk of intracavitary tumor. Indeed, in some cases of widespread metastatic serous carcinoma of the endometrium, the disease in the corpus may be relatively limited but still apparently is the primary tumor. The tumor tissue that lines part or all of the endometrial cavity has an irregular friable granular quality, with varying degrees of hemorrhage, typical

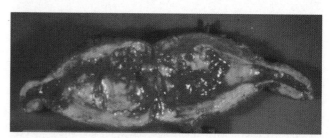

Figure 5–32. Serous carcinoma. The endometrium is extensively involved by a nodular tumor with hemorrhage.

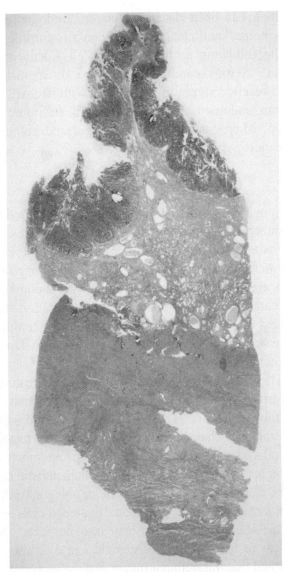

Figure 5–33. Serous carcinoma. The tumor is coating the surface of a polyp.

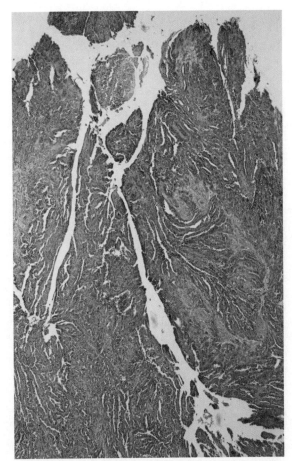

Figure 5–34. Serous carcinoma. There are striking slitlike glands that are common in serous carcinomas of the genital tract.

of most variants of endometrial carcinoma. Occasionally, serous carcinoma is not appreciated grossly, some of these tumors being so small as to not be apparent either on the lining of an apparently normal flat endometrium or on the surface of a polyp that is grossly indistinguishable from a benign polyp (Figure 5–33).

Microscopic examination generally shows the typical morphology of serous carcinoma as seen prototypically in the ovary. In our experience, however, a slit-like glandular pattern (Figure 5–34) is less conspicuous in endometrial neoplasms than in ovarian neoplasms, and the serous designation is usually applied to the endometrial cases on the basis

of a complex papillary pattern (Figure 5–35), with fibrovascular stalks covered by stratified highly atypical epithelial cells forming characteristic cellular buds. The typical irregular slit-like glands of serous carcinoma may be conspicuous in some cases, as may solid sheets of cells. When solid foci are viewed in isolation, the neoplasm would be considered undifferentiated, but when associated with characteristic serous morphology in adjacent zones, they are appropriately considered a component of the serous carcinoma. Psammoma bodies are present in a minority of cases and generally not particularly conspicuous. The nuclear features are typically high grade, at least grade 2 of 3 and usually grade 3 of 3. There is typically marked nuclear pleomorphism with prominent nuclear hyperchromasia, large prominent nucleoli, and numerous mitotic figures. Hobnail-type cells may be seen, indicating that these cells are not diagnostic of clear cell carcinoma.

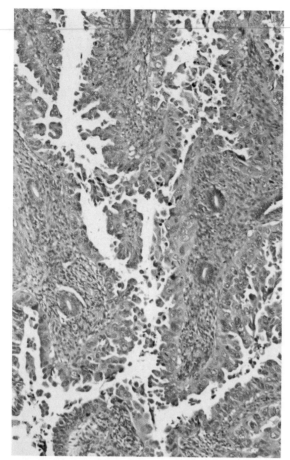

Figure 5–35. Serous carcinoma. There is a striking micropapillary pattern with numerous cellular buds emanating from the surface of the endometrium.

Bizarre mononucleate cells and pleomorphic giant cells may be encountered.

Some serous carcinomas involve part of a polyp, and, in some of these cases, the serous carcinoma is confined to the surface of the polyp.[61] Similarly, a serous carcinoma may be confined to the surface (nonpolypoid) endometrial epithelium. The designation "endometrial intraepithelial carcinoma" or "noninvasive serous carcinoma" has been applied to such cases.[63] The authors do not agree with these terms because these serous carcinoma cells can metastasize, particularly by exfoliation through the fallopian tube in a transcoelomic manner with fatal consequences. Serous carcinomas are typically aneuploid and only rarely express estrogen or progesterone receptors.

The differential diagnosis of serous carcinoma with villoglandular endometrioid carcinoma and endometrioid carcinoma with small nonvillous

papillae has been discussed under "Endometrioid Carcinoma," and clear cell carcinoma is considered in the following section, "Clear Cell Adenocarcinoma." Serous carcinoma must be distinguished from reactive atypia in association with necrosis of benign endometrium, particularly in an infarcted polyp, where striking reactive atypia and hobnail-type cells may be seen.

Clear Cell Adenocarcinoma

Although clear cell carcinoma has been recorded to account for a higher frequency in some studies, in our experience, it represents approximately 1% of endometrial carcinomas.[20,64–74] The presenting features are similar to those of women with endometrioid carcinoma. A history of pelvic irradiation was present in 16% of cases in one study, and in another there was an association with the use of tamoxifen or synthetic progestins.[20,66]

These tumors have no distinctive gross features and are characterized on microscopic examination by the tubulocystic (Figure 5–36), papillary, and solid patterns that characterize this tumor in the female genital system as a whole. Similarly, the endometrial examples show one or more of the characteristic cell types, clear (Figure 5–37), hobnail, or polygonal with abundant eosinophilic cytoplasm. Flattened cells and nonspecific cuboidal cells may also be seen. The nuclear features are typically grade 2 or 3. It should be noted that intraluminal mucin may be seen just as it may in endometrioid carcinoma. In occasional tumors, intracellular mucin takes the form of a dis-

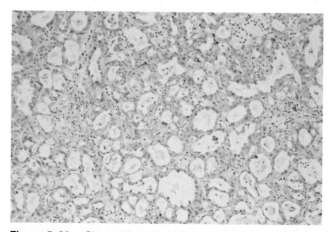

Figure 5–36. Clear cell adenocarcinoma. A typical tubulocystic pattern is shown.

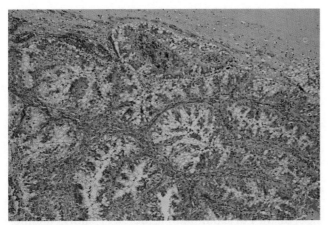

Figure 5–37. Clear cell adenocarcinoma. Most of the tumor cells have a striking clear cytoplasm.

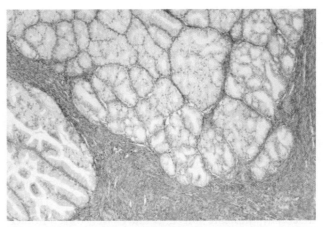

Figure 5–38. Mucinous adenocarcinoma. There is a closely packed glandular pattern, and the cells lining the glands are columnar with conspicuous pale mucin-rich cytoplasm.

tinct eosinophilic "targetoid" globule. Stromal hyalinization with deposition of basement membrane-like material is common, especially in the cores of the papillae, a distinctive feature of clear cell carcinoma compared with serous carcinoma. The cells covering the papillae of clear cell carcinoma are typically not as stratified and do not form cellular buds to the same degree as is seen in serous carcinomas.

Clear cell carcinomas, which are much rarer than serous carcinomas in our experience, commonly share a papillary pattern with serous carcinoma. In the clear cell tumors, the papillae often have hyalinized cores, generally not a feature of serous carcinoma, and a tubulocystic pattern is also typical of clear cell carcinoma. Hobnail cells are more conspicuous in clear cell carcinoma, although not diagnostic on their own; conversely, prominent clear cells are not a feature of serous carcinoma.

Mucinous Adenocarcinoma

In our opinion, mixed endometrioid and mucinous adenocarcinomas are relatively common, and it is even more common to see an endometrioid carcinoma with a minor (less than 10%) component of mucinous cells, where the mucinous component is discounted for purposes of classification. It is our experience that pure or almost pure mucinous carcinomas are distinctly rare and account for no more than 1% of endometrial carcinomas.[12,66,71–75]

Microscopic examination shows endocervical-type columnar cells with pale mucin-rich cytoplasm (Fig-

ure 5–38), the mucinous nature of which can be confirmed with a histochemical stain for mucin. Mucinous metaplasia of the associated nonneoplastic endometrium is present in occasional cases. The cells are usually cytologically bland. The tumors are almost always grade 1 (and focally, the tumor cells may even have a benign appearance) but are occasionally grade 2 and have varied patterns, ranging from complex glandular to cribriform to villous. In some cases there is a microglandular pattern. These small glands and dilated larger glands may contain conspicuous inspissated mucin with neutrophils, a facet of these tumors that contributes to a resemblance of microglandular hyperplasia, as has already been referred to in the "Endometrioid Carcinoma" section.[11,12] Rare mucinous adenocarcinomas have an intestinal-type appearance, containing goblet cells and, in occasional cases, Paneth cells, neuroendocrine cells, or both.[75]

The differential diagnosis of mucinous carcinoma of the endometrium is primarily with mucinous adenocarcinoma of the endocervix. This may be an exceptionally difficult differential diagnosis on morphologic grounds alone but is infrequently encountered because overtly mucinous carcinoma of the endocervix is rare; although it is often considered "mucinous," the usual endocervical adenocarcinoma is not composed of cells with striking mucinous features.[40] When this issue does arise, careful clinical evaluation with hysteroscopy and fractional curettage to discern the exact location of the tumor are often more important than morphology in determining the primary site. However, in a primary endometrial tumor there is more apt to be an admixture with neoplastic or nonneoplastic endometrioid glands or endometrial stroma, and in the endocervical tumors there is more apt to be a dense fibrous stroma. The immunohistochemical findings summarized in the "Endometrioid Carcinoma" section may help but, in our experience, are often not conclusive. The pathologist must be suspicious when benign-appearing mucinous epithelium (particularly if abundant) is present in specimens of definite endometrial origin, a finding that may indicate an unusually well-differentiated mucinous carcinoma of the endometrium. In such cases, the pathologist should evaluate carefully the architectural features and ask for additional specimens or recommend hysteroscopy if the tissue is inadequate for a confident conclusion.

Squamous Cell Carcinoma

These tumors account for 0.25 to 0.5% of endometrial carcinomas.[76,77] Predisposing factors in some cases include cervical stenosis, pyometra, uterine prolapse, and a history of pelvic radiation. On gross examination, the diagnosis may be suggested when a tumor has a uniformly white appearance (Figure 5–39), although in some cases the appearance is nondistinctive. In cases of pyometra, the tumors may be associated with extensive squamous metaplasia of the adjacent endometrial lining ("ichthyosis

uteri"), and this metaplastic squamous epithelium may merge with neoplastic epithelium that in many cases is well differentiated (Figure 5–40). The tissue can, indeed, be so well differentiated that it can pass as benign epithelium in a curettage specimen. If abundant well-differentiated squamous epithelium is obtained with confidence from the endometrial cavity of a postmenopausal patient, it should be considered extremely suspicious for well-differentiated squamous cell carcinoma. In some cases, there is a marked diversity of appearance within the same neoplasm. For example, Figure 5–41 shows another area of the tumor illustrated in Figure 5–40. In the second of the illustrations, the tumor is poorly differentiated in contrast to the extremely well-differentiated keratinizing neoplasm in the other. On the basis of the first view, the differential diagnosis with so-called leukoplakia would be difficult,

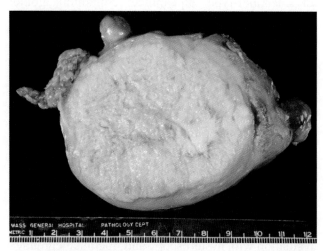

Figure 5–39. Squamous cell carcinoma. The tumor is uniformly white, a frequent feature of squamous cell carcinoma of the corpus that should suggest the diagnosis.

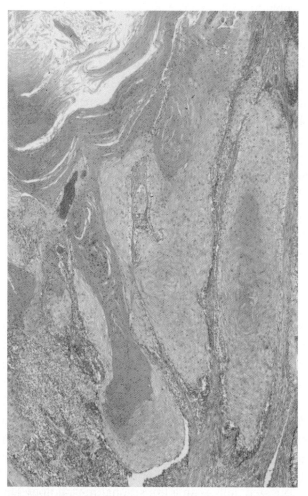

Figure 5–40. Squamous cell carcinoma. The tumor is very well differentiated and associated with abundant keratin production.

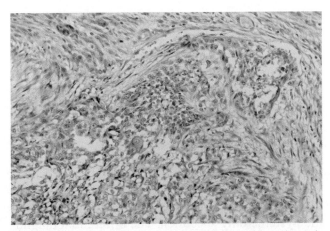

Figure 5–41. Squamous cell carcinoma. This focus of tumor is poorly differentiated. A single keratinizing cell is seen just off center. This focus is from the same tumor as that in the previous figure illustrating the diversity of differentiation that may be seen in individual cases.

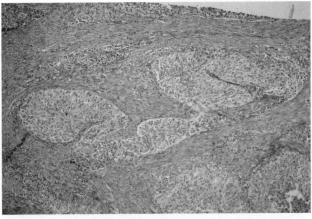

Figure 5–42. Transitional cell carcinoma. The nested pattern is similar to that seen in invasive transitional cell carcinoma of the urinary bladder.

although the mere amount of the squamous epithelium and the somewhat irregular shape of the large columns of epithelial cells is of concern. Extremely rare tumors merit the designation verrucous squamous cell carcinoma if there is the typical pushing border of a very well-differentiated tumor.[78] Rare high-grade tumors have a component of neoplastic spindle cells of the epithelial type.[79] Rare squamous cell carcinomas of the endometrium have been associated with HPV infection.[80]

The differential diagnosis of endometrial squamous cell carcinoma includes extension of a cervical squamous cell carcinoma into the endometrial cavity.[81] Careful clinical evaluation usually readily distinguishes a primary endometrial squamous cell carcinoma from endometrial spread of a cervical carcinoma. The differential diagnosis also includes endometrioid carcinomas with abundant squamous differentiation, in which a biopsy sample may show only the squamous component, but this is a rare occurrence.

Transitional Cell Carcinoma

The small number of these tumors reported have occurred in the typical age group of patients with endometrial cancer.[82,83] Pure primary tumors are rare and typically have a nested (Figure 5–42) or papillary morphology, with the nests and papillae composed of elongated cells with a transitional morphology (Figure 5–43), including appreciable longitudinal nuclear

grooves in well-differentiated tumors. In some cases, transitional cell carcinoma is associated with a carcinoma of another cell type, placing the tumor in the category of a tumor of mixed cell type.

Undifferentiated Carcinoma

This term applies to tumors that are too poorly differentiated to be categorized as belonging to one of the specific categories reviewed above.[84,85] They account for about 1.5% of all endometrial carcinomas. On gross examination, these tumors have no distinctive gross features but typically have ominous features, such as extensive hemorrhage and necrosis. Most of these tumors have a microscopic appearance

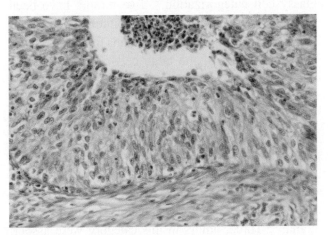

Figure 5–43. Transitional cell carcinoma. The cytologic features are similar to those of a relatively low-grade transitional cell carcinoma of the urinary bladder.

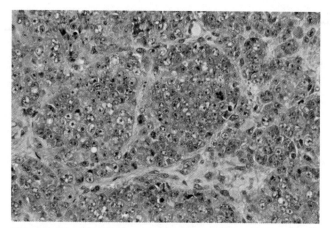

Figure 5–44. Undifferentiated carcinoma. There is a vague nested pattern. The tumor cells have appreciable cytoplasm and large nuclei with prominent nucleoli.

similar to that of undifferentiated carcinoma, not otherwise specified, as seen in many organs of the body, being composed of diffuse sheets and nests (Figure 5–44) and clusters of varying sizes. The cells are typically of moderate to large size, often with appreciable cytoplasm, and with high-grade nuclear atypica. Pleomorphic giant cells may be seen and rarely predominate. Minimal differentiation toward glands and papillae does not exclude a diagnosis of undifferentiated carcinoma. Some tumors have a component of spindled epithelial cells (sarcomatoid carcinoma); such cells typically (but not always) mark with cytokeratin and rarely predominate. Rare tumors resemble the glassy cell carcinoma of the cervix, but, in the authors' opinion, these tumors cannot be consistently distinguished from undifferentiated carcinoma not otherwise specified, and we do not advocate use of glassy cell categorization.[86] Two tumors have been reported that resemble lymphoepithelioma in other sites.[87] Immunohistochemical stains to document the epithelial nature of the large cells in the lymphoid background are diagnostically helpful. In reported cases, there has been no evidence of the presence of Epstein-Barr virus. Rare undifferentiated tumors have differentiated toward choriocarcinoma.[88] A few tumors that would otherwise have been considered large cell undifferentiated carcinoma with eosinophilic cytoplasm have resembled hepatocellular carcinoma and are descriptively designated "hepatoid carcinoma."[89] Three tumors in this category were associated with elevation of the serum alpha-fetoprotein (AFP) level; in a fourth case, the AFP level was not

measured. One patient, with stage IIIA disease, received chemotherapy and was well at 8 years,[89] but the other tumors were fatal. AFP immunoreactivity was documented in all tumors. A component of conventional endometrioid carcinoma was documented in three cases. MMMT often has a component that, in isolation, would be diagnosed as undifferentiated carcinoma, and this is sometimes the only tissue obtained in an initial biopsy or curettage. In such cases, particularly in an elderly woman, the possibility of MMMT should be excluded by examination of the hysterectomy specimen. The differential diagnosis of undifferentiated carcinoma is limited. When there is a uniform diffuse distribution, malignant large cell lymphoma may be an issue, but if the matter cannot be resolved by careful attention to the differing cytologic features of undifferentiated carcinoma and malignant lymphoma, immunohistochemical stains for cytokeratin and lymphoid markers will help. One specific subtype of undifferentiated carcinoma, small cell undifferentiated carcinoma, merits separate consideration.

Small Cell Undifferentiated Carcinoma

These tumors of the endometrium are much less common than those of the uterine cervix and occur in patients at a mean of 60 years of age.[90,91] Approximately two-thirds of the patients have stage II disease or higher. The prognosis is poor. Rare cases are associated with bilateral diffuse uveal melanocytic proliferations.[92]

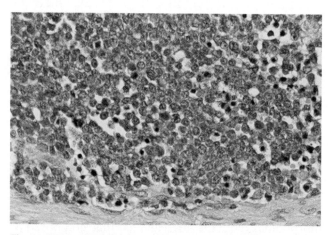

Figure 5–45. Small cell undifferentiated carcinoma. The tumor cells are small with scant cytoplasm and characteristic hyperchromatic nuclei.

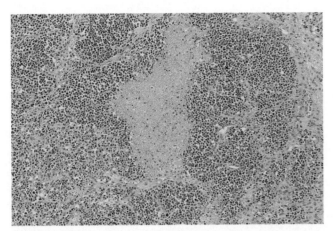

Figure 5–46. Small cell undifferentiated carcinoma. Necrosis is conspicuous.

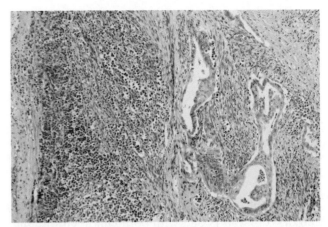

Figure 5–48. Small cell undifferentiated carcinoma (*left*) in a case in which there was a minor component of typical endometrioid carcinoma (*right*).

In most cases, microscopic examination shows sheets of small cells with scant cytoplasm, hyperchromatic nuclei, and a brisk mitotic rate (Figure 5–45). In some cases, the cells grow focally in cords or nests, and rosettes may be seen. Necrosis is often conspicuous (Figure 5–46). Neuroendocrine differentiation has been found with special techniques in most tumors, including immunoreactivity for one or more neuroendocrine markers (Figure 5–47). These tumors may derive from neuroendocrine cells that are present in some endometrioid carcinomas[93] but more likely represent aberrant differentiation of a conventional epithelial cell, and, indeed, many small cell carcinomas are associated with a minor component of endometrioid carcinoma (Figure 5–48), supportive of this contention. Small cell carcinoma is often associ-

ated with prominent vascular invasion in hysterectomy specimens and is typically deeply invasive.

Clinical evaluation generally readily distinguishes these tumors from small cell carcinoma of the cervix. The differential diagnosis with malignant lymphoma or leukemia may be raised, particularly in poorly preserved biopsy or curettage material. In well-fixed routinely evaluated specimens, this differential diagnosis will not usually be a diagnostic problem; if difficulty exists, appropriate immunohistochemical stains for lymphoid markers will be definitive. Rare primitive neuroectodermal tumors may also enter into the differential diagnosis, but they may contain true rosettes or Homer Wright pseudorosettes and occasionally exhibit glial, ependymal, and medulloepithelial differentiation. Immunoreactivity for glial

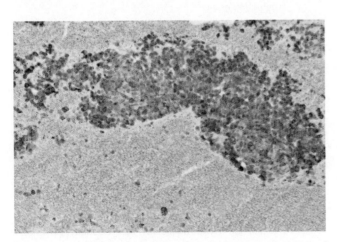

Figure 5–47. Small cell undifferentiated carcinoma. A cluster of tumor cells in a curettage specimen is immunoreactive for chromogranin confirming the neuroendocrine nature of the tumor.

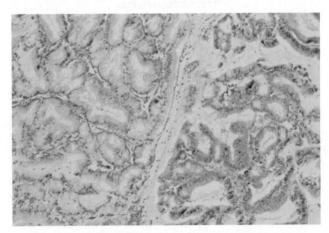

Figure 5–49. Mixed endometrioid and mucinous adenocarcinoma. Endometrioid adenocarcinoma is seen on the *right* and mucinous carcinoma on the *left*.

fibrillary acidic protein may aid in establishing the diagnosis of these rare tumors and their distinction from small cell carcinoma.

CARCINOMAS OF MIXED CELL TYPE

This category is reserved for tumors with 10% or more of a second cell type. The ISGYP-WHO classification notes that by convention, endometrioid carcinomas with squamous elements are not placed in this group. The most common mixed tumor in the authors' opinion is one with both endometrioid and mucinous components (Figure 5–49), each by definition having to account for at least 10% of the tumor. The endometrioid component usually predominates, and the tumors are low grade in the great majority of cases. There are no special clinical features. These tumors may have a microglandular pattern and occasionally cause some confusion with microglandular hyperplasia as described earlier.[11,12]

The next most common admixture of cell types is endometrioid and serous, either of which may predominate.[94] The literature experience is unclear on the issue of how much serous component is needed for a tumor to behave in the adverse manner of a pure serous cancer. In two studies, the behavior was that of a pure serous tumor if the serous component accounted for more than 25% of a mixed tumor.[60,94] Potentially, any other combination of mixed tumors may be seen, and each must be evaluated on the basis of its own particular features.

REFERENCES

1. Scully RE, Bonfiglio TA, Kurman RJ, et al. Histological typing of female genital tract tumors. New York: Springer-Verlag; 1994.
2. Zaino R, Whitney C, Brady MF, et al. Simultaneously detected endometrial and ovarian carcinomas—a prospective clinicopathologic study of 74 cases: a Gynecologic Oncology Group study. Gynecol Oncol 2001;83:355–62.
3. Scully RE, Young RH, Clement PB. Tumors of the ovary, maldeveloped gonads, fallopian tube, and broad ligament. In: Rosai J, editor. Atlas of tumor pathology. 3rd Series, No. 23. Washington (DC): Armed Forces Institute of Pathology; 1998. p. 126.
4. Hachisuga T, Kaku T, Enjoji M. Carcinoma of the lower uterine segment. Clinicopathologic analysis of 12 cases. Int J Gynecol Pathol 1989;8:26–35.
5. Hachisuga T, Fukuda K, Iwasaka T, et al. Endometrioid adenocarcinoma of the uterine corpus in women younger than 50 years of age can be divided into two distinct clinical and pathologic entities based on anatomic location. Cancer 2001;92:2578–84.
6. Jacques SM, Qureshi F, Ramirez NC, et al. Tumors of the uterine isthmus: clinicopathologic features and immunohistochemical characterization of p53 expression and hormone receptors. Int J Gynecol Pathol 1997;16: 38–44.
7. Lee KR, Scully RE. Complex endometrial hyperplasia and carcinoma in adolescents and young women 15 to 20 years of age. A report of 10 cases. Int J Gynecol Pathol 1989;8:201–13.
8. Duska LR, Garrett A, Rueda BR, et al. Endometrial cancer in women 40 years old or younger. Gynecol Oncol 2001;83: 88–93.
9. Pitman MB, Young RH, Clement PB, et al. Endometrioid carcinoma of the ovary and endometrium, oxyphilic cell type: a report of nine cases. Int J Gynecol Pathol 1994;13:290–301.
10. Clement PB, Young RH. Endometrioid carcinoma of the uterine corpus: a review of its pathology with emphasis on recent advances and problematic aspects. Adv Anat Pathol 2002;9:45–84.
11. Young RH, Scully RE. Uterine carcinomas simulating microglandular hyperplasia. A report of six cases. Am J Surg Pathol 1992;16:1092–7.
12. Zaloudek C, Hayashi GM, Ryan IP, et al. Microglandular adenocarcinoma of the endometrium: a form of mucinous adenocarcinoma that may be confused with microglandular hyperplasia of the cervix. Int J Gynecol Pathol 1997; 16:52–9.
13. Jacques SM, Qureshi F, Lawrence, WD. Surface epithelial changes in endometrial adenocarcinoma: diagnostic pitfalls in curettage specimens. Int J Gynecol Pathol 1995; 14:191–7.
14. Schammel DP, Mittal KR, Kaplan K, et al. Endometrial adenocarcinoma associated with intrauterine pregnancy. A report of five cases and a review of the literature. Int J Gynecol Pathol 1998;17:327–35.
15. Connelly PJ, Alberhasky RC, Christopherson WM. Carcinoma of the endometrium. III. Analysis of 865 cases of adenocarcinoma and adenoacanthoma. Obstet Gynecol 1982;59:569–75.
16. Alberhasky RC, Connelly PJ, Christopherson WM. Carcinoma of the endometrium. IV. Mixed adenosquamous carcinoma. A clinical-pathological study of 68 cases with long-term follow-up. Am J Clin Pathol 1982;77:655–64.
17. Abeler VM, Kjorstad KE. Endometrial adenocarcinoma with squamous cell differentiation. Cancer 1992;69:488–95.
18. Zaino RJ, Kurman R, Herbold D, et al. The significance of squamous differentiation in endometrial carcinoma. Data from a Gynecologic Oncology Group study. Cancer 1991; 68:2293–302.
19. Kim KR, Scully RE. Peritoneal keratin granulomas with carcinomas of endometrium and ovary and atypical polypoid adenomyoma of endometrium. A clinicopathological analysis of 22 cases. Am J Surg Pathol 1990;14:925–32.
20. Christopherson WM, Alberhasky RC, Connelly PJ. Carcinoma of the endometrium: I. A clinicopathologic study of clear-cell carcinoma and secretory carcinoma. Cancer 1982;49:1511–23.

21. Silverberg SG, Makowski EL, Roche WD. Endometrial carcinoma in women under 40 years of age: comparison of cases in oral contraceptive users and non-users. Cancer 1977;39:592–8.

22. Tobon H, Watkins GJ. Secretory adenocarcinoma of the endometrium. Int J Gynecol Pathol 1985;4:328–35.

23. Ambros RA, Ballouk F, Malfetano JH, Ross JS. Significance of papillary (villoglandular) differentiation in endometrioid carcinoma of the uterus. Am J Surg Pathol 1994;18:569–75.

24. Zaino RJ, Kurman RJ, Brunetto VL, et al. Villoglandular adenocarcinoma of the endometrium: a clinicopathologic study of 61 cases: a Gynecologic Oncology Group study. Am J Surg Pathol 1998;22:1379–85.

25. Murray SK, Young RH, Scully RE. Uterine endometrioid carcinoma with small nonvillous papillae: an analysis of 26 cases of a favorable-prognosis tumor to be distinguished from serous carcinoma. Int J Surg Pathol 2000;8:279–89.

26. Hendrickson M, Kempson R. Ciliated carcinoma—a variant of endometrial adenocarcinoma: a report of 10 cases. Int J Gynecol Pathol 1983;2:1–12.

27. Eichhorn JH, Young RH, Clement PB. Sertoliform endometrial adenocarcinoma: a study of four cases. Int J Gynecol Pathol 1996;15:119–26.

28. Parkash V, Carcangiu, ML. Endometrioid endometrial adenocarcinoma with psammoma bodies. Am J Surg Pathol 1997;21:399–406.

29. Nogales FF, Gomez-Morales M, Raymundo C, Aguilar D. Benign heterologous tissue components associated with endometrial carcinoma. Int J Gynecol Pathol 1982;1:286–91.

30. Kalir T, Seijo L, Deligdisch L, Cohen C. Endometrial adenocarcinoma with choriocarcinomatous differentiation in an elderly virginal woman. Int J Gynecol Pathol 1995;14:266–9.

31. Jones MA, Young RH, Scully RE. Endometrial adenocarcinoma with a component of giant cell carcinoma. Int J Gynecol Pathol 1991;10:260–70.

32. Zaino RJ, Kurman RJ, Diana KL, Morrow CP. The utility of the revised International Federation of Gynecology and Obstetrics histologic grading of endometrial adenocarcinoma using a defined nuclear grading system. A Gynecologic Oncology Group study. Cancer 1995;75:81–6.

33. Takeshima N, Hirai Y, Hasumi K. Prognostic validity of neoplastic cells with notable nuclear atypia in endometrial cancer. Obstet Gynecol 1998;92:119–23.

34. Taylor RR, Zeller J, Lieberman RW, et al. An analysis of two versus three grades for endometrial cancer. Gynecol Oncol 1999;74:3–6.

35. Lax SF, Kurman RJ, Pizer ES, et al. A binary architectural grading system for uterine endometrial endometrioid carcinoma has superior reproducibility compared with FIGO grading and identifies subsets of advance-stage tumors with favorable and unfavorable prognosis. Am J Surg Pathol 2000;24:1201–8.

36. Hall JB, Young RH, Nelson JH Jr. The prognostic significance of adenomyosis in endometrial carcinoma. Gynecol Oncol 1984;17:32–40.

37. Jacques SM, Lawrence WD. Endometrial adenocarcinoma with variable-level myometrial involvement limited to adenomyosis: a clinicopathologic study of 23 cases. Gynecol Oncol 1990;37:401–7.

38. Longacre TA, Hendrickson MR. Diffusely infiltrative endometrial adenocarcinoma: an adenoma malignum pattern of myoinvasion. Am J Surg Pathol 1999;23:69–78.

39. Silverberg SG, DeGiorgi LS. Histopathologic analysis of preoperative radiation therapy in endometrial carcinoma. Am J Obstet Gynecol 1974;119:698–704.

40. Young RH, Clement PB. Endocervical adenocarcinoma and its variants: their morphology and differential diagnosis. Histopathology 2002;41:185–207

41. Kamoi S, Al Juboury MI, Akin M-R, Silverberg SG. Immunohistochemical staining in the distinction between primary endometrial and endocervical adenocarcinomas: another viewpiont. Int J Gynecol Pathol 2002;21:217–23.

42. Castrillon DH, Lee KR, Nucci MR. Distinction between endometrial and endocervical adenocarcinoma: an immunohistochemical study. Int J Gynecol Pathol 2002;21:4–10.

43. McCluggage WG, Sumathi VP, McBride HA, Patterson A. A panel of immunohistochemical stains, including carcinoembryonic antigen, vimentin, and estrogen receptor, aids the distinction between primary endometrial and endocervical adenocarcinomas. Int J Gynecol Pathol 2002;21:11–5.

44. Hording U, Daugaard S, Visfeldt J. Adenocarcinoma of the cervix and adenocarcinoma of the endometrium: distinction with PCR-mediated detection of HPV DNA. APMIS 1997;105:313–6.

45. Kounelis S, Kapranos N, Kouri E, et al. Immunohistochemical profile of endometrial adenocarcinoma: a study of 61 cases and review of the literature. Mod Pathol 2000;13:379–88.

46. Abeler VM, Kjorstad KE. Endometrial adenocarcinoma in Norway. Cancer 1991;67:3093–103.

47. Carcangiu ML, Chambers JT. Uterine papillary serous carcinoma: a study on 108 cases with emphasis on the prognostic significance of associated endometrioid carcinoma, absence of invasion, and concomitant ovarian carcinoma. Gynecol Oncol 1992;47:298–305.

48. Carcangiu ML, Chambers JT. Early pathologic stage clear cell carcinoma and uterine papillary serous carcinoma of the endometrium: comparison of clinicopathologic features and survival. Int J Gynecol Pathol 1995;14:30–8.

49. Carcangiu ML, Tan LK, Chambers JT. Stage IA uterine serous carcinoma: a study of 13 cases. Am J Surg Pathol 1997;21:1507–14.

50. Chen JL, Trost DC, Wilkinson EJ. Endometrial papillary adenocarcinomas: two clinicopathological types. Int J Gynecol Pathol 1985;4:279–88.

51. Grice J, Ek M, Greer B, et al. Uterine papillary serous carcinoma: evaluation of long-term survival in surgically staged patients. Gynecol Oncol 1998;69:69–73.

52. Eifel PJ, Ross J, Hendrickson M, et al. Adenocarcinoma of the endometrium. Analysis of 256 cases with disease limited to the uterine corpus: treatment comparisons. Cancer 1983;52:1026–31.

53. Hendrickson M, Ross J, Eifel PJ, et al. Adenocarcinoma of the endometrium: analysis of 256 cases with carcinoma limited to the uterine corpus. Pathology review and analy-

sis of prognostic variables. Gynecol Oncol 1982;13: 373–92.

54. Hendrickson M, Ross J, Eifel P, et al. Uterine papillary serous carcinoma: a highly malignant form of endometrial adenocarcinoma. Am J Surg Pathol 1982;6:93–108.

55. Hendrickson MR, Longacre TA, Kempson RL. Uterine papillary serous carcinoma revisited. Gynecol Oncol 1994; 54:261–3.

56. Kato DT, Ferry JA, Goodman A, et al. Uterine papillary serous carcinoma (UPSC): a clinicopathologic study of 30 cases. Gynecol Oncol 1995;59:384–9.

57. Lavie O, Hornreich G, Ben Arie A, et al. BRCA1 germline mutations in women with uterine serous papillary carcinoma. Obstet Gynecol 2000;96:28–32.

58. Lee KR, Belinson JL. Recurrence in noninvasive endometrial carcinoma. Relationship to uterine papillary serous carcinoma. Am J Surg Pathol 1991;15:965–73.

59. Prat J, Oliva E, Lerma E, et al. Uterine papillary serous adenocarcinoma. A 10-case study of p53 and c-erbB-2 expression and DNA content. Cancer 1994;74:1778–83.

60. Sherman ME, Bitterman P, Rosenshein NB, et al. Uterine serous carcinoma. A morphologically diverse neoplasm with unifying clinicopathologic features. Am J Surg Pathol 1992;16:600–10.

61. Silva EG, Jenkins R. Serous carcinoma in endometrial polyps. Mod Pathol 1990;3:120–8.

62. Wheeler DT, Bell KA, Kurman RJ, Sherman ME. Minimal uterine serous carcinoma: diagnosis and clinicopathologic correlation. Am J Surg Pathol 2000;24:797–806.

63. Ambros RA, Sherman ME, Zahn CM, et al. Endometrial intraepithelial carcinoma: a distinctive lesion specifically associated with tumors displaying serous differentiation. Hum Pathol 1995;26:1260–7.

64. Abeler VM, Kjorstad KE. Clear cell carcinoma of the endometrium: a histopathological and clinical study of 97 cases. Gynecol Oncol 1991;40:207–17.

65. Abeler VM, Vergote IB, Kjorstad KE, Trope CG. Clear cell carcinoma of the endometrium. Prognosis and metastatic pattern. Cancer 1996;78:1740–7.

66. Dallenbach-Hellweg G, Hahn U. Mucinous and clear cell adenocarcinomas of the endometrium in patients receiving antiestrogens (tamoxifen) and gestagens. Int J Gynecol Pathol 1995;14:7–15.

67. Kanbour-Shakir A, Tobon H. Primary clear cell carcinoma of the endometrium: a clinicopathologic study of 20 cases. Int J Gynecol Pathol 1991;10:67–78.

68. Kurman RJ, Scully RE. Clear cell carcinoma of the endometrium: an analysis of 21 cases. Cancer 1976;37: 872–82.

69. Malpica A, Tornos C, Burke TW, Silva EG. Low-stage clear-cell carcinoma of the endometrium. Am J Surg Pathol 1995;19:769–74.

70. Webb GA, Lagios MD. Clear cell carcinoma of the endometrium. Am J Obstet Gynecol 1987;156:1486–91.

71. Czernobilsky B, Katz Z, Lancet M, Gaton E. Endocervical-type epithelium in endometrial carcinoma: a report of 10 cases with emphasis on histochemical methods for differential diagnosis. Am J Surg Pathol 1980;4:481–9.

72. Nucci MR, Prasad CJ, Crum CP, Mutter GL. Mucinous endometrial epithelial proliferations: a morphologic spectrum of changes with diverse clinical significance. Mod Pathol 1999;12:1137–42.

73. Ross JC, Eifel PJ, Cox RS, et al. Primary mucinous adenocarcinoma of the endometrium. A clinicopathologic and histochemical study. Am J Surg Pathol 1983;7:715–29.

74. Melham MF, Tobon H. Mucinous adenocarcinoma of the endometrium: a clinico-pathological review of 18 cases. Int J Gynecol Pathol 1987;6:347–55.

75. Zheng W, Yang GCH, Godwin TA, et al. Mucinous adenocarcinoma of the endometrium with intestinal differentiation: a case report. Hum Pathol 1995;26:385–8.

76. Dalrymple JC, Russell P. Squamous endometrial neoplasia—are Fluhmann's postulates still relevant? Int J Gynecol Cancer 1995;5:421–5.

77. Goodman A, Zukerberg LR, Rice LW, et al. Squamous cell carcinoma of the endometrium: a report of eight cases and a review of the literature. Gynecol Oncol 1996;61:54–60.

78. Ryder DE. Verrucous carcinoma of the endometrium—a unique neoplasm with a long survival. Obstet Gynecol 1982;59:78S–80S.

79. Yamashina M, Kobara TY. Primary squamous cell carcinoma with its spindle cell variant in the endometrium. A case report and review of literature. Cancer 1986;57:340–5.

80. Kataoka A, Nishida T, Sugiyama T, et al. Squamous cell carcinoma of the endometrium with human papillomavirus type 31 and without tumor suppressor gene p53 mutation. Gynecol Oncol 1997;65:180–4.

81. Pins MR, Young RH, Crum CP, et al. Cervical squamous cell carcinoma in situ with intraepithelial extension to the upper genital tract and invasion of tubules and ovaries: report of a case with human papilloma virus analysis. Int J Gynecol Pathol 1997;16:272–8.

82. Lininger RA, Ashfaq R, Albores-Saavedra J, Tavassoli FA. Transitional cell carcinoma of the endometrium and endometrial carcinoma with transitional cell differentiation. Cancer 1997;79:1933–43.

83. Spiegel GW, Austin RM, Gelven PL. Transitional cell carcinoma of the endometrium. Gynecol Oncol 1996;60:325–30.

84. Abeler VM, Kjorstad KE, Nesland JM. Undifferentiated carcinoma of the endometrium. A histopathologic and clinical study of 31 cases. Cancer 1991;68:98–105.

85. Alm P, Gudmundsson T, Martensson R, et al. Identification of small areas of solid growth has a strong prognostic impact in differentiated endometrial carcinomas. A histopathologic and morphometric study. Int J Gynecol Cancer 1995;5:87–93.

86. Christopherson WM, Alberhasky RC, Connelly PJ. Glassy cell carcinoma of the endometrium. Hum Pathol 1982;13:418–21.

87. Vargas MP, Merino MJ. Lymphoepithelioma-like carcinoma: an unusual variant of endometrial cancer. A report of two cases. Int J Gynecol Pathol 1998;17:272–6.

88. Pesce C, Merino MJ, Chambers JT, Nogales F. Endometrial carcinoma with trophoblastic differentiation. An aggressive form of uterine cancer. Cancer 1991;68:1799–802.

89. Adams SF, Yamada SD, Montag A, Rotmensch JR. An alpha-fetoprotein-producing hepatoid adenocarcinoma of the endometrium. Gynecol Oncol 2001;83:418–21.

90. Huntsman DG, Clement PB, Gilks CB, Scully RE. Small-cell carcinoma of the endometrium. A clinicopathological study of sixteen cases. Am J Surg Pathol 1994;18:364–75.

91. van Hoeven KH, Hudock JA, Woodruff JM, Suhrland MJ. Small cell neuroendocrine carcinoma of the endometrium. Int J Gynecol Pathol 1995;14:21–9.

92. Chadhud F, Young RH, Remulla JF, et al. Bilateral diffuse uveal melanocytic proliferation associated with extraocular cancers. Review of a process particularly associated with gynecologic cancers. Am J Surg Pathol 2001;25:212–8.

93. Aguirre P, Scully RE, Wolfe HJ, DeLellis RA. Endometrial carcinoma with argyrophil cells: a histochemical and immunohistochemical analysis. Hum Pathol 1984;15:210–7.

94. Williams KE, Waters ED, Woolas, RP, et al. Mixed serous-endometrioid carcinoma of the uterus: pathologic and cytopathologic analysis of a high-risk endometrial carcinoma. Int J Gynecol Cancer 1994;4:7–18.

6

Prognostic and Predictive Factors in the Management of Endometrial Carcinoma

ARLAN F. FULLER JR, MD

The concept of staging of cancer serves the purpose of aggregating patients into comparable groups for the purpose of understanding treatment and for standardization of care. Beyond staging, examination of other attributes related to the patient, treatment, or response to therapy and to the tumor permit a better understanding of the disease process as it interacts with the human host.

Many factors predict the likelihood of occurrence of cancer; others may predict its virulence and propensity for both local invasion or distant metastasis; still other factors may reflect the body's own response to cancer as well as the response to treatment; finally, some factors will indicate the likelihood of patient survival or the risk of recurrence of cancer and death. These factors may be considered prognostic insofar as they delineate risk of success or failure of treatment. A predictive factor, on the other hand, may be more useful, as it not only can indicate likelihood of success or failure but also, by definition, will make the choice among options that will provide the best response. For example, identification of progesterone receptor in a patient with endometrial carcinoma will predict the response to progestin therapy.

In the United States, there were nearly 40,000 reported cases of endometrial carcinoma at the turn of the century. There were over 6,000 deaths as a consequence of this disease, double the number of deaths in the preceding decade. Although there has traditionally been a low case fatality rate for this disease, the declining number of patients with unopposed estrogen-associated endometrial carcinoma and the identification and treatment of women at risk of hyperplasia diminishes the proportion of women with low-grade endometrial carcinoma with a good prognosis.

DEFINITIONS

Prognostic Factors

Prognostic factors have varied origins, are accessible at different times in the patient's course of primary treatment, and will indicate different outcomes. Their purpose is to help identify and classify patients at high risk of these varied outcomes so as to develop protocols of treatment that will modify an outcome. Classification by prognostic risk also permits the comparison of treatment groups in order to assess potential improvements in therapy.

In the simplest and broadest sense, a prognostic factor is a variable associated with disease outcome. Prognostic variables may be derived from demographic factors, disease-related factors, or those associated with the health and well being of the patient (Table 6–1). Prognostic factors may be accessible at different times in the course of the patient's disease; some are available preoperatively, others intraoperatively; still others in the postoperative period (Table 6–2).

Table 6–1. CLASSIFICATION OF PROGNOSTIC FACTORS

Demographic factors
  Age
  Race

Patient factors
  Intercurrent disease (diabetes, hypertension, obesity)
  Duration and severity of symptoms

Tumor factors—gross evaluation
  Preoperative clinicopathologic staging (FIGO and TNM)
    related to clinical examination of the cervix (examination and
    endocervical curettage)
  Operative examination of the adnexa, local extent of disease,
    and regional nodes
  Residual disease following primary surgery for patients with
    stage III and IV disease

Tumor factors—external assessment
  Radiographic studies
  Measurement of tumor markers in patient serum

Tumor factors—microscopic evaluation
  Effect of preoperative positive cervical cytology
  Evaluation of primary tumor histology and grade (type 1
    versus type 2 carcinoma)
  Evaluation of myometrial invasion, lymphovascular invasion
  Microscopic evaluation of regional lymph nodes
  Presence of endocervical mucosal or stromal invasion
  Evaluation of intraoperative peritoneal cytology
  Receptor assays: ER, PR, *HER2/neu* (EGFR)

Tumor factors—molecular assessment
  DNA content (ploidy)
  Evaluation of molecular markers in tumor tissue: *P53, P16,*
    PTEN, BCL2
  Angiogenesis-related factors: VEGF, microvessel density
  Proliferation related: S-phase fraction, *MIB1, PCNA*

EGFR = epidermal growth factor receptor; ER = estrogen receptor; FIGO =
International Federation of Gynecology and Obstetrics; PR = progesterone
receptor; TNM = tumor-node-metastasis; VEGF = vascular endothelial
growth factor.

Table 6–2. AVAILABILITY OF PROGNOSTIC FACTORS

Preoperative
  Demographics (age, race)
  Patient factors (duration and severity of symptoms, method of
    diagnosis)
  Intercurrent disease (obesity, diabetes, hypertension)
  Clinical examination of the cervix, along with assessment of
    uterine size and mobility
  Serologic tumor markers (CA 125)
  Radiographic studies (ultrasonography, computed tomography,
    magnetic resonance imaging)
  Histologic evaluation of the D & C or endometrial biopsy speci-
    men (grade, histologic subtype, presence or absence of
    cervical/endocervical involvement, and molecular markers)

Intraoperative
  Depth of myometrial invasion (visual and frozen section)
  Intra-abdominal exploration (status of omentum, liver
    parenchyma, palpable lymphadenopathy)
  Pelvic exploration (status of adnexa, serosal surfaces, and
    pelvic nodes—both gross and microscopic)
  Extent of residual disease in patients with advanced carcinoma
    (stage III, IV)

Postoperative
  Final histopathology (gross and microscopic evaluations of the
    primary tumor, cervix, adnexa, and resected nodes)
  Status of intraperitoneal washings, examined cytologically
  Evaluation of tumor markers (histologic, such as ER, PR, and
    molecular markers)

CA = cancer antigen; ER = estrogen receptor; PR = progesterone receptor;
D & C = dilatation and curettage.

Prognostic factors may influence different outcomes as follows:

- The extent of disease—defining the risk of occult metastatic disease that, if left untreated, would unfavorably affect the risk of recurrence. For example, the presence and depth of myometrial invasion might be prognostic for the risk of occult nodal metastases.

- The likelihood of tumor recurrence and, ultimately, patient survival. For example, the presence of nodal metastases will increase the risk of recurrence and decrease the chance of survival.

- The site of recurrence—where it may give some insight into the relative risk of recurrence at one site versus another and thereby offer insight into appropriate treatment decisions. Obviously, the patient with a high risk of distant metastases

might benefit by treatment with systemic therapy; alternatively, a patient at risk of nodal metastases would be a candidate for node dissection and further therapy, if positive. The association of a specific prognostic factor and a site of subsequent recurrence in the untreated patient does permit further elaboration as to the mechanisms of invasion and metastases. For example, lymphovascular invasion in the myometrium influences the risk of tumor recurrence at distant sites as well as in pelvic nodes and, hence, the risk of recurrence and death of disease.

- The natural history of untreated disease—in the sense that the evaluation of each patient's extent of disease, or staging, offers a glimpse into the pattern of evolution or spread of disease. Taken as a whole, each glimpse into the evaluation of disease extent in many thousands of patients who have not yet been treated allows us to piece together the continuum of early invasion and subsequent development of metastasis that characterizes the nature of the process of tumor progression and dissemination. For example, the relationship between the depth of invasion and the grade of the tumor in predicting the development of nodal metastases demonstrates that pathophysiologic relationship (Figure 6–1). Further biochemical characterization of the invasiveness of these tumors in the lymphatic and vascular systems not only help identify the time to acquisition of metastatic potential, but also the indications for alterations in treatment that will address the increased risk of regional and distant metastases.

The value of prognostic factors in the treatment of human cancer includes not only the potential ability to better select treatments that may influence survival but also the opportunity to better understand the nature and mechanisms of human malignant disease and to investigate fundamental biologic processes that may shed light on new interventions. The key to better understanding, however, is the ability to look at prognostic factors that are *independently* important in predicting survival or recurrence. Moving from factors that are derivative, for example, duration of symptoms that might be indicative of duration of tumor growth, to independent variables improves the resolution of our observations on the natural history of treated disease.

Insofar as identification of a prognostic factor can influence the choice of treatment, so too can the treatment influence the value of that prognostic factor. Although this may seem intuitive, the review of a recent article is illustrative.[1] Depth of myometrial invasion is prognostic for both lymph-node metastases and risk of local recurrence. If one eliminates patients with nodal metastases by looking only at patients with pathologic stage IB disease and then

treats all patients with vaginal brachytherapy to reduce the small risk of local recurrence, it is not a surprise that depth of myometrial invasion has no prognostic significance in this group.

In the evaluation of potential prognostic variables, the following specific questions should be kept in mind:

1. What is the prevalence of this factor? Is it common enough to be clinically useful and for any conclusions to be made on the basis of a large enough sample to be statistically significant?
2. Is there sufficient data to conclude that the factor operates independently from other common variables?
3. Has the prognostic factor generated from the data on one patient population been *validated* in a second unrelated population with the same disease?
4. Are the data acquired in such a manner as to be easily extended to other patients, or are the study conditions not applicable?
5. Are there opportunities to alter therapy, change the degree or site of surveillance, or provide reassurance for patients, on the basis of the data to be acquired?
6. Is it predictive in its ability to modify therapy and change outcome, not just prognosis?
7. Should this variable be considered in the evaluation of the comparability of groups in clinical trials?
8. Is this an independent variable of such clinical significance that it could be incorporated into a prognostic index for the future management of all patients presenting with this extent of disease?
9. Could this prognostic variable give some insight into the mechanism of carcinogenesis or disease progression that will help us better understand tumor biology? Is there some clinical or basic research suggested by these observations?

Ideally, the identification of prognostic factors may reduce the risk of giving unnecessary treatment to low-risk patients while identifying a subset of patients whose risk of recurrence and death is so great that no standard therapy can be justified.

The ideal prognostic factor would be one that is available preoperatively, prior to any institution of therapy, distinguishes a small subset of patients at

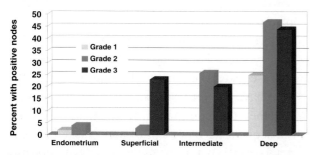

Figure 6–1. The association of tumor grade and depth of myometrial invasion with incidence of pelvic and para-aortic nodal metastases.

very high risk of disease recurrence, and, correspondingly, a very large number of patients with an excellent likelihood of completing standard therapy with a low risk of recurrent disease. The presence of the variable would define a specific site of treatment failure, give an indication as to the mechanism of disease leading to this recurrence, and suggest a therapeutic intervention. The test would identify the patient who would benefit most from referral to a regional treatment center, in contrast to those who could safely remain in the community for standard therapy (Table 6–3). In the specific case of endometrial carcinoma, the clinical utility of preoperative prognostic factors permits identification of patients at low risk of extrauterine disease who do not require an extensive staging procedure (see Chapter 4).

In the United States, there are about 40,100 cases of endometrial carcinoma per year, with approximately 6,800 deaths. It might be anticipated that the case fatality rate may also increase, given the recognition of the association of unopposed estrogen and endometrial cancer risk. Prevention of these estrogen-associated cancers by preventing the occurrence of persistent patterns of unopposed estrogens should decrease the proportion of well-differentiated, good-prognosis cancers and not affect the poor-prognosis, poorly differentiated cancers.

As the majority of patients with endometrial cancer have a fairly good prognosis and are cared for in the community with primary surgical management, assessment of prognostic factors that define the risk of extrauterine disease and the need for more complex surgical staging will help define

which patients should be referred for more comprehensive staging and therapy. Endometrial carcinoma is unusual in that the staging system is not generally applicable to all patients. Complete surgical staging (see Chapter 4) is not applied to all patients but, rather, is applied on the basis of risk of nodal metastases. For this reason, the preoperative assessment of prognostic factors indicating the risk of extrauterine disease is helpful, either for referral or for consultation with a general surgeon to assist the obstetrician/gynecologist in node dissection.

Predictive Factors

Predictive factors are a subset of the group of prognostic factors whose findings can influence the choice of therapy and outcome. For example, progesterone receptor (Tables 1 and 2) is a predictive factor for response to progesterone therapy. The identification of a predictive factor is contingent on the identification of a therapeutic intervention whose efficacy is determined by that factor. The relationship between a predictive factor and response to therapy is dynamic and dependent on the treatment modality. An example of this is the identification of *HER2/neu* as an adverse prognostic factor in breast cancer; it did not become a predictive factor until the development and availability of trastuzumab (Herceptin) as a therapy for HER2/neu-positive tumors. Variables indicating an increased risk of nodal metastases are predictive in that they will influence the decision to carry out a node dissection and, if positive for metastatic disease, the decision to carry out additional therapy for those nodal metastases.

Staging in itself is a prognostic factor and may be a predictive parameter because it defines the morphologic extent of disease as identified preoperatively or, in some cases, postoperatively. Staging may be done clinically (if a large proportion of patients are not treated operatively, eg, cervical cancer) or operatively as surgical-pathologic staging in endometrial cancer. The presence of extensive local disease with findings of a bulky uterus, invasion into the endocervical canal, or high-grade carcinoma may reflect advanced-stage disease. This can be predictive, in addition to being prognostic, as it generally indicates the need for referral to a gynecologic oncologist.

Table 6–3. PROGNOSTIC FACTORS

The "ideal" prognostic factor
  Available preoperatively (fresh or fixed tissue)
  Readily available and reproducible assay
  Identifies a small number of patients with poor outcome as candidates for further intervention
  Indicates biologic mechanisms for intervention or a target for therapy, that is, angiogenesis (mean vessel density [MVD])
  Is an *independent* factor by multivariate analysis

The "problem" prognostic factor
  Identified in a single study as "predictive" of a poor outcome, with a mildly decreased survival
  An esoteric protein, typically associated with proliferation or aneuploidy; generally with a poorly differentiated carcinoma
  No significance or no assessment in the context of multivariate analysis

If one examines the available preoperative prognostic factors, there are several that predict the risk of extrauterine disease; these may also alter the surgical approach in the community setting. As discussed later in greater detail, these additional factors include the cancer antigen (CA) 125 level, clinical examination of the cervix and paracervical ligaments, and radiographic studies that demonstrate either bulky uterine disease with myometrial invasion or evidence of adnexal, parametrial, peritoneal, or nodal metastases. The future development of both prognostic and predictive factors will probably extend to the development of proteomic and transcriptional. These ultimately may provide tissue-specific disease signatures that are based on hundreds of informative genes.[2]

Risk Groups

Risk groups are aggregations of patients whose prognostic factors indicate similar risks of a given outcome. The paradigm for this, of course, is the use of International Federation of Gynecology and Obstetrics (FIGO) and tumor-node-metastasis (TNM) staging, where aggregation of patients with a similar anatomic and histologic extent of disease permits a comparison of outcome between centers and over time within a single center. Another common example is derived from early Gynecologic Oncology Group (GOG) studies of the association of grade and myometrial invasion with risk of nodal metastases. The clinical utility of the combination of two predictive factors yields a risk assessment supporting the decision to carry out pelvic node dissection (Table 6–4). As noted, the clinical utility of prognostic factors available preoperatively is intrinsically greater for the obstetrician–gynecologist faced with the immediate care of the patient with newly diagnosed endometrial cancer (see Table 6–2). Delineation of an algorithm that will minimize risk in the community hospital and maximize the benefit of referral will be helpful to the clinician.

The practical questions that need to be answered (and will be addressed) for the obstetrician-gynecologist and the gynecologic oncologist are given below:

- Is there a group of patients with endometrial cancer for whom primary conservative therapy with total abdominal hysterectomy (TAH) and bilateral salpingo-oophorectomy (BSO) is sufficient?
- Is there a group of young women with endometrial cancer who may be conservatively treated with preservation of reproductive function?
- How does the assessment of the varied histologic types of endometrioid adenocarcinoma affect treatment decisions?
- What is the role of vaginal hysterectomy in the treatment of endometrial cancer?
- Are there any patients who should not undergo primary surgical management?
- What is the prognostic significance of positive peritoneal cytology, and how is this affected by preoperative hysteroscopy?
- How does prognostic information lead to improved outcome?
- Will postoperative therapy reduce the risk of disease recurrence?
- What is the likely site of recurrent cancer in a given individual?

What is the current standard for referral?

- Clinical assessment of uterine size and cervical involvement
- Histologic grade and tumor subtype
- Radiologic studies showing extrauterine disease
  - Ultrasonography showing adnexal disease, ascites, or deep myometrial invasion
  - Computed tomography (CT) demonstrating pelvic or para-aortic nodal metastases
- Evaluation of clinical evidence for omental masses or ascites

Patients with evidence of extrauterine disease, grade 3 histology with histologic subtypes, including serous papillary and clear cell carcinoma, and patients with elevated CA-125s are generally candidates for referral or consultation.

Table 6–4. IDENTIFICATION OF RISK GROUPS BASED ON HISTOLOGIC GRADE AND DEPTH OF MYOMETRIAL INVASION

Grade	Risk of Nodal Metastases Myometrial Invasion			
	M0	M1	M2	M3
1	No	Very low	Low	Moderate
2	Very low	Low	Moderate	High
3	Low	Moderate	High	Very high

DEMOGRAPHIC AND CLINICAL VARIABLES AS PROGNOSTIC FACTORS

Age and Obesity

Young women are traditionally regarded as being at low risk of endometrial carcinoma. The notable exception to this is the young woman with oligo-ovulation secondary to polycystic ovary syndrome or the woman with hyperplasia associated with obesity. Tonic estrogen secretion in the anovulatory woman, uninterrupted by the differentiating effects of progesterone, is associated with the development of grade 1 endometrial carcinoma. The low risk of myometrial invasion and the absence of nodal metastases in this particularly favorable group yields a correspondingly good prognosis for survival and a low risk of recurrence in premenopausal women (see Chapter 9).

These patients, initially treated with hysterectomy for a low-grade cancer associated with atypical endometrial hyperplasia, are now more commonly receiving progestin therapy, in some cases with preservation of fertility.[3–7] In a similar manner, as patients approach menopause, with waning levels of progesterone consistent with an insufficient luteal phase or perimenopausal anovulation, development of hyperplasia and carcinoma may be a transient phenomenon with an equally favorable prognosis. The predominance of low-grade tumors among pre- and perimenopausal women creates a univariate prognostic variable for age, which diminishes when one controls for grade in multivariate analysis.[8]

In a Danish case-control study of young women with endometrial cancer, Parslov and colleagues identified a number of risk factors affecting development of cancer including a positive family history (odds ratio [OR] of 2.1) along with the protective effects of long-term pregnancy (OR of 0.6) and oral contraceptive therapy (OR of 0.2 for 1 to 5 years of use). Surprisingly, body mass index (BMI) was not a risk factor for development of hyperplasia and cancer, though this may have been related to the Danish population studied.[9] This was not the case in a study from Iowa, where Anderson and colleagues demonstrated the association of increased BMI (Quetelet index) with a lower tumor grade, less myometrial invasion, lower stage, and improved outcome. The Quetelet index ranged from 16 to 89; only 5% of those with an index > 40 had nodal metastases; however, 64% of this group did not have node dissection. Given the association of obesity with low tumor grade and lack of invasion, it is not surprising, therefore, that lack of node dissection in this population had no negative effect on survival.[10]

In a second study of obese patients in Japan, Hachisuga and colleagues reported a series of 287 Japanese women; the BMI ranged from 15 to 40 (body weight [kg]/height[m^2]). Twenty-six of 81 premenopausal women and 78 of 206 postmenopausal women were determined to be overweight (BMI > 24.5). In the younger age group, all premenopausal women, there was neither a favorable effect of obesity on survival nor any association of obesity and tumor grade or myometrial invasion. In postmenopausal women, again, there was no association between being overweight and any of the traditional risk factors; however there was a clear survival advantage for overweight postmenopausal women in multivariate analysis. The cumulative 10-year survival rate was 75.2% in normal-weight women compared with 89.4% in overweight subjects.[11]

In the study from Fukuoka, Japan, among premenopausal women, the cumulative 10-year survival was 89%, irrespective of weight.[11] The survival among these young women was significantly better than among their older, postmenopausal counterparts, with a higher proportion of younger women with grade 1 tumors, no myometrial invasion, and no cervical stromal invasion. These findings were similar to those also reported from Japan by Yamazawa and colleagues in Chiba, where Cox regression analysis demonstrated that age ($p = .0001$), stage ($p = .0183$), histology ($p = .0011$), and lymph node metastasis ($p = .0007$) were independent variables related to disease-free survival. In this study, 90% of younger women had early-stage disease and a higher incidence of disease confined to the inner half of the myometrium than in postmenopausal women ($p = .0004$).[12]

Similarly, Nakanishi and colleagues reported on the association of menopausal state and prognosis in endometrial carcinoma. The focus on menopausal state as a surrogate for age demonstrated that the menopausal state was an independent prognostic variable for patients with early-stage disease. As in the studies above, Nakanishi and colleagues from Nagoya, Japan, documented that the poorer survival in postmenopausal patients was associated with an increased risk of myometrial invasion into the outer half of the uterus (41.5% in postmenopausal patients versus 22.5% in premenopausal patients).[13]

Race

Despite the 33% lower incidence of endometrial cancer among African Americans compared with White women in the United States, most clinical studies reveal a higher mortality from endometrial cancer for African American women.[14–18] In the study by Aziz and colleagues that divided groups of White and Black patients by age (60 years or younger versus older than 60 years), there were significant differences in survival between all older and younger patients and Black versus White patients, with the greatest survival among young White patients and the worst among older Black patients (Table 6–5).[14] Analysis of these older patients reveals findings consistent with those described above: higher clinical stage, higher grade, and greater depth of myometrial invasion than in younger patients. In the comparison of Black and White patients, the prevalence of low-grade lesions among White patients may well reflect the increased use of estrogen replacement therapy, as suggested by Plaxe and Saltzstein.[19] Additionally, the greater prevalence of poor-prognosis lesions and a higher frequency of intercurrent comorbid disease (diabetes, hypertension, and coronary artery disease) in Black women might be accounted for by the "dilutional" effect of patients with low-grade, estrogen-associated lesions. Liu and colleagues, in a study from Duke, support this contention with the finding that 13% of Black women with endometrial cancer in their study used exogenous estrogens, in contrast to 44% of White women ($p < .001$), with a corresponding asymmetry in prevalence of low-grade tumors. After correcting for estrogen use, significant racial differences still existed for unfavorable histology, stage, grade, and survival. Although patients with a history of hormone use had a longer (19 weeks versus 10 weeks) delay between onset of symptoms and treatment,

overall, there was no delay in hysterectomy after onset of symptoms for Black women (11.1 weeks) compared with White women (13.7 weeks).[20]

In multivariate analyses, race remains a significant prognostic variable in several studies. Connell and associates at the University of Chicago hospitals identified a hazard ratio (2.0) equivalent to grade (2.6) or stage (1.6), but it was not a significant prognostic variable in a study by Matthews and colleagues who attributed the poorer outcome in Black patients to an increased prevalence of lesions with adverse histologic type.[15,18] It is of note that the distribution of grade was almost identical among 187 Black and 140 White patients with endometrioid histology. Twenty percent of Black women had clear cell or serous papillary histology in contrast to only 5.3% of White women.[18] The prevalence of adverse histology in about 20% of Black women is a fairly consistent observation in most studies.

The papers cited above reflect the experience at single institutions where all patients were treated similarly; the exception to this is a report by Hicks and colleagues from the National Cancer Data Base.[16] This study presented data that were consistent with the observations noted above: more African American patients than White patients were diagnosed with less favorable histologies, more advanced stages of disease, and less tumor differentiation. Although the study noted that African American women were less frequently treated surgically and that surgically treated patients with advanced stages of disease received adjuvant radiotherapy *less* often and chemotherapy *more* often than did White patients, no comment was made about regional variations in care. In fact, twice as many African American patients lived in the South and South Atlantic regions as White patients (60% versus 31%); these

Table 6–5.	AGE AND RACE AS PROGNOSTIC FACTORS IN ENDOMETRIAL CARCINOMA		
		Race	
Age	All	White	Black
All		232 mo	108 mo
< 60 yr	> 200 mo	188 mo 71% 5 yr survival	Median not reached 88% 5 yr survival
> 60 yr	90 mo	155 mo	40 mo

Adapted from Aziz H et al.[14]

differences may well reflect different practices within the geographic regions.[16]

An intriguing report from Washington University evaluated ribosomal deoxyribonucleic acid (rDNA) methylation in African American and White patients with endometrial cancer. The majority of tumors evaluated demonstrated high levels of rDNA methylation (74%). Among 148 women with FIGO stage I–II endometrioid carcinoma, survival was significantly worse for those with low levels of rDNA methylation ($p < .0001$). African American patients were more likely to have low levels of methylation than Whites ($p < .002$). In multivariate analysis, tumor rDNA methylation level was the only significant prognostic factor for both disease-free survival and overall survival with hazard ratios of 11.0 and 26.3, respectively ($p < .01$).[21]

Risk Factors for Hyperplasia-Associated (Type 1) versus Atrophy-Associated (Type 2) Endometrial Carcinoma

Given the association of preexisting endometrial hyperplasia with varying degrees of architectural and cytologic atypia and the development of low-grade endometrial cancer in contrast to high-grade carcinoma arising in from atrophic endometrium, it is not surprising that several authors have proposed that there are two types of endometrial carcinoma. Type 1 disease, arising in association with endometrial hyperplasia, has a more favorable prognosis than type 2 carcinoma, presumably lacking the normal hormonal modulation (Table 6–6). Bokhman proposed that the first type was associated with the endocrinopathy associated with obesity, diabetes, and hypertension. The second type was not associated with this syndrome and represented a smaller proportion of women with high-grade lesions, deep myometrial invasion, and a poor prognosis (60% 5-year survival versus 86% with the classic triad).[8,22] Deligdisch and colleagues were able to classify all their cases studied into one group or the other. Atrophy-associated endometrial cancer, in their studies, was much more likely to be poorly differentiated, to be associated with myometrial invasion, and to have an adverse histologic type (clear cell or serous papillary) with a poor prognosis.[23,24] Westhoff and

colleagues studied factors predisposing to type 1 endometrial carcinoma and found that this was associated with early menarche and late menopause as well as with diabetes, obesity, and hypertension; it was negatively associated with oral contraceptive use and with cigarette smoking.[25] However, division of endometrial cancer into only two types is overly simplistic as it does not take into account the fact that some low-grade endometrioid cancers are not associated with hyperplasia and that some serous and clear cell tumors are hyperplasia associated. Additionally, some endometrial tumors are composed of both endometrioid and nonendometrioid components.

Nulliparity

In an epidemiologic study of 25,000 women ages 40 to 65 years screened for the development of breast cancer, de Waard and colleagues identified an inverse relationship between parity and the risk of developing endometrial carcinoma. A comparison of 147 cases of endometrial cancer with 900 randomly selected controls from the same cohort revealed a significantly increased risk of cancer among nulliparous women, stronger among married women than single women.[26] As to the prognostic effect, the first paper addressing comparative survival among nulliparous and multiparous patients reviewed data on 316 patients treated for endometrial cancer from 1981 to 1990 in Hordaland County, Norway. Salvesen and associates in Bergen, showed a striking

Table 6–6. CLINICAL CONTRAST BETWEEN HYPERPLASIA-ASSOCIATED AND ATROPHY-ASSOCIATED CARCINOMAS OF THE ENDOMETRIUM

(Hyper)Estrogenic Tumors	Nonestrogenic Tumors
Associated with hyperplasia	Associated with atrophic endometrium
Well differentiated (G1, G2)	Poorly differentiated (G3)
Adenocarcinoma with squamous differentiation, or adenocarcinoma	Adenosquamous, or papillary serous histology
Obese patient with diabetes and hypertension	Thin or normal habitus, "shouldn't have endometrial carcinoma"
Anovulatory patient or on HRT	May have normal menstrual periods
Limited myometrial invasion, no nodal metastases	Deep myometrial invasion, with nodal metastases
Good prognosis	Poor prognosis

G = grade; HRT = hormone replacement therapy.

difference in 5-year survival among nulliparous patients compared with their multiparous counterparts. The 5-year survival for nulliparous women was 57% compared with 81% for those women with one or more deliveries ($p = .0001$). In a multivariate Cox proportional hazards regression model, a hazard ratio of 2.81 was found for nulliparous women. They concluded that the decreased survival "may reflect biologic differences between parous and nulliparous endometrial carcinoma patients." Because reliable information about delay in diagnosis was not available, Salvesen and colleagues also recognized that the difference may "be due in part to a greater delay in diagnosing women in the nulliparous group."[27] This latter question was addressed in a study of 328 patients in Japan by Hachisuga and colleagues, who studied the effect of delay in diagnosis. Dividing this patient group into those younger than 50 and over 50 years revealed no effect of nulliparity among the younger patients. Among those over 50 years, in univariate analysis, there was a poorer survival in patients with stage III and IV according to parity. The 10-year survival among nulliparous women, women with one or two pregnancies, or women with three or more was 7.7%, 48%, and 56.2%, respectively. In multivariate analyses, however, these differences did not persist in light of an association with a delay in diagnosis.[28]

Patient Delay in Diagnosis

Menczer and colleagues in Israel studied 181 consecutive patients with endometrial carcinoma between 1970 and 1986, with records that contained details with regard to diagnosis delay and treatment delay. No significant correlation was identified between delay in diagnosis and prognosis. It was of note, however, that only 8.3% of patients had grade 3 disease. If one assumes that delay might be more significant in high-grade, rapidly proliferating lesions, the absence of any significant association may have been due to the preponderance of grade 1 and 2 tumors.[27,29] In a series of 116 patients from Austria with stages I to IV disease, of whom 18% had grade 3 disease and 45% had grade 2 disease, Obermair and colleagues did demonstrate a threefold greater duration of bleeding among patients

with advanced-stage disease in contrast to those with early disease (35.2 ± 69.3 weeks versus 12.7 ± 17.8 weeks).[30] The differences between these two studies can be reconciled in the different proportion of patients with moderate to poorly differentiated tumors. Treatment delay among patients with low-grade tumors seems intuitively less likely to result in progression to more advanced disease than among patients with anaplastic cancers.

POSITIVE CERVICAL CYTOLOGY

Identification of suspicious or malignant cells in the cervical cytology from patients with endometrial carcinoma indicates an increased risk of extrauterine spread. It is intuitively obvious that the positive cytology would be associated with occult or gross cervical metastasis ($p < .001$), but two comprehensive studies also identify an association with tumor grade ($p < .01$) and adverse histologic subtypes ($p < .01$).[31,32] These observations can be interpreted in the context of increased shedding of cells by high-grade nonendometrioid tumors; however, the association of positive cervical cytology with an increased risk of nodal metastases must reflect the innate virulence of the primary tumor shedding these cells. Although univariate analysis associated the presence of positive cervical cytology with poorer survival in patients with endometrial cancer, multivariate analysis demonstrated only stage, grade, and myometrial invasion to be significant.

Of great importance for the clinician is the predictive nature of this variable that is available preoperatively. Identification of malignant cells or, less commonly, atypical glandular cells suspicious for malignancy should lead the clinician to look carefully for occult cervical involvement in the patient with endometrial cancer. Moreover, as shown by both Fukuda and colleagues and Larson and colleagues, the incidence of pelvic nodal metastases is increased threefold with positive cervical cytology, and in Larson and colleagues' study, the incidence of para-aortic nodal metastases was five times greater.[31,32] This preoperative predictive factor can provide the opportunity for referral or consultation so that appropriate and comprehensive retroperitoneal staging may be performed.

Both studies did not show any association of positive cervical cytology with the presence of malignant cells in peritoneal washings. Dissemination of cells through the lower genital tract was apparently not associated with migration of cells through the fallopian tubes into the peritoneal cavity.

TUMOR VARIABLES AS PROGNOSTIC FACTORS—GROSS EVALUATION

Staging: Preoperative Assessment

Anatomic prognostic factors are generally considered part of clinical staging of the "geographic" extent of disease both within the uterus and beyond. The TNM system traditionally is seen as purely anatomic and is the most widely applicable approach to the evaluation of the extent of disease for all cancers (see Chapter 4). It is defined as follows:

T: the extent of the primary tumor (may relate to size and depth of invasion)
N: the involvement of regional (pelvic) nodes, based on preoperative and intraoperative clinical or histopathologic evaluation of nodes
M: the evidence of regional or distant metastases by clinical or radiographic techniques

The TNM system has been subdivided further into the cTNM and pTNM subclassifications, the prefix "c" referring to clinical evaluation and the prefix "p" referring to postsurgical histopathologic classification. Once the malignancy has been classified in the TNM system, the stage is then determined. The TNM Prognostic Factor Project Committee has agreed to defer all staging issues to the FIGO cancer committee; hence, the FIGO staging system is the standard for gynecologic malignancy. The FIGO staging system, specific for endometrial cancer, actually is a hybrid in that grade as a nonanatomic predictive factor, determined by histopathology is used to supplement the assessment of the anatomic extent of disease (Table 6–7). In each case, the purpose of clinical or pathologic stage is to group patients by comparable extent of disease in order to develop treatments appropriate to the anatomic extent of disease and thereafter to establish a basis for comparison of outcomes.

Traditionally, the stage of disease has been the lowest common denominator among the prognostic categories—this information would be available to all caregivers, regardless of the availability of resources in health care. Hence, the distinction between clinical and pathologic stages and the absence of sophisticated radiographic techniques,

Table 6–7. COMPARISON OF FIGO AND TNM NOMENCLATURES

FIGO Stage	Extent of Tumor	TNM Categories
	Primary tumor cannot be assessed	Tx
	No evidence of a primary tumor	T0
0	Carcinoma in situ (preinvasive carcinoma)	Tis
I	Tumor confined to the corpus uteri	T1
IA	Tumor limited to endometrium	T1a
IB	Tumor invades up to less than half of myometrium	T1b
IC	Tumor invades more than one half of myometrium	T1c
II	Tumor invades cervix but does not extend beyond the uterus	T2
IIA	Endocervical gland involvement only	T2a
IIB	Cervical stromal invasion	T2b
III	Local or regional spread beyond the uterus	T3 +/- N1
IIIA	Involves uterine serosa, adnexa, or ascites or washings	T3a
IIIB	Vaginal involvement (by direct extension or metastasis)	T3b
IIIC	Metastasis to pelvic or para-aortic lymph nodes	N1
IVA	Tumor invades bladder or bowel mucosa	T4
IVB	Distant metastasis (excluding metastases to vagina, pelvic serosa or adnexa) (including metastases to intra-abdominal lymph nodes other than para-aortic or inguinal nodes)	M1

Adapted from Benedet JL, Bender H, Jones H III, et al. FIGO staging classifications and clinical practice guidelines in the management of gynecologic cancers. FIGO Committee on Gynecologic Oncology. Int J Gynaecol Obstet 2000;70(2):209–62.
FIGO = International Federation of Gynecology and Obstetrics; TNM = tumor-node-metastasis.

such as magnetic resonance imaging (MRI) and positron emission tomography (PET), from the process. As clinical resources become more plentiful and/or the significance of other prognostic factors becomes greater, additional parameters may be added. At present, however, this is only true for tumor grade in endometrial cancer, where the dominance of grade in prognosis facilitates the decision as to when lymph node dissection as a staging procedure should be carried out (see Table 6–4 and Table 6–8).

Determination of Risk Factors for Nodal Metastases

As discussed in Chapter 4, the decision to perform retroperitoneal dissection of pelvic and/or para-aortic lymph nodes is dependent on the preoperative assessment of risk of nodal metastasis. The data obtained prior to surgery should include the cervical cytology and the histologic grade and subtype of the tumor. An elevated preoperative CA 125 value, an enlarged uterus in the absence of fibroids, a palpable adnexal mass, and/or abnormal radiographic findings will be valuable in formulating preoperative plans for node dissection.

As noted in Table 6–8, patients at low risk of nodal metastases with a mobile uterus and grade 1 tumor can be treated with vaginal hysterectomy and vaginal bilateral salpingo-oophorectomy only. The finding of a higher-grade tumor and/or deep myometrial invasion at the time of final histopathologic review may be an indication for subsequent laparoscopic node dissection. At the time of exploratory laparotomy through an abdominal approach, the decision for node dissection can be based on the operative findings, including evaluation of the excised uterus. This approach can be used even in "elderly" patients $\geq$ 70 years of age with acceptable morbidity.[33]

Residual Disease at the Conclusion of Primary Surgical Therapy

Patients with surgical stage IV disease and bulky residual tumor after laparotomy have a uniformly poor prognosis despite postoperative treatment with either chemotherapy or radiation therapy. In 1994 at the Massachusetts General Hospital, we published our results with surgical cytoreduction in 29 of 47 women presenting with stage IV endometrial carcinoma. Despite the rather heterogeneous postoperative therapy administered to these patients over the previous 15 years of study, the median survival among patients undergoing surgical cytoreduction was 18 months, in contrast to 8 months in patients who did not undergo surgery. By univariate analysis, there was improved survival in those patients who received cyclophosphamide, doxorubicin, and cisplatin (CAP, $p = .0007$) compared with other modalities. Because of the association of CAP chemotherapy with cytoreduction, this association was not significant in multivariate analysis; successful cytoreduction remains as the only statistically significant prognostic variable ($p = .04$).[34]

This work was confirmed in a subsequent study of 55 patients with stage IV endometrial carcinoma at Memorial Sloan-Kettering Cancer Center. In this series, 24 patients had "optimal" (< 2 cm) residual disease at the conclusion of surgical management, 16 of whom required surgical resection of metastatic disease and 8 patients with unresected metastases less than 2 cm in size. Twenty-one additional patients had "suboptimal" resection with bulky residual disease; 10 patients did not undergo resection. The median survival time in the optimal group was 31 months, regardless of whether the 2 cm mass existed de novo or was attained by extensive surgery. Median survival time in the suboptimal group was 12 months and in the group without surgery only 3 months.[35]

Table 6–8. CURRENT SURGICAL MANAGEMENT*
• For endometrioid, low grade: TVH and BSO, if technically possible
• For gross cervical disease: radical abdominal hysterectomy or preoperative brachytherapy
• For all others: laparotomy, TAH, and BSO with the extent of surgical staging determined by subtype and grade and examination of the uterus
• Grade 1: pelvic node dissection if > half invasion
• Grade 2: pelvic node dissection if any invasion
• Grade 3: pelvic and para-aortic node dissection unless contraindicated by extrauterine disease
• Nonendometrioid: generally treated as grade 3

BSO = bilateral salpingo-oophorectomy; TAH = total abdominal hysterectomy; TVH = total vaginal hystrectomy.
*Unusual, particularly nonendometrioid, lesions are individualized.

TUMOR VARIABLES AS PROGNOSTIC FACTORS—EXTERNAL ASSESSMENT

Radiographic Studies

The use of pelvic ultrasonography, CT, MRI, and PET will facilitate the recognition of metastatic disease as well as bulky intrauterine disease, which, in turn, will identify an increased risk of nodal metastases. When indicated, these studies carried out preoperatively will assist in determining the appropriate venue and personnel for surgical staging. Among patients with low-grade cancers with a low risk of nodal metastases, negative radiologic findings will help confirm that comprehensive nodal staging is not necessary. As noted by Reich and colleagues, the size of pelvic lymph nodes does not predict metastatic involvement in patients with endometrial cancer. They measured the size of 125 positive nodes and 160 negative nodes in 32 consecutive patients with node-positive endometrial cancer. Although overall, positive lymph nodes were larger than negative lymph nodes and there was a positive correlation between the size of positive lymph nodes and the size of the metastasis therein, 54% of positive nodes measured less than 10 mm in diameter and 29% of negative nodes measured greater than 10 mm in diameter.[36] On the other hand, with high-grade lesions, in which limited tumor bulk and myometrial invasion can still be associated with nodal metastases, the value of these radiologic studies is limited. Clearly, of patients with nodal metastases, those most likely to be cured are the ones with minimal nodal disease that will not be identified as a mass on CT or MRI (see Chapter 4).

Evaluation of Serum Tumor Markers (CA 125)

An elevated CA 125 level is a marker of advanced endometrial cancer as well as carcinoma of the ovary; the level rises with increasing tumor volume. The clinical utility of a preoperative CA 125 value has been evaluated in order to identify a cutoff value, below which the risk of lymph node metastases is acceptably low so that lymphadenectomy can be avoided and above which lymphadenectomy

becomes a necessity. To that end, Sood and colleagues determined that a CA 125 level in excess of 35 U/mL was associated with advanced-stage, high-grade, deep myometrial invasion and nodal metastases in pelvic and para-aortic sites. At a level of 65 U/mL, there was a 6.5-fold greater risk of extrauterine disease than below that level. A level below 20 U/mL was unlikely to be associated with extrauterine disease in patients with grade 1 histology; carrying out a vaginal hysterectomy avoided surgical staging in 24% of patients and missed only 3% with occult extrauterine disease.[37]

Dotters determined that a CA 125 level > 20 U/mL, a grade 3 tumor, or both, correctly predicted 87% of patients requiring surgical staging. In patients with clinical stage I disease and grade 1 or 2 histology, a CA 125 level > 20 U/mL identified 9 of 12 patients requiring node dissection whereas at a cutoff value of > 35 U/mL, only 6 of 12 were identified.[38] Using the cutoff value of 20 U/mL for patients with grade 1 and 2 tumors, vaginal hysterectomy and vaginal bilateral salpingo-oophorectomy could be carried out for 21 patients, with only 3 subsequently requiring laparoscopic pelvic node dissection. A similar cutoff value was proposed by Kurihara and colleagues, showing similar sensitivity and specificity.[39] Koper and colleagues also combined grade 3 histology and a CA 125 cutoff value of 15 U/mL to detect 39 of 60 (65%) patients requiring lymphadenectomy. The use of those same criteria to exclude patients requiring lymphadenectomy who would be candidates for vaginal surgery yielded a specificity for exclusion of 95% (36 of 38).[40]

Hematologic Effects

The observation of the association of thrombocytosis and malignancy is longstanding. The adverse effect of an elevated platelet count (> 400,000/mm^3) in patients with endometrial cancer was identified by Menczer and colleagues and found to correlate with high-grade, deep myometrial invasion and poorer survival. The lack of statistical significance may well have been due to the small number of patients in his study.[41] A subsequent study of 135 patients with endometrial carcinoma from Graz, Austria, reviewed the association of platelet count with other prognostic factors. In this study, 19 of 135 patients (14%) had thrombocytosis as defined above. These 19 patients had a higher prevalence of advanced disease, unfavorable grade (G2 and G3), as well as deep myometrial invasion and lymphovascular space invasion. Their 5-year survival rate was 61%, in contrast to 96% in patients without thrombocytosis. Gucer and colleagues acknowledged that the pathophysiologic mechanism "is unclear."[42] As far as a humoral mechanism is concerned, tumor-related thrombocytosis is associated with the paraneoplastic release of interleukin-6 (IL-6); this may be the operative mechanism in patients with ovarian cancer. Chopra and colleagues, however, have not found elevated IL-6 levels in endometrial carcinoma.[43] Other potential explanations include elevated levels of granulocyte-macrophage colony-stimulating factor (GM-CSF) and tumor cell–platelet interactions mediated by such agents as thrombospondin 1, which are postulated to play a role in tumor arrest in the vascular bed and metastatic spread of cancer cells.[44]

In a follow-up study, Gucer and colleagues identified an association of poor prognosis and advanced disease with a preoperative low hemoglobin level (< 12 g/dL) and thrombocytosis in 39 (18%) of 212 patients with endometrial carcinoma. The prevalence of thrombocytosis was higher among patients with anemia (36%) than among those with normal hemoglobin levels (8%, $p < .01$). The mechanism for anemia was presumed not to be associated with vaginal bleeding, which was generally minimal, but rather to humoral effects; for example, cytokines produced in association with the tumor mass can induce hemolysis or suppress erythropoiesis. Thrombocytosis, but not anemia, was a significant prognostic factor for survival in multivariate analysis, as anemia was strongly associated with other unfavorable prognostic factors.[45]

TUMOR VARIABLES AS PROGNOSTIC FACTORS—MICROSCOPIC EVALUATION

Evaluation of Tumor Histology

Classification of endometrial cancer as one of two dichotomous lesions, though overly inclusive, categorizes hyperplasia-associated endometrial cancer as

type 1 and atrophy-associated cancer as type 2 (see Table 6–6). The prognostic influence of these two histologic types was evaluated by Gucer and colleagues in Graz, Austria. Patients with hyperplasia-associated endometrial carcinoma were more likely to be pre- or perimenopausal. Body mass index, parity, and the incidence of diabetes were not significantly associated with prognosis. Carcinomas with associated hyperplasia were more likely to be early stage, well differentiated, and less invasive of the myometrium than atrophy-associated carcinomas, which were associated with lymphovascular space invasion, cervical involvement, and spread to the adnexa. The prognostic significance of this histology, present in univariate analysis, was lost in multivariate analysis. Carcinomas that were hyperplasia-associated had a lower frequency of recurrence (4% versus 17%, $p < .004$) and a better 5-year survival (96% versus 85%, $p < .01$).[46]

The great propensity for nonendometrioid (serous papillary and clear cell) carcinoma to present with advanced stage and frequent distant metastases has led to the call for meticulous staging and aggressive therapy.[47,48] Despite the fair survival rate in uterine papillary serous carcinoma (UPSC) patients with surgical stage I and II disease (79%), the 5-year survival of 30 patients in our series was only 30%, with a 25% survival rate in patients with stage III and IV tumors.[47] Given the trends toward more comprehensive staging and more frequent use of chemotherapy, Tay and Ward reviewed the experience at the Royal Women's Hospital in Brisbane, Australia, from 1982 through 1998. Although the patients were more definitively staged and platinum-based chemotherapy more widely used, there was no difference in survival for the group as a whole with superimposable survival curves (Figure 6–2).[49]

At the present time, given this apparent lack of progress, the current therapeutic directions lead toward further investigation of the molecular biology of papillary serous carcinoma, (see below) and trials of whole abdominal radiation therapy in management of advanced disease.[50,51] Recognition of the frequent association of nonendometrioid histology at dilatation and curettage (D & C) with occult disseminated disease at laparotomy (Figure 6–3) and a comparatively poor prognosis (Figure 6–4) has led

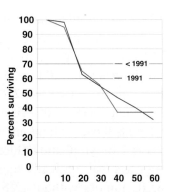

	< 1991	1991 on
Age > 60	46%	51%
FIGO stages I & II	38%	35%
FIGO stages III & IV	62%	65%
Omentectomy	17%	44%
Complete staging	17%	42%
Chemotherapy	33%	63%
Radiation therapy	83%	47%

Figure 6–2. Management of uterine papillary serous carcinoma at the Royal Women's Hospital, Brisbane. FIGO = International Federation of Gynecology and Obstetrics. Reproduced with permission from Tay et al.[49]

to the early recognition of this high-risk subtype and frequent referral.[54]

Evaluation of Grade, Myometrial Invasion, and Lymphovascular Space Involvement

Poorly differentiated tumors are associated with an increased risk of advanced-stage disease (Figure 6–5), myometrial invasion, lymphovascular space invasion, and risk of nodal metastases. The significant association of grade and prognosis (Figure 6–6) and its availability as part of the preoperative evaluation of the patient with endometrial cancer leads to its integration into the FIGO staging system. The impact of grade on prognosis is mediated, in part, by the associated risk of myometrial invasion; together, these two variables predict the risk of nodal metastases (see Table 6–7).

The presence of myometrial invasion as well as cervical stromal invasion can often be identified

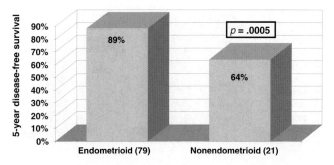

Figure 6–4. The association of nonendometrioid histology and risk of recurrence. Reproduced with permission from Mariani et al.[52]

visually at the time of hysterectomy.[53] As low-grade tumors invade on a broad front, inspection of the cut section of the excised uterus will provide a reliable assessment of the extent and depth of invasion (Figure 6–7 and 8). High-grade tumors, on the other hand, may invade in a more infiltrative, microscopic pattern that is not recognized on gross examination. For this reason, the absence of clinically obvious invasion of a high-grade lesion into the myometrium should not by itself deter the surgeon from consideration of lymph node dissection. Our approach to intraoperative clinical decision making, considering both grade and myometrial invasion, is depicted in Table 6–8.

Deep myometrial invasion is associated with nodal metastases and this trend increases with increasing grade. Among patients with grade 1 and 2 endometrioid carcinomas and negative nodes, however, deep myometrial invasion is associated with a risk of local recurrence at the vaginal apex.

Myometrial invasion is also associated with a risk of hematogenous dissemination. In the series reported by Mariani and colleagues from the Mayo Clinic, pul-

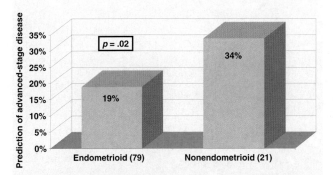

Figure 6–3. Nonendometrioid histology is associated with an increased risk of extrauterine spread of cancer. Reproduced with permission from Mariani et al.[52]

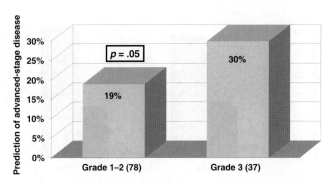

Figure 6–5. The association of tumor grade and risk of extrauterine disease. Reproduced with permission from Mariani et al.[52]

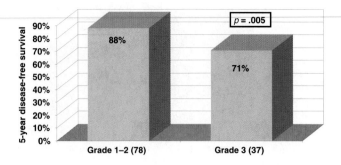

Figure 6–6. The association of increasing tumor grade with decreased survival. Reproduced with permission from Mariani et al.[52]

monary metastases were associated with older age and grade 1 or 2 histology; in contrast, hepatic metastases and other distant disease was associated with grade 3 histology and younger patients (< 65 years). Among patients whose tumors exhibited < 50% myometrial invasion, risk of hematogenous dissemination was 5%; patients with greater than 50% myometrial invasion had a 23% incidence of hematogenous dissemination.[54]

Lymphovascular space involvement (LVSI) is an important prognostic factor for nodal metastases in endometrial carcinoma. In the early GOG study reported by Creasman and colleagues, LVSI was identified in 15% of patients and presented a fourfold increased risk of pelvic nodal metastases and a sixfold increase in risk of para-aortic nodal metastases.[55] Among patients with endometrial carcinoma treated at the Mayo Clinic from 1984 to 1994, there were 142 patients with recurrent cancer, of whom 44 were classified as having lymphatic recurrences. Six of these were identified on the pelvic sidewall, 16 in the para-aortic nodes, 12 in both sites, and

10 involving other nodal groups. In Cox regression analysis, factors predicting lymphatic failure were LVSI (p = .01; relative risk [rr], 4.27), nodal involvement (p = .02; rr, 3.43) and cervical stromal invasion (p = .049; rr, 2.26). Patients with at least one factor had a 30% risk of lymphatic recurrence whereas those without any risk factors had less than 1% risk of lymphatic failure.[56] The latter observation suggests that surgically staged patients with stage IB or IC tumors without LVSI do not require therapy directed toward the pelvic sidewall, that is, whole-pelvic radiation therapy.

For patients with surgical stage I endometrial cancer, the value of pelvic radiation therapy may be questioned, even for patients with LVSI. In a paper presented by Gal and colleagues, 87 patients with surgical stage IB or IC tumors were treated with postoperative pelvic radiation therapy. There were 10 recurrences, all of which were outside the field of radiation. Nine of the 10 patients with recurrence had LVSI and 8 of the 9 died of disease. Overall, 5-year survival for the group was 92%, and LVSI strongly correlated with recurrence (p = .0001).[57] Excluding patients with LVSI, survival in this group was similar to that for a group of stage I patients managed conservatively with pelvic radiation therapy, which was given only for recurrence that was usually local and successfully salvaged.[58]

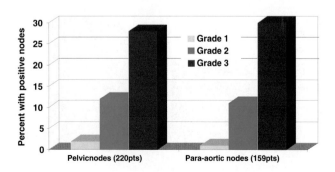

Figure 6–7. Increasing tumor grade is predictive of nodal metastases. Reproduced with permission from Creasman et al.[55]

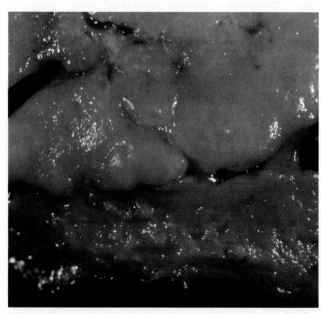

Figure 6–8. Photograph of the incised myometrium demonstrating the gross extent of invasion.

Table 6–9. RISK OF RECURRENCE WITH LYMPHOVASCULAR SPACE INVOLVEMENT

Lymphovascular invasion (LVI) was associated with histologic grade, myometrial invasion, and cervical invasion in a study of 303 women and was prognostic for survival and lymph node metastasis in multivariate analysis

- Effect on nodal metastases

No LVI	1/63	(1.6%)
Mild LVI	1/13 (pelvic)	(7.7%)
Severe LVI	13/27 (pelvic)	(48%)
	5/27 (para-aortic) (2 had both)	

- Effect on survival

No LVI	98.9% 10-year survival
Mild LVI	88.6%
Severe LVI	55.4%

Mild = a focus of LVI around a tumor; Severe = diffuse and multifocal. Adapted from Hachisuga T et al.[59]

Hachisuga and colleagues in Fukuoka, Japan, have provided a semiquantitative assessment of lymphovascular space involvement with a grading system that is predictive of both nodal metastases and tumor recurrence (Table 6–9). The presence of diffuse or multifocal LVSI is associated with a 50% incidence of pelvic nodal metastases and a 50% 5-year survival.[59]

Prognostic Significance of Nodal Metastases

The identification of patients at risk of nodal metastases from endometrial carcinoma and the dissection or sampling of nodes in pelvic and para-aortic nodal regions constitutes an important part of the surgical pathologic staging of endometrial carcinoma. As this component in the management of the patient with endometrial cancer is not usually part of the surgical experience of the generalist obstetrician–gynecologist, these patients generally require referral or further consultation.

Once the nodal metastases have been identified, clarification of the nature and local extent of nodal spread is essential to the formulation of further treatment plans. As described above, Mariani and colleagues have identified the presence of nodal metastases as a risk factor for lymphatic failure.[56] Although this may be considered intuitive, the pattern of recurrence may vary with the extent of nodal metastases as well as with treatment. Nelson and colleagues, for example, identified the patterns of

treatment failure among patients with positive pelvic nodes and negative para-aortic nodes who received postoperative pelvic radiation therapy. Among 77 patients with stage IIIC disease involving isolated pelvic nodes, the actuarial 5-year disease-free survival was 81%. In univariate analysis, the presence of positive peritoneal cytology increased the risk of treatment failure, but no failure occurred in the peritoneal cavity. Two patients developed a recurrence at para-aortic nodal sites, and two distant recurrences involved the lung, brain, and bone.[60]

McMeekin and colleagues in Oklahoma examined the prognostic effect of nodal metastases in the context of the extent of disease in 47 patients with FIGO stage IIIC disease.[61] This group was identified from 607 patients with endometrial carcinoma who were selectively staged with node dissection. Patients with low-grade, clinical stage I endometrial carcinoma with limited myometrial invasion of less than one-third did not undergo node dissection. Forty-two of the group had both para-aortic and pelvic node dissection. Associated intraperitoneal disease (adnexal involvement and/or positive cytology) was identified in 12 patients with survival at 3 years of 39% in contrast to 93% in the 35 patients without extranodal metastasis. Only one patient developed an intra-abdominal recurrence.

Analysis of the distribution of nodal metastases in the group revealed that 17 patients had pelvic nodal metastases alone, 15 had both pelvic and para-aortic nodal metastases, and 10 had only para-aortic nodal metastases. Increasing numbers of pelvic nodal metastases and bilateral pelvic nodal metastases were highly associated with the risk of para-aortic nodal spread. Sites of recurrence were not associated with the extent of nodal metastases. Neither the total number of positive lymph nodes nor the proportion of lymph nodes removed was indicative of prognosis.[62]

In a study from Roswell Park, 109 patients with endometrial carcinoma clinically limited to the uterus underwent para-aortic node dissection or sampling at the time of hysterectomy and bilateral salpingo-oophorectomy. Nineteen of the 109 were identified with either microscopic or macroscopic para-aortic nodal metastases. Subsequent treatment consisted of pelvic radiation therapy with either adjuvant progestin treatment or para-aortic irradiation. All patients with progestin therapy and those with macroscopic nodal disease treated with pelvic and para-aortic radiation therapy developed recurrent cancer. Twenty-seven percent of patients with para-aortic nodal radiation (only among the group with microscopic disease) had 5-year disease-free survival.[63]

Evidence of a therapeutic role for para-aortic node dissection is revealed in another study from the Mayo Clinic in which 51 patients with positive pelvic or para-aortic nodes were followed up for recurrence. Of these, the group with para-aortic node dissection, defined as removing at least five nodes, had a significant improvement in survival compared with those without para-aortic node dissection. The 5-year overall survival for patients with para-aortic node dissection was 77%, in contrast to a 42% survival in those without para-aortic node dissection. Moreover, lymph node recurrences were detected in 37% of those without para-aortic dissection but in none of those who had undergone therapeutic para-aortic node dissection.[64]

The adverse effect of *any* metastatic nodal involvement is evident in multiple studies of meticulous surgical staging demonstrating that patients with disease limited to the uterus but having *negative* nodes have an excellent outcome.[58,65–67] The present goal in preoperative treatment planning remains the identification of patients at risk of nodal metastases who will have definitive staging, as well as that group with *no significant risk* of metastases who can be treated by hysterectomy and bilateral salpingo-oophorectomy alone (see Chapter 4).

Significance of Gross and Microscopic Cervical Involvement

The identification of clinically evident cervical metastasis from endometrial carcinoma is an increasingly uncommon event. The identification of gross, bulky cervical extension requires exclusion of a primary cervical cancer and then typically either radical hysterectomy or preoperative brachytherapy or external pelvic radiation therapy. Prior to the revision of the FIGO staging system in 1988, gross cervical involvement would have been classified clinically as stage II disease. In our recent report, there were few patients with gross metastatic disease to the cervix, as

most of these patients were found to have other sites of metastasis in the pelvis and beyond at the time of laparotomy.[68] One might expect that very few patients, indeed, will have bulky metastases of endometrial carcinoma to the cervix *alone*. In our patients with surgically staged disease, all of whom had negative nodes and cervical involvement by definition, LVSI was the strongest predictor of disease recurrence (p = .002). Ten of 65 patients with endometrial adenocarcinoma developed recurrence of disease with a mean time to recurrence of 25 months. The 5-year disease-specific survival was 93%. Neither the surgical procedure (radical versus extrafascial hysterectomy) nor the extent of cervical involvement (gross versus microscopic) affected survival or recurrence. Two of 10 recurrences were local and developed after postoperative vaginal brachytherapy only; postoperative external pelvic radiation therapy potentially could have prevented these two recurrences.

In a second recent study from the Netherlands, Jobsen and colleagues reported on the treatment results of 42 patients with clinical stage I tumors who were found to have cervical involvement (pathologic stage II disease). Twenty-one patients had mucosal cervical involvement only; an equal number had cervical stromal invasion. All patients received external pelvic radiation therapy alone. Nine of 42 patients developed recurrence; 7 of these had a distant component of recurrence. The depth of myometrial invasion and the presence of LVSI correlated with distant metastasis (p = .03). Seven of 9 recurrences developed in patients with stage IIB disease (7 of 21 patients, 33%). Patients with grade 3 tumor and cervical stromal invasion had a 5-year survival of 48.6% (p = .003); consideration of more aggressive therapy was recommended for these patients.[69]

Given the adverse prognostic effect of cervical stromal invasion, the significance of involvement of the lower uterine segment (LUS) has been addressed in a recent study by Phelan and colleagues. Among 98 surgical stage I cases reviewed, 41 (42%) had evidence of LUS involvement. No differences were seen in clinico-pathologic features, extent of surgical staging, or adjuvant therapies among patients with and those without LUS involvement. Although the 5-year actuarial disease-free survival was worse in women with LUS involvement (80.3% versus 94.0%), multivariate analysis demonstrated no significance with patient outcome ($p = .98$) or pelvic recurrence.[70]

The Evaluation of Intraoperative Peritoneal Cytology

Cytologic washings are routinely obtained as part of the FIGO staging protocol for all patients undergoing surgery. Patients with positive washings, irrespective of the presence of ascites, are classified as having stage IIIA disease. The controversy regarding the prognostic significance of positive peritoneal cytology and its treatment are discussed in Chapter 10. The role of hysteroscopy and its potential for increasing the prevalence of positive peritoneal cytology has been addressed in Chapter 4.

Expression of Hormone Receptors and Epidermal Growth Factor Receptor with Prognosis

Epidermal Growth Factor and Epidermal Growth Factor Receptor: Relationship to Extent of Disease and Prognosis

One explanation for tumor growth and progression is an alteration in the presence of growth factors or their receptors. Tumors may secrete growth factors for which they already have cytoplasmic or nuclear receptors (autocrine stimulation) or there may be growth factors produced in adjacent tissue, such as stroma that can facilitate local tumor growth (paracrine stimulation). The epidermal growth factor (EGF) "system" comprises EGF receptor (EGFR), "normal" EGF, and altered forms of both transforming growth factor (TGF)-α, a tumor-produced form of EGF, and *HER2/neu*, of the EGF receptor family. *HER2/neu* has been infrequently identified in the endometrioid histologic subtype but is more frequently associated (as is *P53*) with poor-prognosis subtypes, such as papillary serous and clear cell endometrial carcinoma.[71] Khalifa and colleagues described a series of 69 patients, of whom 16 had papillary serous carcinoma and 8 a clear cell histology; in this group, EGFR overexpression was associated with a significant decline in 5-year survival, from 86 to 27%. In contrast, there was only a modest

but significant decline in survival among patients with endometrioid histology (89 to 69%, $p = .04$). Seventy-seven percent of patients with metastatic disease were determined to be EGFR positive (again this was predominantly in the group with nonendometrioid histology) in contrast to only 36% positivity among those with localized disease ($p < .002$). In subsequent studies, EGFR has been identified in normal proliferative endometrium as well as in endometrial cancer, with higher levels in the proliferative endometrium.[72] The presence of EGFR was not associated with grade or prognosis, sex steroid hormone levels, or the presence of estrogen receptor (ER) and progesterone receptor (PR).[73,74]

Support for autocrine or paracrine activity in endometrial carcinoma comes from the work of Yokoyama and colleagues who found evidence of immunohistochemically localized estradiol and TGF-α in poorly differentiated tumors of endometrioid histology.[75] The presence of TGF-α appeared to correlate with high-grade, early-stage lesions. Consistent with the observations above, the presence of EGF or EGFR did not correlate with grade, clinical stage, or survival.

Relationship of Sex Steroid Hormone Receptors to Treatment and Prognosis

As suggested in Table 6–6, steroid hormone receptors have been identified in association with type 1 endometrial carcinoma associated with hyperplasia.[76] Although both ER and PR are commonly identified in patients with endometrial cancer (35% and 32%, respectively), usually co-expressed ($p < .0001$), and their loss is highly associated with nonendometrioid histology, deep myometrial invasion, and increased angiogenesis, they are highly associated with tumor grade and not independently prognostic.[77] Halperin and colleagues divided 64 cases of endometrial carcinoma into three prognostic groups on the basis of the expression of ER/PR, *bcl-2*, *P53*, and *HER2/neu*.[78] Group 1 represented 28 patients with grade 1 or grade 2 tumors: 86% expressed ER, 79% expressed PR, and 43% expressed the apoptotic protein **bcl-2**; there was low level expression of *P53* and *HER2/neu* (14.3%). Group 3 comprised 22 patients with uterine papillary serous carcinoma: there was no expression of ER, PR, or *bcl-2*; there was marked overexpression of *P53* (82%) and *HER2/neu* (45%). The intermediate group, group 2, consisted of 14 patients with grade 3 tumors, with no expression of ER, PR, or *HER2/neu*; there was low level *bcl-2* expression (7.1%) but relatively high *P53* expression at 57.1%. As one might expect, this immunohisto-chemical profile can help identify patients at high risk of extrauterine disease, nodal metastases, and disease recurrence, thereby adding additional prognostic information in marginal situations where grade and histologic type are not sufficient.

TUMOR VARIABLES AS PROGNOSTIC FACTORS—MORPHOMETRY

In search of objective risk factors that could be applied to broad groups of patients, the use of morphometric and DNA cytometric features have been studied in order to identify patients at risk of recurrent disease. In one series, 137 women from northern Norway were treated for endometrial cancer between 1980 and 1993; all patients were treated by total abdominal hysterectomy and bilateral salpingo-oophorectomy without lymphadenectomy. All patients with stage IB and IC received postoperative radiation therapy, irrespective of prognostic factors. Morphometric analysis of nuclear parameters was prognostically superior to subjectively assessed grade.[79] Measurement of the nuclear perimeter along with the presence of lymphovascular invasion were shown to be the most useful prognostic factors; because of considerable interobserver variation of lymphovascular invasion, they recommended the use of immunohistochemical staining for vascular endothelium to improve reliability. Consistent with another study, also from Norway, nuclear perimeter appeared to be the most important morphometric factor, in combination with stage and grade.[80] Given the fact that lymphovascular invasion was difficult to evaluate, morphometric analysis of the nuclear perimeter was identified as the most valuable prognostic factor in this group of patients, second only to FIGO stage.

A similar study from Denmark of 68 patients with clinical stage I endometrial cancer (without lymphadenectomy as well) revealed that the mean nuclear volume was second only to the FIGO pathologic stage in predicting risk of recurrence. "Patients who had localized tumors or tumors with small nuclei had better probability of surviving than did women with advanced tumors or tumors with large nuclei." Of the 68 patients, 42 were postsurgically classified as having pathologic stage I high-risk carcinoma, another 11 had pathologic stage II tumors, and 15 had pathologic stage III tumors. At the end of the observation period (observed for a median of 6.4 years), 65% were survivors. Using a mean nuclear volume of 500 cubic microns as a threshold, the survival of 17 patients above that threshold was 29%, and in 51 patients with small nuclei, it was 80% ($p = .0001$).[81]

These two studies offer the advantage of objective measurement of tumor virulence. Given the large numbers of patients with pathologic stage I endometrial carcinoma at relatively low risk of recurrence, the opportunity to identify a high-risk subset remains. The use of some morphometric measurements remains to be investigated in patients with disease histologically confirmed to be confined to the uterus. In both studies reviewed, the clinical utility of morphometric analysis, once generated in the study population, still remains to be evaluated in a second, unrelated target population.

TUMOR VARIABLES AS PROGNOSTIC FACTORS—DNA CONTENT AND PROLIFERATION RELATED

DNA Ploidy and S-Phase Fraction

As one of the characteristic behaviors of cancer is uncontrolled proliferation, measurement of nuclear DNA content (DNA ploidy, determined as diploid versus nondiploid or aneuploid) and S-phase fraction have been considered potentially useful prognostic factors. Britton, in a report from the Mayo Clinic, determined that flow cytometric analysis of endometrial carcinoma provided a more accurate estimate of risk of recurrence and histologic grade.[85] In the era of clinical staging, retrospective analysis of 203 cases of endometrial carcinoma limited to the uterus (without lymphadenectomy) were evaluated. In this study of paraffin-embedded tissue, diploid DNA patterns were identified in 171 cases and

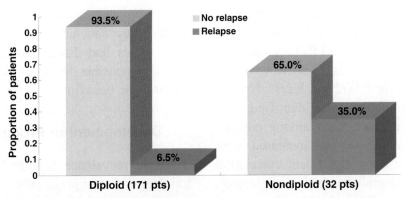

Figure 6–9. Association of nondiploid status with increased risk of relapse. pts = patients. Reproduced with permission from Britton LC, et al.[82]

nondiploid in the remaining 32 specimens. Diploid tumors had a 6.5% risk of relapse versus a 35% relapse rate among nondiploid tumors (Figure 6–9). Although nondiploid DNA specimens were found in only 16% of all stage I patients, they represented 50% of all recurrences. Of 7 patients with positive peritoneal cytology, 5 patients with a diploid pattern did not experience recurrence whereas both patients with nondiploid cytology had relapses.

Although DNA ploidy is customarily studied by flow cytometry, Lundgren and colleagues in Stockholm used image cytometry, which is stated to be more sensitive in the detection of aneuploid populations in fixed tissue. Three hundred fifty-eight patients with stage I to IV cancer treated over 2 years (1994–1995) and thought to be tumor free following primary treatment were evaluated by DNA ploidy, *MIB1*, and *P53* analysis. Although all patients were staged pathologically by the 1988 FIGO criteria, routine node sampling was not carried out. In multivariate analysis, after pathologic stage and histopathologic subtype, DNA ploidy was the strongest predictor of outcome whereas histologic grade and *P53* lost significance.[83]

The relationship between DNA ploidy and S-phase fraction and endometrial carcinoma was investigated by Gudmundsson and colleagues in a retrospective evaluation of tumor material from 243 patients treated throughout 1980 to 1985.[84] Of a group of 351 low-risk patients with well-differentiated and moderately differentiated tumors without solid areas, 24 patients died of disease compared with 52 representative survivors. S-phase fraction ≥ 8.0% was the only independent prognostic factor in multi-

variate analysis, including age, clinical stage, and degree of differentiation, with an odds ratio (OR) of 18.2 (*p* = .0001). In contrast, among high-risk patients with moderately differentiated tumors and solid areas or poorly differentiated tumors, there was a difference in ploidy in multivariate analysis but not in S-phase fraction. The 5-year survival was 75% for 106 patients with diploid tumors compared with 44% of those with nondiploid tumors (*p* = .0001). These two variables appear to have different prognostic significance depending on tumor grade.[84]

Microsatellite Instability

Endometrial carcinoma is the second most common malignancy arising in women with the hereditary nonpolyposis colorectal cancer syndrome. The identification of the germline mutation or epigenetic alterations in *MSH2* or *MLH1*, results in numerous replication errors throughout the genome with evidence of microsatellite instability (MSI) (see also Chapter 3). As a consequence, several investigators have identified MSI in patients with sporadic endometrial carcinoma, raising the question as to its role in carcinogenesis. Microsatellite instability is recognized as electrophoretic shifts in allele sizes of microsatellite DNA sequences. Wong and colleagues screened 50 patients with sporadic primary endometrial carcinoma, identifying 15 cases (30%) with MSI at one of five loci studied. Two additional cases exhibited MSI at two or more loci. No statistical significance with respect to survival was identified.[85] Baldinu and colleagues reported on examination of 116 consecutive samples from patients with endometrial carcinoma; MSI was identified by polymerase chain reaction (PCR)-based microsatellite analysis.[86] Thirty-nine patients (34%) showed evidence of MSI; 25 tumor samples (64%) showed negative immunostaining for *MSH2* and *MLH1*. No significant germline mutation was identified, and although MSI was more common among patients with advanced-stage disease and increased with tumor grade, there was no significant correlation with disease-free or overall survival.[86] In contrast, Fiumicino and colleagues identified 11 tumors in 65 patients with instability at two or more loci. This was a greater degree of MSI than that seen by Wong and colleagues; Fiumicino and colleagues actually classified patients with MSI at only one locus as "microsatellite stable." He correlated this greater degree of MSI with tumor grade and disease-free survival. The 5-year disease-free survival rate of patients with MSI at two loci was 63% versus 96% in those with microsatellite stability (p = .0004).[87]

A molecular distinction between hyperplasia-associated and atrophy-associated endometrial cancers might facilitate preoperative discrimination between these two diseases and help determine the intensity of therapy appropriate to the risk of recurrence. Progress in that direction was reported by Koul and colleagues, who noted that MSI was present in 21% of 53 sporadic endometrial tumors. All MSI tumors were diploid and had a significantly higher rate of *PTEN* mutations. All *PTEN* mutations occurred in diploid tumors; *P53* mutations were more often found with nondiploid tumors and never in tumors with *PTEN* mutations.[88] The absence of *P53* overexpression and MSI were also correlated with *PTEN* mutation, which are favorable molecular features associated with better prognosis.[89,90] *PTEN* inactivation has been shown in endometrial hyperplasia, a precursor of invasive endometrial adenocarcinoma, which suggests that *PTEN* mutation is an early event in endometrial carcinogenesis.[91,92]

In papillary serous carcinoma of the endometrium, Lax and colleagues identified no cases of MSI in 34 patients from Graz, Austria, and the Johns Hopkins Hospital. *P53* mutations were identified in 25 of 27 (93%) evaluable cases compared with 7 of 42 (17%) cases of endometrioid malignancy. Microsatellite instability was present in 16 of 57 (28%)

cases with endometrioid histology as well. These results, they concluded, suggested that these two tumor types had distinct molecular genetic alterations responsible for their differing morphology and biologic behavior.[93]

Development of Prognostic Indices

Given the prevalence of stage I endometrial cancer and the number of prognostic factors available postoperatively that might be of use in planning subsequent treatment, one goal has been to correlate a number of potentially independent prognostic factors into a therapeutic index that might help determine which patients would be candidates for postoperative treatment. Baak and colleagues from the Netherlands have developed a prognostic score using myometrial invasion, DNA ploidy, and mean shortest nuclear axis (MSNA) based on the evaluation of 77 "FIGO stage I" patients with long-term follow-up of 10 to 15 years. In multivariate analysis, the MSNA was easily reproducible and the best discriminating variable between surviving and nonsurviving patients. Of lesser, but independent, significance were DNA ploidy and depth of myometrial invasion. Unfortunately, the FIGO staging employed was the pre-1988 system, and none of these patients was surgically staged.

The endometrial carcinoma prognostic index stage I (ECPI-I) is calculated as follows:

ECPI-1 = 0.6494 × (mean shortest nuclear axis) + 0.6939 × (DNA code) + 02398 × (myometrial invasion) − 5.7283

In this formula, the MSNA is expressed in micrometers to one decimal place; DNA code as: 1 = diploid, 2 = peritetraploid, 3 = aneuploid; and myometrial invasion is 1 if the depth of invasion was less than half and 2 if the depth of invasion was more than one-half of the myometrial wall thickness.

The ECPI-I demonstrated in this group of patients, from which it was derived using a threshold of 0.87, that only 2 of 64 patients below the threshold had died (at 14 and 62 months). In contrast, 11 of 13 patients with an ECPI-1 of > 0.87 died of disease.[94] Although quantitative assessment of prognostic risk is an attractive strategy that eliminates a lot of observer variability, this specific approach was not validated in a second group of patients, and it does not address the 1988 changes in FIGO staging. It would be impractical in the routine setting, particularly in a large group of relatively good-prognosis patients (such as surgical stage IB and IC patients) to identify a small subset at risk of recurrence.

TUMOR VARIABLES AS PROGNOSTIC FACTORS—MOLECULAR ASSESSMENT

Oncogenes and Tumor Suppressor Genes as Prognostic Factors

PTEN Mutation

The tumor suppressor gene *PTEN* has been cloned and mapped to chromosome 10q23 and is reportedly associated with the regulation of cellular migration, invasion, and tumor cell proliferation. Investigation of sporadic endometrial carcinoma reveals loss of heterozygosity at chromosome 10q23 in 40% of tumors and *PTEN* mutations in 30 to 50% of patients.[89] Salvesen and colleagues identified loss of cytoplasmic PTEN protein expression in 56 of 279 (20%) evaluable patients.[89,95]

In other types of cancers, *PTEN* mutation has been associated with metastatic disease and poor prognosis. The role of *PTEN* mutation in endometrial cancer is not as clear. In several studies, *PTEN* mutation has been shown to be a positive prognostic factor associated with endometrioid histology ($p = .004$), early stage, and nonmetastatic disease ($p = .01$).[89,96,97] In the 1998 study by Risinger and colleagues, *PTEN* mutation was also associated with more favorable survival within the endometrioid subset.[89] Lower recurrence rates ($p = .003$) and more favorable survival were seen in tumors with *PTEN* mutations compared with tumors without *PTEN* mutations.

A recent immunohistochemical study looking at protein expression of PTEN in endometrial carcinomas showed an association between loss of PTEN expression and metastatic disease ($p = .05$). There were no significant differences in 5-year survival or 5-year recurrence-free survival rates between tumors that lacked and those that retained PTEN expression, even in the subset of endometrioid

tumors. Heterogeneity in PTEN expression also did not influence survival. A trend toward a greater proportion of nonendometrioid tumors lacking PTEN expression was observed but did not reach statistical significance.[95] It is possible that the antibodies used in immunohistochemistry might have stained mutant or inactive forms of *PTEN* in addition to normal *PTEN*, thereby combining samples with mutant PTEN expression with wild-type PTEN expression. The tumors lacking PTEN expression altogether could also contain other mutations that might influence the course of disease and FIGO stage. The same research group earlier found that methylation of the PTEN promoter was significantly associated with metastatic disease and MSI.[98]

The varied sites of *PTEN* mutation may well be associated with varied prognostic effects. According to a study by Minaguchi and colleagues, which analyzed the sequences of *PTEN* mutations in 67 endometrial carcinoma specimens to determine the prognostic significance of mutations in specific exons, *PTEN* mutations outside exons 5–7 correlate with better 5-year survival ($p = .04$). Fifty-five percent of specimens contained *PTEN* mutations, with 9 cases containing multiple mutations. The same trend was seen within the subset of advanced-stage disease (stage III/IV), although it did not reach statistical significance ($p = .13$). There were no differences in treatment between the group with *PTEN* mutations outside exons 5–7 and the remaining patients. Interestingly, *PTEN* wild type and *PTEN* mutants within exons 5–7 had similar 5-year survival rates of 66% and 65%, respectively. Both univariate and multivariate analyses confirmed that grade 1, stage I/II, and *PTEN* mutation outside exons 5–7 were significant predictors of increased survival ($p = .001, .0007, .02$, respectively). Unlike previous studies, no significant relationship was found between *PTEN* mutation and any clinicopathologic feature, such as age, menopausal status, gravidity/parity, BMI, diabetes, histologic grade, peritoneal cytology, muscular invasion, cervical/adnexal/peritoneal involvement, lymph node metastases, or FIGO stage.[99]

Exons 5–7 in the *PTEN* gene contain regions central to tumor suppressor function. Exons 5 and 6 contain the WPD, P, and TI loops that form the phosphatase domain active site. Exon 7 contains the

CBR3 loop that may aid in phospholipid membrane binding of the C2 domain.[100] It is possible that mutation of these domains disturbs the tumor suppressor function of *PTEN* more than the mutation of other domains outside of exons 5–7, which would account for the favorable prognosis for patients with *PTEN* mutations outside of exons 5–7. This model, however, does not account for the fact that patients with wild-type *PTEN* had similar survival rates to patients with mutations in exons 5–7. Simpkins and colleagues suggest that more than 60% of tumors with loss of heterozygosity of chromosome 10q do not contain *PTEN* mutations, so it is possible that other mutations are present in wild-type PTEN tumors that affect survival rates.[101] Exon 8 also contains an element that is important for tumor suppressor function; it is the $c\alpha_2$ element associated with membrane binding. Mutations in this element have previously been shown to result in intermediate growth suppression.[100] Mutations on exon 7 often truncate both the CBR3 loop and the $c\alpha_2$ element and would presumably affect membrane binding to a greater degree than $c\alpha_2$ truncation alone, which would explain why patients with *PTEN* mutations outside exons 5–7 have higher survival rates.[102]

The study by Minaguchi and colleagues evaluating prognosis associated with *PTEN* mutations in specific exons may serve to explain some of the contradictory reports of *PTEN*'s association with metastatic versus nonmetastatic endometrial carcinoma. Further study of the role of *PTEN* in endometrial tumors would be useful prior to using this information in treatment decisions for patients with endometrial carcinoma.[98]

P53 and HER2/neu Overexpression

Many authors have reported on overexpression of the *P53* gene in patients with both endometrioid carcinoma of the endometrium and its more aggressive variant, papillary serous carcinoma.[52,74,93,103–110] The function of *P53* in the process of DNA repair is to induce apoptosis in the presence of unsuccessful repair. Mutations in the *P53* gene are common in many human tumors, and the defective gene is often overexpressed. These alterations are associated with extent of disease, LVSI, pathologic staging, and prognosis.

In a paper from the University of California Los Angeles (UCLA) by Pisani and colleagues, overexpression of P53 was documented in 15% of tumors and was associated with a 12% probability of 5-year survival, compared with a 90% probability among those without mutation and overexpression ($p = .0001$).[111] Eleven percent of these patients were found to have HER2/neu overexpression that showed a nonsignificant trend toward poor prognosis. Had there been a higher proportion of tumors with HER2/neu overexpression, this might well have reached significance. Hamel and associates at the Mayo Clinic identified HER2/neu overexpression in 15% of their patients and P53 overexpression in 10% with a similar adverse prognosis. Along with histologic subtype and DNA ploidy, there were four independent prognostic factors. When no one factor was present, 4-year progression-free survival was 96%; when one or more factors were present, the survival was 63% ($p < .001$), and with two or more factors, survival dropped to 40% ($p < .001$).[112]

Angiogenesis-Related Substances and Prognosis

The angiogenic pathway associated with tumor proliferation and stromal vascularization can be identified at three levels in endometrial cancer: (1) the gross level with increased intratumoral blood flow measured by Doppler in the intact uterus, (2) the microscopic level with measurement of microvessel density in histologic sections, and (3) the molecular level, measuring vascular endothelial growth factor (VEGF) and its receptor by immunohistochemistry in tumor sections.

Intratumoral Blood Flow

If one makes the assumption that angiogenesis is associated with tumor progression and that the more advanced disease in aggregate will have greater blood flow, one would then expect that color Doppler studies of advanced endometrial carcinoma will show a lower intratumoral resistance index (RI). Cheng and associates in Taipei evaluated 66 patients preoperatively to evaluate RI and then correlated the lowest RI recorded with the extent of tumor at laparotomy. They identified an inverse linear relationship between RI and tumor size with a correlation coefficient = 0.47 ($p < .001$). Lower RI was significantly correlated with higher stage (stage I versus > I), histologic grade (grade 1/2 versus grade 3), myometrial invasion (< 50% versus > 50%), and pelvic lymph node metastases (negative versus positive), all at the $p < .001$ level.[113]

Alcazar and colleagues have expanded on this observation with transvaginal color Doppler ultrasonography, demonstrating both low arterial RI and high peak systolic velocity (PSV) with advanced endometrial cancer. This paper presented a preoperative study of 45 patients with findings of a significantly lower RI with an infiltrative growth pattern ($p = .013$), grade 3 histology ($p = .001$), > 50% myometrial invasion ($p = .006$), cervical involvement ($p = .009$), LVSI ($p = .008$), lymph node metastasis ($p = .049$), stage $\geq$ IC ($p = .004$), and a high risk of recurrence ($p = .001$). In addition, a significantly higher PSV was found in tumors that were grade 3 ($p = .034$), invasive of > 50% of the myometrium ($p = .029$), stage $\geq$ IC ($p = .015$), and at high risk of recurrence ($p = .002$).[114]

In both these studies, further validation of their applicability to routine preoperative assessment of patients with early endometrial carcinoma may be helpful in identifying patients at risk of extrauterine disease who are candidates for consultation or referral.

Microvessel Density

At the microscopic level, measurement of microvessel density (MVD) in the primary tumor has been demonstrated to be of prognostic benefit in several solid tumors, including breast and prostate cancers. Lee and colleagues in Taipei have correlated their ultrasound data with MVD and VEGF levels, demonstrating a linear relationship among these three prognostic factors and correlating them with the adverse histopathologic outcome described above. This comprehensive study places the clinical, microscopic, and molecular observations of angiogenesis into a precise relationship.[115] Salvesen in Norway identified a cutoff threshold for microvessel density at 68 mm^{-2} or less. Patients with increased mean MVD above this threshold

had a significantly shorter 5-year survival (57%) compared with those with less vascularity (90%) ($p < .004$). Mean microvessel density was an independent prognostic value in multivariate analysis along with FIGO stage, histologic type, histologic grade, and nuclear p53 protein expression.[116]

Vascular Endothelial Growth Factor

Given the significance of MVD in prognosis, it is not surprising to see various components of the VEGF angiogenic pathway associated with tumor invasion and prognosis. Variation in these observations and their prognostic significance relate to the methodology and to the particular targets studied. Overall, although VEGF serum levels do not correlate to tumor burden, assessment in tumor tissue of VEGF, its congeners, and its receptors is associated with grade, stage, metastases, and outcome.[116–118]

SUMMARY

Of the prognostic factors that are available preoperatively, the grade, presence of nonendometrioid histology, and clinical stage are the most useful for planning the extent of surgical staging. The potential roles of intratumoral blood flow, *P53* overexpression, and tumor ploidy remain to be determined in prospective studies. Overall, in the evaluation of patients for postoperative management, the status of regional lymph nodes and lymphovascular invasion significantly affect outcome. Patients without adverse prognostic factors generally have an excellent survival without adjunctive therapy or, at most, vaginal brachytherapy.

The optimal therapy for patients with extrauterine disease remains to be determined; patients with isolated nodal metastases appear to do well with radiation therapy. The majority of patients with extrauterine disease, however, have a substantial risk of distant metastases, and further clinical trials are needed for these patients.

REFERENCES

1. Alektier KM, McKee A, Lin O, et al. The significance of the amount of myometrial invasion in patients with stage IB endometrial carcinoma. Cancer 2002;95:316–21.

2. Mohr S, Leikauf GD, Keith G, Rihn BH. Microarrays as cancer keys: an array of possibilities. J Clin Oncol 2002; 20(14):3165–75.

3. Imai M, Jobo T, Sato R, et al. Medroxyprogesterone acetate therapy for patients with adenocarcinoma of the endometrium who wish to preserve the uterus-usefulness and limitations. Eur J Gynaecol Oncol 2001;22(3):217–20.

4. Wang CB, Wang CJ, Huang HJ, et al. Fertility-preserving treatment in young patients with endometrial adenocarcinoma. Cancer 2002;94(8):2192–8.

5. Leo L, Arduino S, Febo G, et al. Endometrial carcinoma in women 45 years of age or younger. Eur J Gynaecol Oncol 1996;17(5):403–5.

6. Pinto AB, Gopal M, Herzog TJ, et al. Successful in vitro fertilization pregnancy after conservative management of endometrial cancer. Fertil Steril 2001;76(4):826–9.

7. Kim YB, Holschneider CH, Ghosh K, et al. Progestin alone as primary treatment of endometrial carcinoma in premenopausal women. Report of seven cases and review of the literature. Cancer 1997;79(2):320–7.

8. Ludwig H. Prognostic factors in endometrial cancer. Int J Gynaecol Obstet 1995;49 Suppl:S1–7.

9. Parslov M, Lidegaard O, Klintorp S. Risk factors among young women with endometrial cancer: a Danish case-control study. Am J Obstet Gynecol 2000;182:23–9.

10. Anderson B, Connor JP, Andrews JI, et al. Obesity and prognosis in endometrial cancer. Am J Obstet Gynecol 1996; 174(4):1171–8.

11. Hachisuga T, Kawarabayashi T, Hirakawa T, Fukuda K. The effect of being overweight on survival in endometrioid carcinoma of the endometrium at different ages. Int J Gynecol Cancer 2000;10:228–32.

12. Yamazawa K, Seki K, Kihara M, Sekiya S. Prognostic factors in young women with endometrial carcinoma: a report of 20 cases and review of the literature. Int J Gynecol Cancer 2000;10:212–22.

13. Nakanishi T, Ishikawa H, Suzuki Y, et al. Association between menopausal state and prognosis of endometrial cancer. Int J Gynecol Cancer 2001;11(6):483–7.

14. Aziz H, Hussain F, Edelman S, et al. Age and race as prognostic factors in endometrial carcinoma. Am J Clin Oncol 1996;19(6):595–600.

15. Connell PP, Rotmensch J, Waggoner SE, Mundt AJ. Race and clinical outcome in endometrial carcinoma. Obstet Gynecol 1999;94(5 Pt 1):713–20.

16. Hicks ML, Kim W, Abrams J, et al. Racial differences in surgically staged patients with endometrial cancer. J Natl Med Assoc 1997;89(2):134–40.

17. Hicks ML, Phillips JL, Parham G, et al. The National Cancer Data Base report on endometrial carcinoma in African-American women. Cancer 1998;83(12):2629–37.

18. Matthews RP, Hutchinson-Colas J, Maiman M, et al. Papillary serous and clear cell type lead to poor prognosis of endometrial carcinoma in black women. Gynecol Oncol 1997;65(2):206–12.

19. Plaxe SC, Saltzstein SL. Impact of ethnicity on the incidence of high-risk endometrial carcinoma. Gynecol Oncol 1997;65:8–12.

20. Liu JR, Conaway M, Rodriguez GC, et al. Relationship between race and interval to treatment in endometrial cancer. Obstet Gynecol 1995;86(4 Pt 1):486–90.

21. Powell MA, Mutch DG, Rader JS, et al. Ribosomal DNA methylation in patients with endometrial carcinoma. Cancer 2002;94(11):2941–52.

22. Bokhman JV. Two pathogenic types of endometrial carcinoma. Gynecol Oncol 1983;15:10–7.

23. Deligdisch L, Cohen C. Histologic correlates and purulence implications of endometrial carcinoma associated with adenomatous hyperplasia. Cancer 1985;56:1452–5.

24. Deligdisch L, Holinka C. Endometrial carcinoma: two diseases? Cancer Detect Prev 1987;10:237–46.

25. Westhoff C, Heller D, Drosinos S, Tancer L. Risk factors for hyperplasia-associated versus atrophy-associated endometrial carcinoma. Am J Obstet Gynecol 2000;182:506–8.

26. de Waard F, de Ridder CM, Baanders-van Halewyn EA, Slotboom BJ. Endometrial cancer in a cohort screened for breast cancer. Eur J Cancer Prev 1996;5(2):99–104.

27. Salvesen HB, Akslen LA, Albrektsen G, Iversen OE. Poorer survival of nulliparous women with endometrial carcinoma. Cancer 1998;82(7):1328–33.

28. Hachisuga T, Fukuda K, Hirakawa T, Kawarabayashi T. The effect of nulliparity on survival in endometrial cancer at different ages. Gynecol Oncol 2001;82(1):122–6.

29. Menczer J, Krissi H, Chetrit A, et al. The effect of diagnosis and treatment delay on prognostic factors and survival in endometrial carcinoma. Am J Obstet Gynecol 1995;173 (3 Pt 1):774–8.

30. Obermair A, Hanzal E, Schreiner-Frech I, et al. Influence of delayed diagnosis on established prognostic factors in endometrial cancer. Anticancer Res 1996;16(2):947–9.

31. Fukuda K, Mori M, Uchiyama M, et al. Preoperative cervical cytology in endometrial carcinoma and its clinicopathologic relevance. Gynecol Oncol 1999;72(3):273–7.

32. Larson DM, Johnson KK, Reyes CN Jr, Broste SK. Prognostic significance of malignant cervical cytology in patients with endometrial cancer. Obstet Gynecol 1994; 84(3):399–403.

33. Giannice R, Susini T, Ferrandina G, et al. Systematic pelvic and aortic lymphadenectomy in elderly gynecologic oncologic patients. Cancer 2001;92(10):2562–8.

34. Goff BA, Goodman A, Muntz HG, et al. Surgical stage IV endometrial carcinoma: a study of 47 cases. Gynecol Oncol 1994;52(2):237–40.

35. Chi DS, Welshinger M, Venkatraman ES, Barakat RR. The role of surgical cytoreduction in stage IV endometrial carcinoma. Gynecol Oncol 1997;67(1):56–60.

36. Reich O, Winter R, Pickel H, et al. Does the size of pelvic lymph nodes predict metastatic involvement in patients with endometrial cancer? Int J Gynecol Cancer 1996;6: 445–7.

37. Sood AK, Buller RE, Burger RA, et al. Value of preoperative CA 125 level in the management of uterine cancer and prediction of clinical outcome. Obstet Gynecol 1997; 90(3):441–7.

38. Dotters DJ. Preoperative CA 125 in endometrial cancer: is it useful? Am J Obstet Gynecol 2000;182(6):1328–34.

39. Kurihara T, Mizunuma H, Obara M, et al. Determination of a normal level of serum CA 125 in postmenopausal women as a tool for preoperative evaluation and postoperative surveillance of endometrial carcinoma. Gynecol Oncol 1998;69(3):192–6.

40. Koper NP, Massuger LF, Thomas CM, et al. Serum CA 125 measurements to identify patients with endometrial cancer who require lymphadenectomy. Anticancer Res 1998;18(3B):1897–902.

41. Menczer J, Geva D, Schejter E, Zakut H. Elevated platelet count in patients with endometrial carcinoma: correlation with selected prognostic factors and with survival. Int J Gynecol Cancer 1996;6:463–6.

42. Gucer F, Moser F, Tamussino K, et al. Thrombocytosis as a prognostic factor in endometrial carcinoma. Gynecol Oncol 1998;70(2):210–4.

43. Chopra V, Dinh TV, Hannigan EV. Serum levels of interleukins, growth factors and angiogenin in patients with endometrial cancer. J Cancer Res Clin Oncol 1997;123:167–72.

44. Nathan FE, Hernandez E, Dunton CJ, et al. Plasma thrombospondin levels in patients with gynecological malignancies. Cancer 1994;73:2853–8.

45. Gucer F, Tamussino KF, Reich O, et al. Pretreatment hemoglobin, platelet count, and prognosis in endometrial carcinoma. Int J Gynecol Cancer 2001;11(3):236–40.

46. Gucer F, Reich O, Tamussino K, et al. Concomitant endometrial hyperplasia in patients with endometrial carcinoma. Gynecol Oncol 1998;69(1):64–8.

47. Kato DT, Ferry JA, Goodman AK, et al. Uterine papillary serous carcinoma (UPSC): a clinicopathologic study of 30 cases. Gynecol Oncol 1995;59:384–9.

48. Cirisano FD, Robboy SJ, Dodge RK, et al. Epidemiologic and surgicopathologic findings of papillary serous and clear cell endometrial cancers when compared to endometrioid carcinoma. Gynecol Oncol 1999;74(3):385–94.

49. Tay EH, Ward BG. The treatment of the uterine papillary serous carcinoma (UPSC): are we doing the right thing? Int J Gynecol Cancer 1999;9:463–9.

50. Sasano H, Comerford J, Wilkinson DS, et al. Serous papillary adenocarcinoma of the endometrium. Cancer 1990;65:1545–51.

51. Grice J, Ek M, Greer B, et al. Uterine papillary serous carcinoma: evaluation of long-term survival in surgically staged patients. Gynecol Oncol 2002;69:69–73.

52. Mariani A, Sebo TJ, Katzmann JA, et al. Pretreatment assessment of prognostic indicators in endometrial cancer. Am J Obstet Gynecol 2000;182(6):1535–44.

53. Vorgias G, Hintipas E, Katsoulis M, et al. Intraoperative gross examination of myometrial invasion and cervical infiltration in patients with endometrial cancer: decision-making accuracy. Gynecol Oncol 2002;85:483–6.

54. Mariani A, Webb MJ, Keeney GL, et al. Hematogenous dissemination in corpus cancer. Gynecol Oncol 2001;80(2):233–8.

55. Creasman WT, Morrow CP, Bundy BN. Surgical pathologic spread patterns of endometrial cancer: a gynecologic oncology group study. Cancer 1987;60:2035–41.

56. Mariani A, Webb MJ, Keeney GL, et al. Predictors of lymphatic failure in endometrial cancer. Gynecol Oncol 2002;84(3):437–42.

57. Gal D, Rush S, Lovecchio J, et al. Lymphvascular space involvement—a prognostic indicator in patients with surgical stage I endometrial adenocarcinoma treated with postoperative radiation. Int J Gynecol Cancer 1996;6:135–9.

58. Straughn JM Jr, Huh WK, Kelly FJ, et al. Conservative management of stage I endometrial carcinoma after surgical staging. Gynecol Oncol 2002;84(2):194–200.

59. Hachisuga T, Kaku T, Fukuda K, et al. The grading of lymphovascular space invasion in endometrial carcinoma. Cancer 1999;86(10):2090–7.

60. Nelson G, Randall M, Sutton G, et al. FIGO stage IIIC endometrial carcinoma with metastases confined to pelvic lymph nodes: analysis of treatment outcomes, prognostic variables, and failure patterns following adjuvant radiation therapy. Gynecol Oncol 1999;75(2):211–4.

61. McMeekin DS, Lashbrook D, Gold M, et al. Analysis of FIGO stage IIIc endometrial cancer patients. Gynecol Oncol 2001;81(2):273–8.

62. McMeekin DS, Lashbrook D, Gold M, et al. Nodal distribution and its significance in FIGO stage IIIc endometrial cancer. Gynecol Oncol 2001;82(2):375–9.

63. Hicks ML, Piver MS, Puretz JL, et al. Survival in patients with paraaortic lymph node metastases from endometrial adenocarcinoma clinically limited to the uterus. Int J Radiat Oncol Biol Phys 1993;26(4):607–11.

64. Mariani A, Webb MJ, Galli L, Podratz KC. Potential therapeutic role of para-aortic lymphadenectomy in node-positive endometrial cancer. Gynecol Oncol 2000;76(3):348–56.

65. Seago DP, Raman A, Lele S. Potential benefit of lymphadenectomy for the treatment of node-negative locally advanced uterine cancers. Gynecol Oncol 2001;83(2):282–5.

66. Fanning J. Long-term survival of intermediate risk endometrial cancer (stage IG3, IC, II) treated with full lymphadenectomy and brachytherapy without teletherapy. Gynecol Oncol 2001;82(2):371–4.

67. Sainz de la Cuesta R, Goff BA, Nikrui N, et al. Postoperative management of patients with stage Ib endometrial carcinoma. Eur J Gynaecol Oncol 1996;17(5):338–41.

68. Feltmate CM, Duska LR, Chang Y, et al. Predictors of recurrence in surgical stage II endometrial adenocarcinoma. Gynecol Oncol 1999;73(3):407–11.

69. Jobsen JJ, Schutter EM, Meerwaldt JH, et al. Treatment results in women with clinical stage I and pathologic stage II endometrial carcinoma. Int J Gynecol Cancer 2001;11(1):49–53.

70. Phelan C, Montag AG, Rotmensch J, et al. Outcome and management of pathological stage I endometrial carcinoma patients with involvement of the lower uterine segment. Gynecol Oncol 2001;83(3):513–7.

71. Khalifa MA, Mannel RS, Haraway SD, et al. Expression of EGFR, HER-2/neu, P53, and PCNA in endometrioid, serous papillary, and clear cell endometrial adenocarcinomas. Gynecol Oncol 1994;53(1):84–92.

72. Miturski R, Semczuk A, Postawski K, Jakowicki JA. Epidermal growth factor receptor immunostaining and epidermal growth factor receptor-tyrosine kinase activity in proliferative and neoplastic human endometrium. Tumour Biol 2000;21(6):358–66.

73. Nagai N, Oshita T, Fujii T, et al. Prospective analysis of DNA ploidy, proliferative index and epidermal growth factor receptor as prognostic factors for pretreated uterine cancer. Oncol Rep 2000;7(3):551–9.

74. Athanassiadou P, Petrakakou E, Liossi A, et al. Prognostic significance of p53, bcl-2 and EGFR in carcinoma of the endometrium. Acta Cytol 1999;43(6):1039–44.

75. Yokoyama Y, Takahashi Y, Hashimoto M, et al. Immunohis-

tochemical study of estradiol, epidermal growth factor, transforming growth factor alpha and epidermal growth factor receptor in endometrial neoplasia. Jpn J Clin Oncol 1996;26(6):411–6.

76. Ohkawara S, Jobo T, Sato R, Kuramoto H. Comparison of endometrial carcinoma coexisting with and without endometrial hyperplasia. Eur J Gynaecol Oncol 2000;21(6): 573–7.

77. Sivridis E, Giatromanolaki A, Koukourakis M, Anastasiadis P. Endometrial carcinoma: association of steroid hormone receptor expression with low angiogenesis and bcl-2 expression. Virchows Arch 2001;438(5):470–7.

78. Halperin R, Zehavi S, Habler L, et al. Comparative immuno-histochemical study of endometrioid and serous papillary carcinoma of endometrium. Eur J Gynaecol Oncol 2001; 22(2):122–6.

79. Orbo A, Rydningen M, Straume B, Lysne S. Significance of morphometric, DNA cytometric features, and other prognostic markers on survival of endometrial cancer patients in northern Norway. Int J Gynecol Cancer 2002;12(1):49–56.

80. Salvesen HB, Iversen OE, Akslen LA. Prognostic impact of morphometric nuclear grade of endometrial carcinoma. Cancer 1998;83(5):956–64.

81. Mogensen O, Sorensen FB, Bichel P, Jakobsen A. Mean nuclear volume: a supplementary prognostic factor in endometrial cancer [record supplied by publisher]. Int J Gynecol Cancer 1999;9(1):72–9.

82. Britton LC, Wilson TO, Goffey TA, et al. Flow cytometric DNA analysis of stage I endometrial carcinoma. Gynecol Oncol 1989;34:317–22.

83. Lundgren C, Auer G, Frankendal B, et al. Nuclear DNA content, proliferative activity, and p53 expression related to clinical and histopathologic features in endometrial carcinoma. Int J Gynecol Cancer 2002;12(1):110–8.

84. Gudmundsson TE, Hogberg T, Alm P, et al. The prognostic information of DNA ploidy and S-phase fraction may vary with histologic grade in endometrial carcinoma. Acta Oncol 1995;34(6):803–12.

85. Wong YF, Ip TY, Chung TKH, et al. Clinical and pathologic significance of microsatellite instability in endometrial cancer. Int J Gynecol Cancer 1999;9:406–10.

86. Baldinu P, Cossu A, Manca A, et al. Microsatellite instability and mutation analysis of candidate genes in unselected Sardinian patients with endometrial carcinoma. Cancer 2002;94:3157–68.

87. Fiumicino S, Ercoli A, Ferrandina G, et al. Microsatellite instability is an independent indicator of recurrence in sporadic stage I-II endometrial adenocarcinoma. J Clin Oncol 2001;19(4):1008–14.

88. Koul A, Willen R, Bendahl PO, et al. Distinct sets of gene alterations in endometrial carcinoma implicate alternate modes of tumorigenesis. Cancer 2002;94(9):2369–79.

89. Risinger JI, Hayes K, Maxwell GL, et al. PTEN mutation in endometrial cancers is associated with favorable clinical and pathologic characteristics. Clin Cancer Res 1998; 4(12):3005–10.

90. Maxwell GL, Risinger JI, Alvarez AA, et al. Favorable survival associated with microsatellite instability in endometrioid endometrial cancers. Obstet Gynecol 2001;97(3):417–22.

91. Maxwell GL, Risinger JI, Gumbs C, et al. Mutation of the PTEN tumor suppressor gene in endometrial hyperplasias. Cancer Res 1998;58(12):2500–3.

92. Levine RL, Cargile CB, Blazes MS, et al. PTEN mutations and microsatellite instability in complex atypical hyperplasia, a precursor lesion to uterine endometrioid carcinoma. Cancer Res 1998;58(15):3254–8.

93. Lax SF, Kendall B, Tashiro H, et al. The frequency of p53, K-ras mutations, and microsatellite instability differs in uterine endometrioid and serous carcinoma. Cancer 2000; 88(4):814–24.

94. Baak JP, Snijders WP, Van Diest PJ, et al. Confirmation of the prognostic value of the ECPI-1 score (myometrial invasion, DNA-ploidy and mean shortest nuclear axis) in FIGO stage I endometrial cancer patients with long follow-up [record supplied by publisher]. Int J Gynecol Cancer 1995;5(2):112–6.

95. Salvesen HB, Stefansson I, Kalvenes MB, et al. Loss of PTEN expression is associated with metastatic disease in patients with endometrial carcinoma. Cancer 2002;94(8): 2185–91.

96. Tashiro H, Blazes MS, Wu R, et al. Mutations in PTEN are frequent in endometrial carcinoma but rare in other common gynecological malignancies. Cancer Res 1997; 57(18):3935–40.

97. Risinger JI, Hayes AK, Berchuck A, Barrett JC. PTEN/ MMAC1 mutations in endometrial cancers. Cancer Res 1997;57(21):4736–8.

98. Salvesen HB, MacDonald N, Ryan A, et al. PTEN methylation is associated with advanced stage and microsatellite instability in endometrial carcinoma. Int J Cancer 2001; 91(1):22–6.

99. Minaguchi T, Yoshikawa H, Oda K, et al. PTEN mutation located only outside exons 5, 6, and 7 is an independent predictor of favorable survival in endometrial carcinomas. Clin Cancer Res 2001;7(9):2636–42.

100. Lee JO, Yang H, Georgescu MM, et al. Crystal structure of the PTEN tumor suppressor: implications for its phosphoinositide phosphatase activity and membrane association. Cell 1999;99(3):323–34.

101. Simpkins SB, Peiffer-Schneider S, Mutch DG, et al. PTEN mutations in endometrial cancers with 10q LOH: additional evidence for the involvement of multiple tumor suppressors. Gynecol Oncol 1998;71(3):391–5.

102. Backe J, Gassel AM, Hauber K, et al. p53 protein in endometrial cancer is related to proliferative activity and prognosis but not to expression of p21 protein. Int J Gynecol Pathol 1997;16(4):361–8.

103. Coronado PJ, Vidart JA, Lopez-asenjo JA, et al. P53 overexpression predicts endometrial carcinoma recurrence better than HER-2/neu overexpression. Eur J Obstet Gynecol Reprod Biol 2001;98(1):103–8.

104. Geisler JP, Geisler HE, Wiemann MC, et al. p53 expression as a prognostic indicator of 5-year survival in endometrial cancer. Gynecol Oncol 1999;74(3):468–71.

105. Ito K, Watanabe K, Nasim S, et al. Prognostic significance of p53 overexpression in endometrial cancer. Cancer Res 1994;54(17):4667–70.

106. Kohlberger P, Gitsch G, Loesch A, et al. p53 protein overexpression in early stage endometrial cancer. Gynecol Oncol 1996;62(2):213–7.

107. Kohler MF, Carney P, Dodge R, et al. p53 overexpression in advanced-stage endometrial adenocarcinoma. Am J Obstet Gynecol 1996;175(5):1246–52.

108. Powell B, Soong R, Grieu F, et al. p53 protein overexpression is a prognostic indicator of poor survival in stage I endometrial carcinoma. Int J Oncol 1999;14(1):175–9.

109. Sherman ME, Bur ME, Kurman RJ. p53 in endometrial cancer and its putative precursors: evidence for diverse pathways of tumorigenesis. Hum Pathol 1995;26(11):1268–74.

110. Pisani AL, Barbuto DA, Chen D, et al. HER-2/neu, p53, and DNA analyses as prognosticators for survival in endometrial carcinoma. Obstet Gynecol 1995;85(5 Pt 1):729–34.

111. Hamel NW, Sebo TJ, Wilson TO, et al. Prognostic value of p53 and proliferating cell nuclear antigen expression in endometrial carcinoma. Gynecol Oncol 1996;62(2):192–8.

112. Cheng WF, Chen TM, Chen CA, et al. Clinical application of intratumoral blood flow study in patients with endometrial carcinoma. Cancer 1998;82(10):1881–6.

113. Alcazar JL, Galan MJ, Jurado M, Lopez-Garcia G. Intratumoral blood flow analysis in endometrial carcinoma: correlation with tumor characteristics and risk for recurrence. Gynecol Oncol 2002;84(2):258–62.

114. Lee CN, Cheng WF, Chen CA, et al. Angiogenesis of endometrial carcinomas assessed by measurement of intratumoral blood flow, microvessel density, and vascular endothelial growth factor levels. Obstet Gynecol 2000; 96(4):615–21.

115. Salvesen HB, Iversen OE, Akslen LA. Independent prognostic importance of microvessel density in endometrial carcinoma. Br J Cancer 1998;77(7):1140–4.

116. Fine BA, Valente PT, Feinstein GI, Dey T. VEGF, flt-1, and KDR/flk-1 as prognostic indicators in endometrial carcinoma. Gynecol Oncol 2000;76(1):33–9.

117. Fujisawa T, Watanabe J, Akaboshi M, et al. Immunohistochemical study on VEGF expression in endometrial carcinoma—comparison with p53 expression, angiogenesis, and tumor histologic grade. J Cancer Res Clin Oncol 2001;127(11):668–74.

118. Hirai M, Nakagawara A, Oosaki T, et al. Expression of vascular endothelial growth factors (VEGF-A/VEGF-1 and VEGF-C/VEGF-2) in postmenopausal uterine endometrial carcinoma. Gynecol Oncol 2001;80(2):181–8.

7

Radiotherapy and Postsurgical Management of Endometrial Cancer

THOMAS F. DELANEY, MD
RICHARD T. PENSON, MD, MRCP

The majority of the 40,000 new cases of endometrial cancer will present with tumor confined to the uterine corpus and a 5-year disease-free survival in excess of 75%.[1,2] Certain features, such as depth of myometrial invasion, lymph node metastases, histologic subtype and grade, and presence or absence of vascular invasion, can be correlated with the risk of relapse and, thus, be used to assess the need for adjuvant treatment (see Chapter 6). The decision to use postoperative adjuvant radiotherapy is based on the pathologic findings in the uterus, the status of the pelvic and para-aortic lymph nodes, and peritoneal washings taken at the time of laparotomy. Available radiation modalities include adjuvant vaginal cuff brachytherapy, pelvic radiotherapy with or without para-aortic radiotherapy, and whole abdominal radiotherapy. Treatment recommendations are based on failure patterns noted after surgery alone, an assessment of the patient's risk of recurrence based on pathologic findings and other features of the patient's presentation, results of the few randomized prospective studies that have been performed, and data from retrospective studies. The goal of adjuvant therapy for patients with early-stage, low-risk disease is to maintain excellent clinical outcome while minimizing treatment morbidity. For patients with more advanced disease at presentation, pelvic and nodal disease control can be improved with adjuvant radiotherapy. These patients are at risk of systemic metastatic disease, and investigations into the efficacy of systemic adjuvant therapies are ongoing. Radiotherapy also has an important role in the prevention of and treatment of patients with vaginal or pelvic recurrences of endometrial cancer after surgery. In contrast to carcinoma of the uterine cervix, irradiation alone without surgery is not an optimal therapy for endometrial carcinoma. Nevertheless, it is the primary local therapy for patients who are medically inoperable, and this treatment will also be discussed.

HISTORY OF THERAPY FOR ENDOMETRIAL CANCER

During the past 50 years, treatment has evolved from preoperative intracavity radium or external beam radiotherapy followed by hysterectomy, to the use of intrauterine tandem and vaginal ovoids, and, increasingly, hysterectomy with surgical staging as primary intervention with adjuvant radiotherapy for patients with significant myometrial invasion or nodal involvement. During the past 30 years, a number of hormonal and chemotherapy regimens have been tested as adjuvant therapy. Such modalities remain investigational.

RISK STRATIFICATION

Numerous prognostic factors have been identified for endometrial cancer. On the basis of these risk factors, patients have been grouped into low, intermediate, and high risk of development of recurrent disease. For those patients with tumor confined to the uterus (stages I and II), the primary risk factors for development of recurrent disease are tumor histology (mainly endometrioid versus papillary serous, clear cell and other rare aggressive subtypes), tumor grade, depth of myometrial invasion, lymphovascular space invasion, and patient age. Endometrioid adenocarcinoma has been identified as having the most favorable outcome and uterine serous carcinoma the least (see Chapter 11).[3] On the basis of the risk factors present, patients with uterine-confined tumor can be classified as at low risk or intermediate risk of developing recurrent disease.

RADIOTHERAPY

Risk of Recurrence and Radiotherapy Treatment Algorithms

The risk of pelvic and aortic lymph node metastases in patients with pathologic stage I disease was defined in a Gynecologic Oncology Group (GOG) study. The relationship among grade, depth of invasion, and nodal metastases is shown in Tables 7–1 and 7–2. The anticipated 5-year recurrence-free survival for patients with negative pelvic lymph node metastases in one study was 85%, compared with 70% for those with positive pelvic nodes and negative para-aortic nodes and 36% when the para-aortic nodes were involved.[4] Multivariate analysis of multiple factors has also been used to predict lymph node involvement, as shown in Table 7–3.

The incidence of lymph-vascular invasion (LVI) is 16 to 20%. This pathologic finding is associated with a higher rate of lymph node metastases and a worse prognosis.[5,6] Creasman reported the incidence of pelvic and para-aortic lymph node metastases as 27% and 19%, respectively, when LVI was present, compared with 7% and 3% when not present.[5] The

Table 7–2. GRADE, DEPTH OF MYOMETRIAL INVASION, AND AORTIC LYMPH NODE METASTASIS

Depth of Invasion	Grade		
	1	2	3
Confined to endometrium	0%	0.5%	1.9%
Inner half	0.17%	0.76%	2.42%
Outer half	3.5%	6.0%	10.2%

Adapted from International Federation of Gynecology and obstetrics. Annual report on the results of treatment in gynecological cancer. *J Epidemiol Boistat* 1998;3:1.

GOG reported 5-year survival of 61% among clinical stage I/II patients with LVI compared with 86% among patients without LVI.[7]

Patients whose tumors show pathologic evidence of lower uterine involvement also have more frequent lymph node involvement with associated worse prognosis.[5] Increasing tumor size is also associated with a higher frequency of lymph node metastases. Schinck and colleagues reported that stage I patients with tumors ≤ 2 cm had lymph node metastases in only 6% of cases compared with 21% for tumors > 2 cm and 35% for those that involved the entire endometrium.[8] Positive peritoneal cytology occurs in approximately 15% of patients and is generally associated with other known unfavorable prognostic factors; indeed, fewer than 5% of patients with positive cytology have no evidence of extrauterine disease (see Chapter 10).[5] Creasman reported that 6 of 13 patients (46%) who had positive peritoneal cytology as the only extrauterine finding died due to disseminated intraperitoneal carcinomatosis.[9] Because this study predated the recognition of uterine serous carcinoma, a histologic subtype frequently associated with positive cytology, the significance of positive cytology as an independent prognostic factor in endometrioid carcinoma remains uncertain.

Other factors associated with a higher risk of recurrence include aneuploidy, progesterone receptor, HER2/neu oncogene overexpression, and *P53* mutation.[10–13]

In order to better estimate the clinical outcome of patients, multivariate models that include these multiple risk factors have been created. Algan and colleagues studied 98 surgical stage I/II patients who had all received radiation therapy.[14] Four prognostic

Table 7–1. GRADE, DEPTH OF MYOMETRIAL INVASION, AND PELVIC LYMPH NODE METASTASIS

Depth of Invasion	Grade		
	1	2	3
Confined to endometrium	0.4%	0.46%	2.97%
Inner half	1.2%	3%	5.4%
Outer half	15%	15.7%	23.8%

Adapted from International Federation of Gynecology and obstetrics. Annual report on the results of treatment in gynecological cancer. *J Epidemiol Boistat* 1998;3:1.

Table 7–3. RISK FACTORS FOR NODAL METASTASIS USING MULTIVARIATE ANALYSIS

Risk Factor	Lymph Node Metastasis	
	Pelvic	Aortic
Low risk (No moderate or high risk factors) Grade 1, endometrium only, no intraperitoneal disease	0/44 (0%)	0/44 (0%)
Moderate risk (Inner or midinvasion, grade 2 or 3, no intraperitoneal disease)		
Only one factor	4/158 (3%)	3/158 (2%)
Both factors	15/268 (6%)	6/268 (2%)
High risk (Intraperitoneal disease, and/or deep myometrial invasion)		
Deep invasion only	21/116 (18%)	17/116 (15%)
Intraperitoneal disease only	4/12 (33%)	1/12 (8%)
Both factors	14/23 (61%)	7/23 (30%)

Adapted from Creasman WT et al.[5]

variables—grade, lymphatic invasion, depth of invasion, and cervical stromal involvement—were evaluated. Patients with 0/1 versus 2 versus 3/4 risk factors had progressively decreased survival rates at 5 years, of 88, 76, and 60%, respectively. The GOG surgical pathologic study also evaluated the frequency of recurrence based on individual and multiple risk factors.[4] Their analysis is shown in Table 7–4.

Patients with stage IA, grades 1 and 2 endometrial adenocarcinomas are at low risk of developing recurrent disease after primary surgery without adjuvant radiotherapy. No prospective, randomized controlled trial of adjuvant therapy has been performed in this patient group because the risk of recurrence is less than 10%, and an informative phase III trial would be prohibitively large. Retrospective studies and pathologic models of survival, however, suggest that postoperative adjuvant radiotherapy should not be routinely administered to this group of patients.[7] Our own institutional algorithm for postoperative adjuvant therapy for stages I and II disease is shown in Figure 7–1.

Patients with surgical stages IB, IC, and IIA disease are at intermediate risk of recurrent disease. The GOG-99 study is the one prospective, randomized study that has evaluated the issue of adjuvant, postoperative external beam radiotherapy in this patient population.[15] Patients were randomized to receive either surgery alone or surgery with postoperative pelvic radiation. The surgery was a transabdominal hysterectomy and bilateral salpingo-oophorectomy (TAH/BSO), pelvic and para-aortic lymph node sampling, and peritoneal cytology. Patients included in the study had surgical stage I or IIA disease, with no tumor seen in the sampled lymph nodes. The adjuvant postoperative radiotherapy was delivered to the pelvis at 1.8 Gray (Gy) daily to a total dose of 50.4 Gy. Vaginal cuff brachytherapy was not given. This study, currently only reported in abstract form with a median follow-up of 56 months, randomized 392 patients, of whom 58% were stage IB, 33% stage IC, and 9% stage IIA. Eighty-two percent of tumors were grades 1 or 2, and 18% were grade 3. Indeed, the majority of the patients accrued to the trial had either stage IB or

Table 7–4. RISK OF RECURRENCE BY SINGLE AND MULTIPLE RISK FACTORS

Risk Factor	% Recurrence
Single factor	
Aortic node metastases	40.0
Pelvic node metastases	27.7
Lymphatic vessel invasion	26.5
Positive cytology	18.8
Isthmus/cervix involvement	16.0
Adnexa	14.3
Multiple factors	
One factor	20.1
Two factors	43.1
Three or more factors	63.3

Adapted from Morrow CP et al.[4]

MANAGEMENT ALGORITHM FOR STAGE I ENDOMETRIOID ENDOMETRIAL CANCER

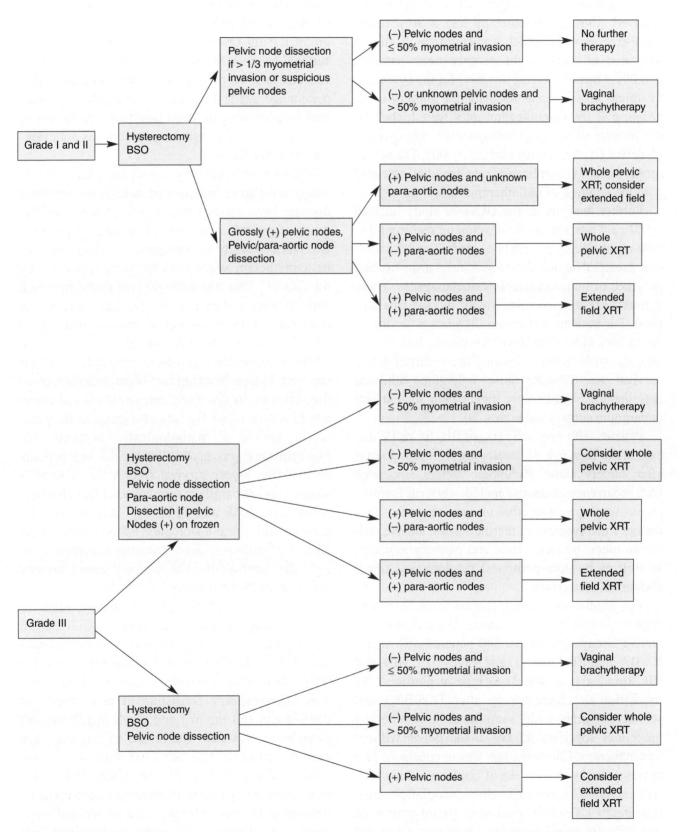

Figure 7–1. Management algorithm for postoperative adjuvant radiotherapy for stages I and II endometrial cancer. BSO = bilateral salpingo-oophorectomy; XRT = radiotherapy.

grade 1 and 2 tumors, rendering them at low risk of recurrent disease after surgery alone. Patients who received adjuvant radiotherapy had a 96% recurrence-free survival, which was significantly higher than that of 88% in the surgery-alone patients, $p = .001$. Overall survival was 94% for the combined treatment group versus 89% for the surgery-alone group, $p = .09$. Complication rates were higher for the patients undergoing postoperative radiotherapy, 15 versus 6% for surgery alone, $p = .007$. The severe (grade 3 and 4) complication rate was also increased with the addition of radiotherapy.

Further analysis of the GOG-99 study defined significant risk factors for developing recurrent disease as advancing patient age, grade 2 and 3 histology, greater than one-third myometrial invasion, and presence of tumor in lymphovascular spaces. These factors were also correlated with disease-free survival. For patients older than 70 years with one of the factors, older than 50 years with two factors, and any age with all three factors, the recurrence-free survival was 87% for those undergoing adjuvant radiotherapy, significantly higher than for patients undergoing surgery alone, $p < .01$.

Patients with surgically staged IIB, III, or IV disease are at high risk of developing recurrent disease after surgery alone. Pathologic factors associated with recurrence of disease include cervical involvement, tumor beyond the uterus, or both. This includes involvement of uterine serosa, adnexa, fallopian tubes, ovaries, pelvic and para-aortic nodes, as well as positive peritoneal cytology and upper abdominal metastases.

Few studies of adjuvant therapy have been conducted in these high-risk patients. The Italian Cooperative Group randomized 340 patients with stages IC, IIA, and IIB (grade 3) and stages IIIA, IIIB, and IIIC (grades 1, 2, and 3) to receive postoperative irradiation or chemotherapy after TAH/BSO and selective lymph node sampling.[16] Radiotherapy guidelines specified 45 Gy to the pelvis without brachytherapy. Chemotherapy was to consist of five cycles given every 4 weeks of cisplatin (50 mg/m^2), Adriamycin (45 mg/m^2), and cyclophosphamide (600 mg/m^2). The rate of pelvic or distant recurrence was 27% for those receiving irradiation compared with 29% for those receiving chemotherapy, with no significant difference in outcome. The rate of isolated pelvic recurrence was 5% for those receiving irradiation and 10% for those in the chemotherapy group, $p = .09$. Overall survival and progression-free survival have not yet been reported from this study. An analysis of prognostic factors indicated that patient age, grade 3 histology, and depth of myometrial invasion were the most significant predictors of recurrence. Lymph-vascular invasion was not evaluated as a risk factor.

Patients with papillary serous and clear cell histology are also at high risk of developing recurrent disease. Most series report a poor outcome in this group of patients, regardless of the stage. A prospective phase II study of postoperative whole abdominal radiotherapy was conducted in these patients by the GOG.[17] This was a single-arm study, in which patients with stages I to IV papillary serous and clear cell carcinoma as well as patients with stages III and IV endometrioid endometrial cancer received 30 Gy whole abdominal radiotherapy at 150 cGy per day with kidney blocking and boost radiotherapy to the pelvis to 50 Gy. Supplemental boost radiotherapy to a dose of 45 Gy was also given to the para-aortic nodes, if pathologically positive. No brachytherapy was given. Among the 165 patients accrued, the 5-year survival figures for those with stages I and II papillary serous and clear cell carcinoma were 65% and 33%, for stage III and IV patients with these histologies. Patients with stages III and IV endometrioid endometrial carcinoma had a 5-year survival of 31%. Chronic bowel toxicity was seen in 7% of patients.

This study was followed by a two-arm randomized, prospective phase III study, GOG-122, in which patients with stage III or IV endometrial cancer of any histology were randomized to receive whole abdominal radiotherapy as above or postoperative chemotherapy consisting of eight cycles of doxorubicin (60 mg/m^2) and cisplatin (50 mg/m^2) given every 3 weeks. The results of this study are currently pending. The GOG has initiated a subsequent randomized phase III study (GOG-184) in this same patient population comparing tumor-volume–directed pelvic radiotherapy with or without para-aortic radiotherapy, followed by cisplatin and doxorubicin with or without paclitaxel in patients with surgical stage III or IV endometrial carcinoma following TAH/BSO and pelvic lymph node sampling. End points are survival and progression-free survival. Intracavitary vaginal cuff irradiation is also delivered for those patients with deep myometrial invasion or involvement of the lower uterine segment or cervix.

Radiotherapy for Patients with Incomplete Surgical Staging

Prior to the adoption of the surgical staging system for endometrial cancer by the International Federation of Gynecologists and Obstetricians (FIGO), patients rarely underwent lymph node sampling. A significant proportion of patients still undergo TAH/BSO without lymph node staging. The results of several large randomized trials of patients not undergoing lymph node sampling are applicable to this group of patients. These include the Norwegian Radium Hospital study, in which 540 patients with clinical stage I endometrial cancer were randomized to postoperative treatment after TAH/BSO with vaginal cylinder brachytherapy alone or combined brachytherapy and pelvic nodal irradiation.[18] Brachytherapy consisted of 6,000 cGy delivered with low-dose-rate radium insertion to the vaginal mucosa. Pelvic irradiation was specified as 4,000 cGy over 4 weeks in five daily fractions of 200 cGy. Central blocking was used after 2,000 cGy. The obturator and external iliac lymph nodes received another 300 to 400 cGy from the brachytherapy. No significant difference in survival was noted between the two groups, with 90% in the brachytherapy-alone group and 87% in the combined brachytherapy and external beam group being alive at 10 years. The death and recurrence rate was 12.3% in the former group and 11.8% in the latter. When the entire patient population was analyzed according to risk factors, it was noted that a higher death and recurrence rate was noted in patients 60 years or older, seemingly related to a higher frequency of deeply infiltrating tumors. The death and recurrence rate was also significantly higher in patients with grade 3 disease compared with those with grade 1 or 2 disease, $p = .02$. Although vaginal and pelvic recurrences were reduced from 6.9 to 1.9% by the addition of pelvic radiation to vaginal brachytherapy, this was outweighed by the higher frequency of distant metastases in the group receiving pelvic radiotherapy, 9.9% versus 5.4%, resulting in no significant difference in overall survival. Analysis of subgroups by risk factors demonstrated that patients with grade 1 or 2 tumors and patients with grade 3 tumors invasive of $< 50\%$ of the myometrium did not benefit from pelvic radiotherapy. There were fewer vaginal/pelvic recurrences as well as deaths from cancer, however, in grade 3, deeply invasive tumors with the addition of pelvic radiotherapy. The vaginal/pelvic recurrence rate in these patients was lowered from 19.6 to 4.5% with the external radiation, and the death from cancer rate fell from 27.5 to 18.5%.

A recent randomized phase III European trial addressed postoperative pelvic radiotherapy in patients who did not undergo lymph node sampling.[19] They included patients with grade 1 disease and $> 50\%$ myometrial invasion, grade 2 disease with any myometrial invasion, and grade 3 disease with $< 50\%$ myometrial invasion. Patients were randomized to receive postoperative radiotherapy of 46 Gy or no further therapy after TAH/BSO. The study enrolled 715 patients and was reported with a median follow-up of 52 months. The actuarial 5-year locoregional recurrence rates were lowered in the radiotherapy group from 14 to 4% ($p < .001$); 73% of the locoregional recurrences were vaginal. Salvage treatment of vaginal relapse was often successful. After vaginal recurrence, the 3-year survival was 69% in contrast to 13% after pelvic or distant relapse ($p < .001$). No difference in distant metastases was noted, with 8% in the radiotherapy group and 7% in the control group. No difference was seen in the overall survival rates of 85% in the control group at 5 years compared with 81% in the irradiated patients, $p = .31$. Deaths from endometrial cancer occurred in 9% of the irradiated patients and 6% of the control patients, $p = .37$. Most deaths were not related to endometrial cancer. Of the 105 deaths seen, 41 were related to endometrial cancer, 19 from another cancer, and 45 from other causes, primarily cardiovascular. Complications of any severity were seen in 25% of the patients in the irradiated group compared with 6% in the control group, $p < .001$.

Most complications were gastrointestinal. Grade 3 or 4 complications were only seen in 7 of the 715 patients; 6 of these 7 patients had been irradiated. The four-field box technique was associated with a lower risk of radiation-related complications, 20%, compared with 30% for anterior posterior/posterior anterior (AP/PA) fields and 36% for three fields.[20] A Cox multivariate regression analysis revealed that prognostic factors for pelvic recurrence or death were patient age > 60 years old, > 50% myometrial invasion, and grade 3 histology. Lymph-vascular space invasion was not examined. Patients with grade 3 tumors invading < 50% of the myometrium had a locoregional recurrence risk that was similar to that of patients with grade 1/2 tumors with more than 50% invasion. The death rate was highest in women with grade 3 tumors.

Preoperative Radiation Therapy

Although primary surgery with postoperative adjuvant radiation therapy is the primary treatment sequence currently employed, there are situations where preoperative radiotherapy has been given. Preoperative radiation therapy can be given by external beam, by brachytherapy, or a combination of the two. Preoperative intracavitary brachytherapy was first described by Heyman and colleagues.[21] It may produce fewer complications than postoperative radiation therapy.[21] Furthermore, it may provide a survival advantage for patients with deeply invasive or grade 3 tumors when compared with postoperative external beam radiation therapy.[22] A prospective, randomized phase III trial compared external pelvic irradiation with brachytherapy prior to surgery.[23] Those undergoing the intracavitary brachytherapy experienced fewer local recurrences, improved survival, and fewer complications. The complication rates were 11% with external beam radiotherapy compared with 3% with brachytherapy. As the strategy of preoperative radiotherapy commits some women with relatively low risk of locoregional recurrence to unnecessary radiation therapy, its use has been abandoned for patients with stage I/IIA disease in favor of surgery followed by postoperative radiation of women at risk of locoregional recurrence.

Preoperative radiotherapy is given in many centers for patients with clinical stage II endometrial cancer with cervical stromal involvement, with external radiotherapy, intracavitary brachytherapy, or both.[24,25] No prospective randomized trial of this approach has been conducted in this patient population, but retrospective studies indicate that survival rates for this group of patients ranges from 70 to 85%. Preoperative radiation may be the best approach for patients with gross cervical involvement; alternatively, radical hysterectomy has also been used in lieu of radiotherapy.[26]

Radiotherapy for Salvage of Postoperative Vaginal and/or Pelvic Recurrence

When recurrence is noted in the vagina and/or pelvis, restaging with chest computed tomography (CT) and abdominopelvic magnetic resonance imaging (MRI) or CT should be performed to determine sites of recurrent disease (see Chapter 8). For a substantial proportion of patients with disease confined to the vagina or the pelvis, radiation can provide effective salvage treatment. It is worth emphasizing that different anatomic configurations of locoregional recurrent disease will have different prognoses. Isolated vaginal cuff recurrence is the most favorable scenario.[19] Outcome in this setting will depend on multiple factors, including age, tumor size and vaginal stage of disease, time interval from hysterectomy, initial tumor grade, and radiation boost technique.[27] Three-year survival figures as favorable as 69% have been reported.[19] Kuten and colleagues evaluated 51 patients with locoregional recurrence of endometrial cancer.[28] They reported that 40% of patients with isolated vaginal cuff recurrence were alive and free of disease at 5 years. Their figures fall into the 20 to 50% range that others have reported. They, however, noted no survivors beyond 1.5 years with pelvic lymph node recurrence. Sears and colleagues reported local control of isolated vaginal disease of 58% at 5 years, compared with only 20% for pelvic disease, $p = .0119$.[27] They identified other factors in their study which were significant for local control by univariate analysis. These included vaginal stage with 77%, 51%, and 17% local control at 5 years as they progressed, respectively, from stage I to II to

III/IV, p = .006. Seventy-four percent of those with tumors $\leq$ 2 cm were locally controlled compared with only 30% with larger tumors (p = .007). Those patients whose locoregional recurrence occurred more than 1 year following surgery fared better than those with earlier recurrences, with local control achieved in 70% and 39%, respectively (p = .0004). Younger patients with recurrent disease had an inferior outcome, p < .0001. Forty-four of their 45 patients were treated by external beam pelvic radiation therapy, median dose of 5,000 cGy. Additional brachytherapy boost was given in 27 patients, external beam boost in 6 patients, and no boost in 12 patients. Local control was highest in those boosted with brachytherapy at 64% compared with only 44% in those undergoing external beam boost and 28% in those not boosted (p = .0118). Multivariate analysis demonstrated that only boost technique and age were significantly associated with local control, both at the p < .0001 level.

Radiation Therapy Techniques

Pelvic radiation therapy is given with high-energy photons ($\geq$ 10 MV) delivered with a four-field technique, AP/PA, and laterals (Figure 7–2). When vaginal brachytherapy is planned, 45 Gy is delivered in 25 fractions of 1.8 Gy daily. A boost of 5.4 Gy is delivered to the vaginal cuff with external beam radiation if vaginal brachytherapy is not given. If patients are able to lie prone on a belly-board, this may reduce the amount of small bowel in the lateral beams. As many of these patients are obese, however, with a recent surgical incision, prone positioning may be uncomfortable. Treating with a full bladder can also help minimize the amount of small bowel in the beam. Customized blocking is used to shield normal tissues. At the time of simulation, vaginal and rectal markers are employed. Small bowel contrast can be used in situations where boost doses above 45 Gy are contemplated. The superior border is set at the L5-S1 interspace, and the inferior border is generally at the bottom of the obdurator foramen, including at least two-thirds of the vagina, using a radiographic marker in the vagina for verification. On the anterior/posterior fields, the lateral borders are placed 2 cm lateral to the bony pelvic rim. On the lateral fields, the anterior border is set at the pubic symphysis and the posterior border should include S3.

When common iliac and/or para-aortic nodes are involved, the pelvic field is extended superiorly to the L1-L2 interspace to cover the para-aortic nodes

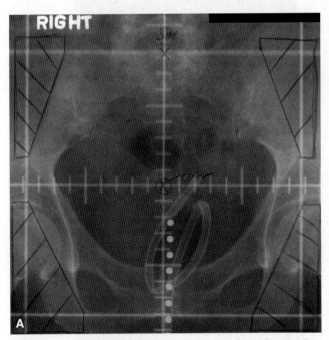
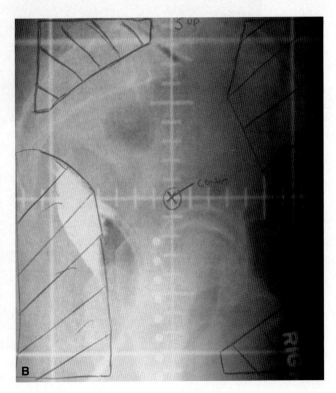

Figure 7–2. Postoperative pelvic radiotherapy fields for a patient with endometrial cancer. Four-field technique (anterior, posterior, and laterals) is used. *A,* Anterior and *B,* lateral fields are shown here.

(Figure 7–3). Customized blocking of small bowel in the para-aortic region should maintain at least a 1-cm margin from the para-aortic nodes. Kidney dose must be kept at less than 1,800 cGy; this can be facilitated by weighting the AP/PA:lateral fields in a 2:1 ratio, with the kidneys completely blocked on the AP/PA fields.

For patients with high-risk histologies, such as papillary serous carcinoma or clear cell carcinoma, and for patients with positive peritoneal washings who are going to receive whole abdominal radiation therapy, radiation is given in daily doses of 125 to 150 cGy to the whole abdomen up to a dose of 25 to 30 Gy (Figure 7–4). Posterior renal shielding (five half-value layers) is used to limit the kidney dose. Pelvic boost radiotherapy to 45 to 50 Gy follows the whole abdominal treatment; para-aortic nodal boosts up to 45 Gy can be given when the common iliac and/or para-aortic nodes are involved.

Vaginal brachytherapy can be given with either high-dose-rate or low-dose-rate brachytherapy. Low-dose-rate treatment is generally given with a cylinder loaded with cesium sources. Low-dose-rate brachytherapy requires hospital admission, with the patient bed-bound and immobilized for 50 to 60 hours. This is associated with a 30-day morbidity rate of 6.4% and mortality of 1.5% and a deep venous thrombosis rate of 1.2%. For this reason, high-dose-rate brachytherapy is preferred. A high-activity iridium-192 source is employed that delivers the dose over a period of approximately 5 minutes in the outpatient setting. Remote after-loading equipment is used to deliver the sources into the applicator once the patient is in a shielded room, thus eliminating any significant radiation exposure to medical personnel (Figure 7–5). The preferred applicator is a vaginal cylinder, as shown in Figure 7–6. These are available in diameters that range from 2 to 4 cm in 0.5 cm increments. There is a dosimetric advantage to using the largest cylinder that is comfortable for the patient. When, as is generally done, dose is prescribed to a depth of 0.5 cm, the vaginal mucosal dose for any

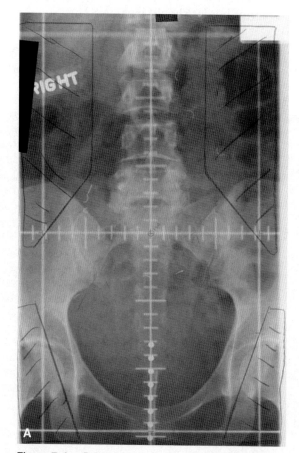
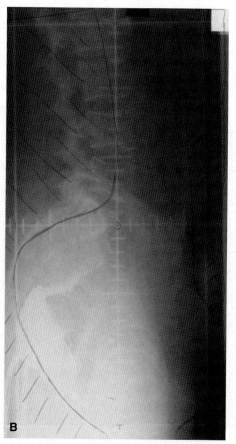

Figure 7–3.   Pelvic and para-aortic radiotherapy (ie, extended) fields for patient with common iliac and/or para-aortic nodal involvement. Four-field technique is employed with *A*, anterior and *B*, lateral fields shown here.

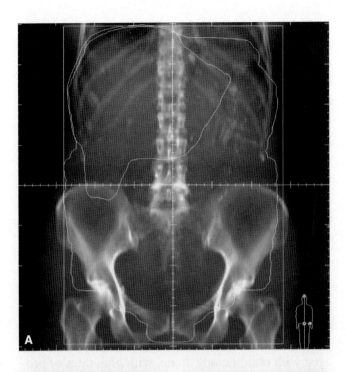

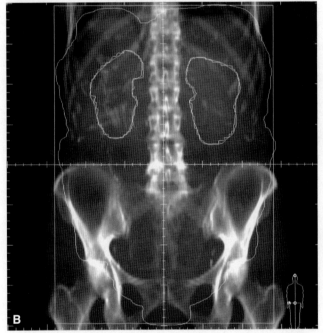

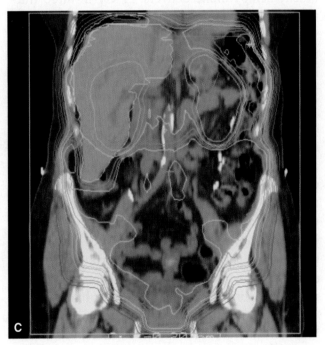

Figure 7–4. *A* and *B*, Whole abdominal anterior and posterior radiotherapy portals and *C*, dose-distribution display for patients with high-risk endometrial cancer. Note the full-thickness posterior kidney blocks.

given prescribed dose at 0.5 cm will be lower with the larger cylinder because of the inverse square law. The lower vaginal dose will reduce the risk of treatment-related complications. Ideal application requires that the cylinder be in contact with the vaginal vault mucosa. Hence, gentle pressure should be applied to the cylinder to ensure appropriate contact before the applicator is secured. An alternative applicator system is vaginal ovoids.

Because the majority of treatment failures in patients who are treated with surgery alone occur in the vaginal vault, the target for vaginal brachytherapy is the proximal third to half of the vagina.[19,29,30] This can spare patients the increased risk of complications associated with treating the entire vagina.[31] Radiation dose schedules that are associated with high rates of vaginal control and low rates of morbidity have been published. The most com-

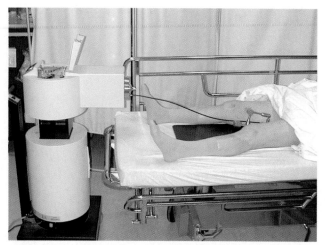

Figure 7–5. Patient with endometrial cancer undergoing outpatient, high-dose-rate brachytherapy for adjuvant treatment of the vaginal cuff.

monly employed high-dose-rate schedule for brachytherapy alone delivers 21 Gy in three fractions of 7 Gy prescribed to a depth of 0.5 cm at weekly intervals. When combined with pelvic radiation doses not exceeding 45 Gy in 25 fractions, the brachytherapy dose is reduced to 15 Gy in three fractions of 5 Gy.

Patients with medically inoperable endometrial cancer are treated with intracavitary brachytherapy, alone or in combination with external radiation therapy based on the uterine size, grade of tumor, and extent of disease. Magnetic resonance imaging and ultrasonographic evaluations are helpful in assessing the depth of myometrial invasion (see Chapter 4). Brachytherapy alone is usually used for very elderly patients and patients with grade 1 or 2 disease with superficial myometrial invasion. Patients with deep invasion, poorly differentiated tumors, bulky uterine tumors, or extrauterine disease are treated with combination external beam and brachytherapy.

External beam pelvic radiotherapy fields are, as noted above, determined with consideration of a midline AP/PA block for patients who undergo brachytherapy. Low-dose-rate brachytherapy is delivered by a low-dose-rate Simon after-loading system. This consists of multiple Teflon tubes inserted into the uterine cavity and afterloaded with cesium. High-dose-rate brachytherapy is most commonly delivered with a double-tandem applicator as shown in Figure 7–7. Dose prescriptions for these systems are described in the literature.

THERAPY FOR MEDICALLY INOPERABLE PATIENTS

Some patients with endometrial cancer present with comorbidities that preclude hysterectomy and surgical staging. These patients, often elderly, can be managed with radiotherapy alone, with high rates of progression-free survival and overall survival rates of 70 to 80%.[21,32] Patients can be treated with brachytherapy alone or combined external beam radiotherapy and intracavitary insertions, based on the depth of invasion. For patients with clinical stage I disease, MRI or ultrasonography and tumor grade are used to assess the depth of tumor invasion and the risk of pelvic lymph node metastases.[33] This information is used to decide whether pelvic radiotherapy is needed in addition to brachytherapy. Grigsby and colleagues reported that the 5-year progression-free survival for patients with clinical stage I disease stratified by grade was 94% for those with grade 1 tumors, 92% for grade 2, and 78% for grade 3 tumors, if the patients received both external irradiation and intracavitary brachytherapy.[32] Brachytherapy in this patient population can be given with either low-dose or high-dose techniques. There is a low risk of com-

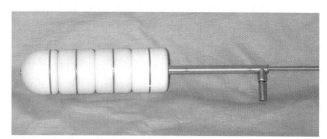

Figure 7–6. High-dose-rate brachytherapy vaginal cylinder for treatment of the vaginal cuff.

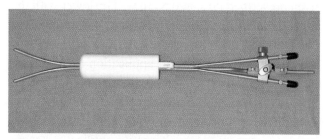

Figure 7–7. High-dose-rate double-tandem and cylinder for brachytherapy treatment of the intact uterus and vagina.

plications with these procedures. One series evaluating low-dose-rate brachytherapy in medically inoperable patients reported a 2.1% mortality rate in 96 patients (1 myocardial infarction and 1 pulmonary embolus) and a life-threatening complication rate of 4.2%.[34] Similar complication rates have been reported after outpatient high-dose-rate brachytherapy in this patient population.[35–37]

Patients with medically inoperable clinical stage II endometrial carcinoma are generally treated with combined pelvic irradiation and intracavitary brachytherapy. The 5-year survival rates for these patients is in the 50 to 60% range, lower than that reported for preoperative radiation and surgery.[32,38] Patients with clinical stage III endometrial cancer are uncommon, comprising 5 to 10% of patients, and generally are patients with vaginal or adnexal involvement. This is a different group of patients from those with surgical stage III disease, most of whom are stage IIIC on the basis of nodal involvement noted at the time of lymph node sampling. The published 5-year survival figures for patients managed with external radiation and intracavitary brachytherapy range from 16 to 42%.[39–42] Because of these poor survival rates with radiotherapy alone, these patients are commonly managed by surgical resection and postoperative radiation, although controlled data comparing the two approaches are not available.

Stage IV endometrial carcinoma is found in fewer than 5% of patients. In patients with disease confined to the pelvis and involving the bladder or rectum, irradiation alone can be used, although long-term survivors are rare. Goff and colleagues reported a median survival of 18 months in patients undergoing cytoreductive surgery compared with 8 months for those who did not.[43] In patients with symptomatic, locally advanced, unresectable disease in the pelvis, radiotherapy is often an effective palliative agent. Spanos and colleagues reported the results of a Radiation Therapy Oncology Group (RTOG) study evaluating a convenient, accelerated, hypofractionated schedule for palliation of symptomatic pelvic disease in such patients with advanced and recurrent endometrial carcinoma.[44] Radiotherapy can also provide effective palliation for symptomatic retroperitoneal lymphadenopathy, as well as bone or lung metastases.

ADJUVANT HORMONAL THERAPY

History of Hormonal Therapy for Endometrial Cancer

It has been known for a long time that some cancers have hormone-dependent growth and differentiation. In 1836, Cooper observed a correlation between tumor growth and the menstrual cycle, and in 1896, Beatson reported the regression of metastatic breast cancer after oophorectomy in premenopausal patients.[45,46] Huggins and Bergenstal demonstrated, with Nobel Prize–winning research in 1952, that the excision of the adrenal glands of postmenopausal women can provide significant remission of metastatic disease.[47] In the 1970s, it became clear that the estrogen-receptor content of hormonally sensitive tumors determined the response to endocrine therapy.[48] The presence of cytoplasmic estrogen receptor and progesterone receptor has been associated with histologic differentiation and with response to hormonal treatment for endometrial cancer and associated with better prognosis.[49–51]

Kelley and Baker in 1961 reported the profound effect of progesterone on endometrial cancer with six objective responses in 21 patients that were durable between 9 months and $4^1/_2$ years and suggested that adjuvant hormonal therapy might reduce the risk of recurrence.[52]

Clinical Trials of Hormonal Therapy for Endometrial Cancer

The overall response rate of recurrent or metastatic endometrial cancer to progestins is approximately 25%, with a range from 18 to 34%, and lower response rates reported in multi-institutional studies with rigorous response criteria (reviewed in Chapter 8).[53,54] These response rates are lower than those reported in estrogen-receptor–positive metastatic breast cancer, and formal evaluation of the potential role of adjuvant endocrine therapy for early-stage endometrial cancer is ongoing, with no clear evidence that this intervention yields an overall survival or disease-free survival advantage. Although adjuvant hormonal treatment is rarely recommended, 28% of the 39 North American cancer centers that responded in one recent questionnaire study reported the addition of hormonal therapy to primary treatment for FIGO stage III/IV endometrial cancer.[55] Despite the poor response rates, early uncontrolled studies suggest that progestin therapy after initial therapy, surgery, or radiation was associated with a decreased risk of recurrence in patients with clinical stage I or II endometrial cancer.[56,57]

A number of randomized studies that demonstrated no benefit were too small (only 35 patients),[58] with too short a follow-up (22 months),[59] or too complex (excessive exclusions in a study of four treatment arms[58–61] to be informative.

A multi-institutional trial by Lewis and colleagues in 1974 compared 5 mg medroxyprogesterone acetate given intermuscularly weekly for 14 weeks with placebo.[60] At the end of 4 years, the recurrence rate was approximately 9% in both groups of patients, with no statistically significant advantage for therapy. MacDonald and colleagues randomized 429 patients with initial surgery or radiation therapy to observation of hydroxyprogesterone caproate followed by medroxyprogesterone acetate for 5 years.[61] The overall survival was 76% for both treated and control patients.

Subsequently, Vergote and colleagues from Norway studied 1,084 patients with stages I and II endometrial cancer treated with surgery (TAH/BSO) comparing 1 g of hydroxyprogesterone caproate given intermuscularly twice weekly for 1 year with observation.[62] At a median follow-up of 72 months, overall survival and relapse rates were not different between the two groups (Figure 7–8). Cancer related mortality was worse in the control arm (22 versus 30 month median survival, $p = .03$, [Figure 7–9]). However, noncancer-related mortality was significantly higher in the progestin group ($p = .04$), despite a similar initial incidence of diabetes and hypertension resulting in a nonsignificant difference in overall mortality ($p = .10$). Kneale and colleagues from Australia also neatly framed the issue in a letter criticizing the study by MacDonald and colleagues of 429 patients with stages I to III endometrial cancer (Figure 7–10).[61,63] Given an expected survival of 75%, with approximately 40% of the mortality being unrelated to cancer, detecting a treatment-related benefit in survival of 5% would require randomization of 2,000 patients.[63]

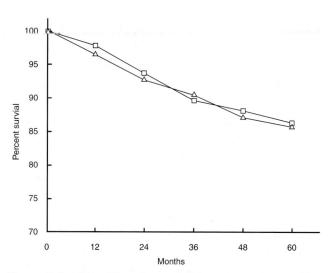

Figure 7–8. Actuarial crude survival in 553 patients receiving 1-year adjuvant hydroxyprogesterone caproate compared with 531 control patients. Controls (*triangles*) treatment group (*squares*). Reproduced with permission from Vergote I et al.[63]

Subsequent randomized studies have replicated these results. Krafft and colleagues randomized 196 patients (93 postoperatively and 103 irradiated) to norethisteronacetate (NEA) 50 mg/d in alternating 6-month periods as a continual adjuvant for 5 years.[64] Five-year survival in the operation group was 92% without NEA and 82% with NEA, and in the irradiated group, 43% and 45%, respectively. Side effects of NEA were at least twice as common (47.9%) compared with the control group.

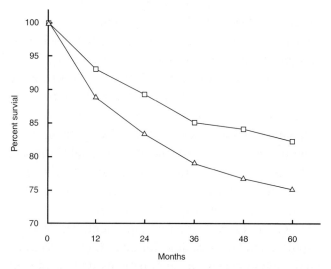

Figure 7–9. Actuarial disease-free survival in 233 high-risk patients treated 1-year with adjuvant hydroxyprogesterone caproate compared with that in 228 control patients. Patients with intercurrent death are excluded. The difference seen in favor of the treatment group is not significant ($p = .10$). Controls (*triangles*) treatment group (*squares*). Reproduced with permission from Vergote I et al.[62]

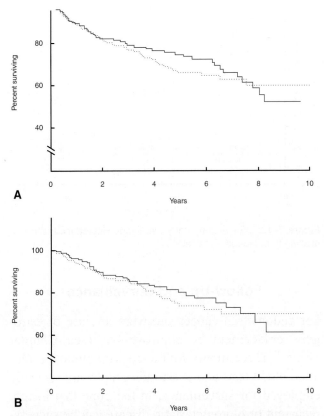

Figure 7–10. Survival rate. *A,* Overall: (*solid line*) control (*n* = 215); (*broken line*) progestogen (*n* = 214); *p* = .6248. *B,* After removal of withdrawals: (*solid line*) control (*n* = 168); (*broken line*) progestogen (n = 178); *p* =.7116. Reproduced with permission from MacDonald RR et al.[61]

A prospective randomized study of 195 patients with endometrial cancer, randomized to medroxy-progesterone acetate 100 mg alone or in combination with tamoxifen 20 mg, demonstrated no statistical difference between the two groups.[65]

Last, in a prospective randomized study of 540 surgical and irradiated patients, the influence of adjuvant hormone therapy by oxyprogesterone caproate (OPC), alone and in combination with tamoxifen, for 6 to 36 months appeared to increase the corrected 5-year survival rates by 19%.[66] However, this Russian study has not been replicated.

In summary, the role of adjuvant hormonal therapy in the adjuvant treatment of endometrial cancer is unproven. Critical review suggests that despite numerous randomized studies, there still has never been an appropriately powered study evaluating a group of women with hormone-receptor–positive tumors. Since this group enjoys a more favorable prognosis than do patients with receptor-negative

tumors, it would require a very large study to address it definitively. In the absence of such data, it is difficult to ignore the increased risk of cardiovascular mortality associated with these therapies.

CHEMOTHERAPY

History of Adjuvant Chemotherapy for Endometrial Cancer

With the dominant role of adjuvant radiation therapy for stages I and II endometrial cancer, chemotherapy for patients with endometrial cancer has only recently been investigated as an option for treatment. Indeed, in his 1974 review, Donovan reported only 126 patients treated with 16 different agents.[67] Subsequently, the investigation of different cytotoxic agents has followed advances in the use of chemotherapy for metastatic breast and ovarian cancers. There is a conflicting body of data about the combination of endocrine therapy and chemotherapy within the breast cancer literature, without the clear benefit seen with the combination, and it is generally felt that the addition of progestin to chemotherapy does not enhance response and may exacerbate thromboembolic complications. Although adjuvant chemotherapy is rarely recommended, 54% of the 49 North American cancer centers that responded in one recent questionnaire study reported the addition of chemotherapy to the primary treatment for FIGO stage III/IV endometrial cancer.[55]

In many of the studies, and perhaps best illustrated in the Morrow study, survival was shown to be much more significantly influenced by age, depth of muscle invasion, FIGO stage, and differentiation than adjuvant therapy (Figure 7–11).[68]

Clinical Trials of Adjuvant Chemotherapy for Moderate-Risk Endometrial Cancer

Two studies have been commonly cited to inform on this issue. Stringer and colleagues from the M.D. Anderson Cancer Center evaluated cisplatin (Platinol), doxorubicin (Adriamycin), and cyclophosphamide (PAC) chemotherapy, and the GOG protocol investigating the role of single-agent doxorubicin.[68–70]

In the PAC study, 31 patients with stage I endometrial cancer and 2 patients with occult stage II disease with poor prognostic features—deep myometrial invasion, high-grade, and nonendometrioid histology or extrauterine disease that was completely resected—were treated postoperatively with cisplatin (platinol) 30 mg/m^2, doxorubicin (Adriamycin) 50 mg/m^2, and cyclophosphamide 500 mg/m^2 (PAC) every four weeks to six cycles.[69] The 2-year progression-free interval was 79% and 2-year survival was 83%. The median survival for patients with disease confined to the uterus was not reached at 45 months. Comparing these results with the historic control from the same institution, the authors considered this superior, and PAC chemotherapy has been used by a number of institutions for high-risk disease.[69]

The GOG treated 181 patients in clinical stage I and stage II disease with poor prognostic features using postoperative whole pelvic irradiation with or without doxorubicin (Figures 7–11 and 7–12).[68] These patients were randomized to receive doxorubicin 40 to 60 mg/m^2 every 3 weeks to a cumulative dose of 500 mg/m^2 following completion of radiotherapy. There was no difference in progression-free survival or overall survival. Patients with disease limited to the uterus had a 63% survival with radiation alone. Survival with doxorubicin was not statistically significantly different at 72%. Until larger randomized studies are completed, cytotoxic chemotherapy cannot be recommended as an adjuvant for high-risk stage I/II endometrial cancer.

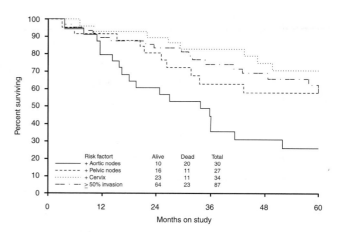

Figure 7–12. Survival by entry risk factor. Reproduced with permission from Morrow CP et al.[68]

Follow-Up and Surveillance

For endometrial cancer survivors, the use of estrogen replacement is controversial (see Chapter 12).[72–75] Three-month follow-up with clinical evaluation blood tests and chest radiography are typically employed for surveillance, in the hope that locally recurrent or oligometastatic disease can be successfully treated. However, data from the breast cancer literature casts doubt on whether close follow up improves outcomes.

SEXUAL HEALTH AND SURVIVORSHIP ISSUES

Generally, sexual health appears to improve with definitive treatment. Relief from heavy bleeding and pain is thought to contribute to the observed improvement in sexual health following hysterectomy, with 39% experiencing intercourse as "much improved" or "better" and 40% as unchanged after hysterectomy for benign disease in one study.[76] However, this has been reported as lower in other studies (27% reporting increased sexual interest), and good data are only available on the psychosexual outcomes following hysterectomy for benign disease and treatment for cervical cancer.[77–79]

There are no data on the postoperative quality of life for patients with endometrial cancer. Studies focusing on sexual health and overall quality of life are important and should be the focus of future studies.[80]

Health-related quality of life is starting to be assessed using validated instruments such as the

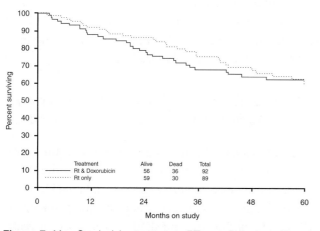

Figure 7–11. Survival by treatment. RT = radiotherapy. Reproduced with permission from Morrow CP et al.[68]

European Organization for Research and Treatment of Cancer questionnaire, EORTC QLQ-C30. Klee and Machin reported that 10% of patients free of recurrence at 2 years, following external irradiation for endometrial cancer, had chronic local symptoms, and a large number of the patients continue to be anxious about their treatment.[81]

Regular vaginal dilation is widely recommended to these women as a way to maintain vaginal health and good sexual function.[82] For those women who have had vaginal cuff brachytherapy, it also reduces upper vaginal stenosis and facilitates follow-up examinations. However, the compliance rate with this recommendation is low. One group reported an apparent increase in the use of vaginal dilation from 5.6% in the control group to 44.4% with written information and brief counseling with a concomitant reduction in fear about sex after cancer treatment. Sexual health impacts quality of life, and treatment for gynecologic cancer threatens physical comfort, sexual satisfaction, and feelings of intimacy.[83]

Human sexuality encompasses more than the endocrinology and anatomy of gender. Before the Kinsey and colleagues' reports, the sexual lives of most people were shaped in a social vacuum and were determined to a large extent by tacit dogma, personal experiment, and uninformed gossip.[84,85] Human sexuality is shrouded in myth. The four most insidious myths are (1) Sexuality cannot be understood; "it is a mystery"; (2) the opposite extreme: love is "natural," simple, and does not require any thought or effort; (3) once it goes, it is gone; and (4) our personal worth is solely dependent on how much sex appeal we possess.[856] Cancer treatments often cause physical and psychological disruptions to sexual health.[87] Cancer's threat to one's sexuality may range from disfigurement, infertility, and impotence to fatigue and alopecia. The existential vulnerability caused by a diagnosis of cancer changes patients' view of themselves and their relationships with others.[88]

Cancer compounds the fatigue and distraction that blunts sexual arousal among healthy partners. Masters and Johnson found that the sexual response cycle was identical for homosexuals and heterosexuals.[89] Within the sexual arousal circuit, there are three important potential break points. The first is *physical* discomfort. Second, in the *emotional* arena,

insecurity over image, fear of failure, pressure to perform, unresolved conflict or undisclosed resentment, and guilt are potentially the most powerful blocks. The third is *mental* "preoccupation," with either intrusive distractions or by being an anxious spectator of the event.

Three influential studies color our perception of sexuality after radiotherapy to the pelvis or after surgery.[77,78,90] Bergmark and colleagues conducted a well-controlled anonymous questionnaire survey of 247 women with a history of early-stage cervical cancer aged 26 to 80 years treated in Sweden between 1991 and 1992. Twenty-six percent of the women who had cancer reported moderate to severe distress owing to vaginal changes compared with 8% of the women in the control group.[78] The frequency of orgasms and orgasmic pleasure was similar in the two groups. In age-matched groups within this study, little difference was observed between surgery and irradiation. The second study was in men. A prospective study of 279 men with early prostate cancer appeared to show greater sexual dysfunction and urinary incontinence in the year following radical prostatectomy than after radiotherapy but that the effects increased with time following radiotherapy.[90] Lastly, Rhodes and colleagues reported Maryland Women's Health Study of hysterectomy in 1,101 women interviewed prior to and during 2 years of follow-up following hysterectomy for benign disease.[77] The percentage of women who engaged in sexual relations increased significantly from 70.5% before hysterectomy to 77.6%, and the rate of frequent dyspareunia dropped significantly from 18.6% before hysterectomy to 3.6% after hysterectomy. The authors concluded that sexual functioning and activity increased after hysterectomy and problems with sexual functioning decreased.

Under stress, both staff and patients may limit how much information is exchanged.[91] In a recent study that investigated the use of sexual activity questionnaires in gynecologic clinical trials, women were supportive of the research and did not find the questionnaire intrusive.[92] Frustratingly, issues of sexuality are often written out of quality of life scales.[93] Sexual dysfunction is common among cancer patients because of anxiety, ill health, and a broad spectrum of

Table 7–5. PROSPECTIVE RANDOMIZED TRIALS OF ADJUVANT HORMONAL THERAPY FOR ENDOMETRIAL CANCER

Author and Year	Eligibility	N	Intervention	FU	5 yr Overall Survival (Rx vs No Rx)	Criticisms
MacDonald 1988	Stage I–III Prior surgery or RT	429	IM HPC 5 d preop MPA 100 mg tid 1 yr Then qd for 5 yr	$1/2$ pts more than 5 yr postop	73 vs. 80% $p = 0.63$	Interim analysis at 382 patients showed no benefit. Withdrawals ($n = 83$) Unknown number of protocol violations
Vergote 1989	Stage I–III Prior surgery	1148	IM HPC 10 mg biweekly 1 yr	72 mo	Approx 87% $p =$ NS	Withdrawals ($n = 64$) Protocol violations ($n = 31$)

HPC = hydroxyprogesterone caproate; MPA = medroxyprogesterone acetate; IM = intramuscular; RT = radiation therapy; FU = follow up; NS = not significant; Rx = therapy.

specific organic causes and treatment. The message has been aptly put: *talk about it*.[80] Patients often do not volunteer sexual problems, and health professionals should inquire of sexual function. This is often met with relief rather than embarrassment.[94]

FUTURE DIRECTIONS

Ongoing Radiotherapy Studies

Ongoing studies of interest include the Canadian National Cancer Institute (NCI) study evaluating the role of adjuvant radiotherapy in intermediate-risk endometrial cancer following laparoscopically assisted vaginal hysterectomy or TAH/BSO. Patients are randomized after surgery to observation or pelvic radiotherapy with or without brachytherapy. Postoperative pathologic stage IA/IB (grade 3) or stage IC (grade 1–3) are eligible. Patients with more than 50% myometrial invasion (grade 1 or 2) or less than 50% myometrial invasion (grade 3) but with positive peritoneal cytology are also eligible.

The Medical Research Council in the United Kingdom is conducting a randomized study evaluating the efficacy of lymphadenectomy in addition to hysterectomy in patients with stage I endometrial cancer preoperatively thought to be confined to the uterine corpus. High-risk patients in both arms of the study receive postoperative radiotherapy. Treatment outcome and quality of life will be assessed.

RTOG 9905 is testing the value of adjuvant chemotherapy in patients with intermediate-risk endometrial cancer. Patients with grade 2 or 3 endometrial adenocarcinoma with organ-confined disease with myometrial invasion > 50% (stages IC

or IIA) or cervical stromal invasion (stage IIB) are randomized after surgery to either postoperative pelvic radiotherapy of 50.4 Gy or radiotherapy concurrent with cisplatin and subsequent adjuvant chemotherapy with four cycles of cisplatin and taxol.

GOG-137A is a phase III randomized study of estrogen replacement therapy versus placebo in women with stage I or II endometrial adenocarcinoma. GOG-189 is a phase III randomized study of doxorubicin, cisplatin, paclitaxel, and filgrastim (granulocyte colony-stimulating factor [G-CSF]) versus tamoxifen and megestrol in patients with stage III or IV or recurrent endometrial cancer.

Novel Therapy

Given the impressive results with chemoradiation therapy in cervical cancer, the possibility of combining cisplatin with radiation therapy is attractive; however, there are no data to inform on the use of this, and toxicity will be greater. Given the benefit demonstrated by concurrent hormonal radiation therapy and neoadjuvant hormonal manipulation for locally advanced prostate cancer, similar approaches have been attempted in patients with endometrial cancer, with pathologic complete remission seen in 17 of 42 patients prior to surgery when treated with intracavity progestin.[95]

As information becomes available about the potential prognostic value of molecular factors, these may identify a high-risk population for targeted adjuvant initiatives. Given the low mortality from endometrial cancer, more accurate staging with tumor markers or novel imaging, such as positron emission tomography (PET), are only in the preliminary stages of investigation.

REFERENCES

1. Landis SH, Murray T, Bolden S, Wingo PA. Cancer statistics, 1999. CA Cancer J Clin 1999;49:8–31.

2. International Federation of Gynecology and Obstetrics. Annual report on the results of treatment in gynecologic cancer. Stockholm: FIGO; 1985.

3. Abeler VM, Kjorstad KE, Berle E. Carcinoma of the endometrium in Norway: a histopathological and prognostic survey of a total population. Int J Gynecol Cancer 1992;2:9–22.

4. Morrow CP, Bundy BN, Kurman RJ, et al. Relationshiop between surgical-pathological risk factors and outcome in clinical stage I and II carcinoma of the endometrium: a Gynecologic Oncology Group study. Gynecol Oncol 1991;40:55–65.

5. Creasman WT, Morrow CP, Bundy BN, et al. Surgical pathologic spread patterns of endometrial cancer: a Gynecologic Oncology Group study. Cancer 1987;60:2035–41.

6. Ambros RA, Kurman RJ. Combined assessment of vascular and myometrial invasion as a model to predict prognosis in stage I endometrioid adenocarcinoma of the uterine corpus. Cancer 1992;69:1424–31.

7. Zaino RJ, Kurman RJ, Diana KL, Morrow CP. Pathologic models to predict outcome for women with endometrial adenocarcinoma: the importance of the distinction between surgical stage and clinical stage—a Gynecologic Oncology Group study. Cancer 1996;77:1115–21.

8. Schink JC, Rademaker AW, Miller DS, Lurain JR. Tumor size in endometrial cancer. Cancer 1991;67:2791–4.

9. Creasman WT, Disaia PJ, Blessing J, et al. Prognostic significance of peritoneal cytology in patients with endometrial cancer and preliminary data concerning therapy with intraperitoneal radiopharmaceuticals. Am J Obstet Gynecol 1981;141:921–9.

10. Zaino RJ, Davis AT, Ohlsson-Wilhelm BM, Brunetto VL. DNA content is an independent prognostic indicator in endometrial adenocarcinoma. A Gynecologic Oncology Group study. Int J Gynecol Pathol 1998;17:312–9.

11. Kleine W, Maier T, Geyer, H, Pfleiderer A. Estrogen and progesterone receptors in endometrial cancer and their prognostic relevance. Gynecol Oncol 1990;38:59–65

12. Hetzel DJ, Wilson TO, Keeney GL, et al. HER-2/neu expression: a major prognostic factor in endometrial cancer. Gynecol Oncol 1992;47:179–85.

13. Lukes AS, Kohler MF, Pieper CF, et al. Multivariable analysis of DNA ploidy, p53, and HER-2/neu as prognostic factors in endometrial cancer. Cancer 1994;73:2380–5.

14. Algan O, Tabesh T, Hanlon A, et al. Improved outcome in patients treated with postoperative radiation therapy for pathologic stage I/II endometrial cancer. Int J Radiat Oncol Biol Phys 1996;35:925–33.

15. Roberts JA, Brunetto VL, Keys HM, et al. A phase III randomized study of surgery vs. surgery plus adjunctive radiation therapy in intermediate risk endometrial adenocarcinoma (GOG 99) [abstract]. Gynecol Oncol 1998; 68:135.

16. Maggi R, Cagnazzo G, Atlante G, et al. Risk groups and adjuvant therapy in surgical staged endometrial cancer patients. A randomized multicentre study comparing chemotherapy with radiation therapy (abstract). In: 7th Biennial Meeting of the International Gynecologic Cancer Society; 1999; Rome, Italy.

17. Axelrod J, Bundy J, Roy T, et al. Advanced endometrial carcinoma (EC) treated with whole abdominal irradiaiton (WAI): a Gynecologic Oncology Group (GOG) study [abstract]. Gynecol Oncol 1995;56:135–6.

18. Aalders J, Abeler V, Kolstad P, Onsrud M. Postoperative external irradiation and prognostic parameters in stage I endometrial cancer. Obstet Gynecol 1980;56:419–27.

19. Creutzberg CL, van Putten WL, Koper PC, et al. Surgery and postoperative radiotherapy versus surgery alone for patients with stage-1 endometrial carcinoma: multicentre randomised trial. PORTEC Study Group. Post Operative Radiation Therapy in Endometrial Carcinoma. Lancet 2000;355:1404–11.

20. Creutzberg CL, van Putten WL, Koper PC, et al. The morbidity of treatment for patients with stage I endometrial cancer: results from a randomized trial. Int J Radiat Oncol Biol Phys 2001;51:1246–55.

21. Heyman J, Reuterwall O, Benner S. The Radiumhemmet experience with radiotherapy of the corpus of the uterus: classification, method of treatment and results. Acta Radiol 1941;22:11–98.

22. Sause WT, Fuller DB, Smith W, et al. Analysis of preoperative intracavitary cesium application versus postoperative external beam radiation in stage I endometrial carcinoma. Int J Radiat Oncol Biol Phys 1990;18:1011–7.

23. Weigensberg IJ. Preoperative radiation therapy in stage I endometrial adenocarcinoma. II. Final report of a clinical trial. Cancer 1984;53:242–7.

24. Lanciano RM, Curran WJ Jr, Greven KM, et al. Influence of grade, histologic subtype, and timing of radiotherapy on outcome among patients with stage II carcinoma of the endometrium. Gynecol Oncol 1990;39:368–73.

25. Grigsby PW, Perez CA, Camel HM, et al. Stage II carcinoma of the endometrium: results of therapy and prognostic factors. Int J Radiat Oncol Biol Phys 1985;11:1915–23.

26. Homesley HD, Boronow RC, Lewis JL Jr. Stage II endometrial adenocarcinoma. Memorial Hospital for Cancer, 1949-1965. Obstet Gynecol 1977;49:604–8.

27. Sears JD, Greven KM, Hoen HM, Randall ME. Prognostic factors and treatment outcome for patients with locally recurrent endometrial cancer. Cancer 1994;74:1303–8.

28. Kuten A, Grigsby P, Perez C, et al. Results of radiotherapy in recurrent endometrial cancer. A retrospective analysis. Int J Radiat Oncol Biol Phys 1987;17:29–34.

29. Elliott P, Green D, Coates A, et al. The efficacy of postoperative vaginal irradiation in preventing vaginal recurrence in endometrial cancer. Int J Gynecol Cancer 1994;4:84–93.

30. MacLeod C, Fowler A, Duval P, et al. High-dose-rate brachytherapy alone post-hysterectomy for endometrial cancer. Int J Radiat Oncol Biol Phys 1998;42:1033–9.

31. Nag S, Erickson B, Parikh S, et al. The American Brachytherapy Society recommendations for high-dose-rate brachytherapy for carcinoma of the endometrium. Int J Radiat Oncol Biol Phys 2000;48:779–90.

32. Grigsby PW, Perez CA. Radiotherapy alone for medically inoperable carcinoma of the uterus. Int J Radiat Oncol Biol Phys 1991;21:375–8.

33. Hricak H. Cancer of the uterus: the value of MRI pre- and post-irradiation. Int J Radiat Oncol Biol Phys 1991;21:1089–94.

34. Chao CK, Grigsby PW, Perez CA, et al. Brachytherapy-related complications for medically inoperable stage I endometrial carcinoma. Int J Radiat Oncol Biol Phys 1995;31:37–42.

35. Kucera H, Knocke TH, Kucera E, Potter R. Treatment of endometrial carcinoma with high-dose-rate brachytherapy alone in medically inoperable stage I patients. Acta Obstet Gynecol Scand 1998;77:1008–12.

36. Nguyen TV, Petereit DG. High-dose-rate brachytherapy for medically inoperable stage I endometrial cancer. Gynecol Oncol 1998;71:196–203.

37. Sorbe B, Frankendal B, Risberg B. Intracavitary irradiation of endometrial carcinoma stage I by a high dose-rate afterloading technique. Gynecol Oncol 1989;33:135–45.

38. Kupelian PA, Eifel PJ, Tornos C, et al. Treatment of endometrial carcinoma with radiation therapy alone. Int J Radiat Oncol Biol Phys 1993;27:817–24.

39. Grigsby PW, Perez C, Kuske RR, et al. Results of therapy, analysis of failures, and prognostic factors for clinical and pathologic stage III adenocarcinoma of the endometrium. Gynecol Oncol 1987;27:44–57.

40. Aalders JG, Abeler V, Kolstad P. Clinical (stage III) as compared to subclinical intrapelvic extrauterine tumor spread in endometrial carcinoma: a clinical and histopathological study of 175 patients. Gynecol Oncol 1984;17:64–74.

41. Greven K, Curran W, Whittington R, et al. Analysis of failure patterns in stage III endometrial carcinoma and therapeutic implications. Int J Radiat Oncol Biol Phys 1989;17:35–9.

42. Mackillop W, Pringle J. Stage III endometrial cancer: a review of 90 cases. Cancer 1985;56:2519–23.

43. Goff BA, Goodman A, Muntz HG, et al. Surgical stage IV endometrial cancer: a study of 47 cases. Gynecol Oncol 1994;552:137–40.

44. Spanos W, Perez C, Marcus S, et al. Effect of rest interval on tumor and normal tissue response—a report of phase III study of accelerated split course palliative radiation for advanced pelvic malignancies (RTOG 8502). Int J Radiat Oncol Biol Phys 1993;25:399–403.

45. Cooper A. The principles and practice of surgery. London: Cox; 1836. p. 333–5.

46. Beatson G. On the treatment of inoperable cases of carcinoma of the mamma: suggestions for a new method of treatment with illustrative cases. Lancet 1896;ii:104–7.

47. Huggins C, Bergenstal D. Inhibition of human mammary and prostatic cancers by adrenalectomy. Cancer Res 1952;12:134–41.

48. Englesman E, Persijn J, Korsten C, Cleton F. Estrogen receptors in human breast cancer tissue in response to endocrine therapy. BMJ 1973;2:750–2.

49. Ehrlich CE, Young PC, Cleary RE. Cytoplasmic progesterone and estradiol receptors in normal, hyperplastic, and carcinomatous endometria: therapeutic implications. Am J Obstet Gynecol 1981;141:539–46.

50. Creasman WT, McCarty KS Sr, Barton TK, McCarty KS Jr. Clinical correlates of estrogen- and progesterone-binding proteins in human endometrial adenocarcinoma. Obstet Gynecol 1980;55:363–70.

51. Creasman WT, Soper JT, McCarty KS Jr, et al. Influence of cytoplasmic steroid receptor content on prognosis of early stage endometrial carcinoma. Am J Obstet Gynecol 1985;151:922–32.

52. Kelley R, Baker W. Progestational agents in the management of carcinoma of the endometrium. N Engl J Med 1961;264:215–22.

53. Sall S, DiSaia P, Morrow CP, et al. A comparison of medroxy-progesterone serum concentrations by the oral or intra-muscular route in patients with persistent or recurrent endometrial carcinoma. Am J Obstet Gynecol 1979;135:647–50.

54. Thigpen JT, Brady MF, Alvarez RD, et al. Oral medroxy-progesterone acetate in the treatment of advanced or recurrent endometrial carcinoma: a dose-response study by the Gynecologic Oncology Group. J Clin Oncol 1999;17:1736–44.

55. Maggino T, Romagnolo C, Landoni F, et al. An analysis of approaches to the management of endometrial cancer in North America: a CTF study. Gynecol Oncol 1998;68:274–9.

56. Kauppila A, Kujansuu E, Vihko R. Cytosol estrogen and progestin receptors in endometrial carcinoma of patients treated with surgery, radiotherapy, and progestin. Clinical correlates. Cancer 1982;50:2157–62.

57. Kauppila A, Gronroos M, Nieminen U. Clinical outcome in endometrial cancer. Obstet Gynecol 1982;60:473–80.

58. Malkasian GD Jr, Bures J. Adjuvant progesterone therapy for stage I endometrial carcinoma. Int J Gynaecol Obstet 1978;16:48–9.

59. DePalo G, Mersom M, Vecchio MD, et al. A controlled clinical study of adjuvant medroxyprogesterone acetate (MPA) therapy in pathological stage I endometrial cancer with myometrial invasion. Proc Am Soc Clin Oncol 1985;4:121.

60. Lewis GC Jr, Slack NH, Mortel R, Bross ID. Adjuvant progestogen therapy in the primary definitive treatment of endometrial cancer. Gynecol Oncol 1974;2:368–76.

61. MacDonald RR, Thorogood J, Mason MK. A randomized trial of progestogens in the primary treatment of endometrial carcinoma. Br J Obstet Gynaecol 1988;95:166–74.

62. Vergote I, Kjorstad K, Abeler V, Kolstad P. A randomized trial of adjuvant progestagen in early endometrial cancer. Cancer 1989;64:1011–6.

63. Kneale BL, Quinn MA, Rennie GC. A randomized trial of progestogens in the primary treatment of endometrial carcinoma. Br J Obstet Gynaecol 1988;95:828.

64. Krafft W, Steuckardt R, Konig EM, et al. [Efficacy of an adjuvant norethisterone acetate therapy (NEA) of endometrial carcinoma treated with primary surgery or irradiation.] Zentralbl Gynakol 1990;112:1023–30.

65. Vavra N, Salzer H, Sevelda P, et al. Adjuvant hormone therapy in endometrial carcinoma: medroxyprogesterone acetate versus tamoxifen-medroxyprogesterone acetate sequential therapy Gynakol Geburtshilfliche Rundsch 1990;30:133–43.

66. Vishnevsky AS, Bokhman Ya V, Loutfi G. Favourable influence of adjuvant hormone therapy by oxyprogesterone caproate (OPC) and by its combination with tamoxifen on 5-year survival rate of surgical and combined treatment of primary endometrial carcinoma patients. Eur J Gynaecol Oncol 1993;14:150–3.

67. Donovan J. Non-hormonal chemotherapy of endometrial carcinoma: a review. Cancer 1974;34:1587–92.

68. Morrow CP, Bundy BN, Homesley HD, et al. Doxorubicin as an adjuvant following surgery and radiation therapy in patients with high-risk endometrial carcinoma, stage I and occult stage II: a Gynecologic Oncology Group Study. Gynecol Oncol 1990;36:166–71.

69. Stringer CA, Gershenson DM, Burke TW, et al. Adjuvant chemotherapy with cisplatin, doxorubicin, and cyclophosphamide (PAC) for early-stage high-risk endometrial cancer: a preliminary analysis. Gynecol Oncol 1990;38:305–8.

70. Goff BA, Goodman A, Muntz HG, et al. Surgical stage IV endometrial carcinoma: a study of 47 cases. Gynecol Oncol 1994;52:237–40.

71. Randall ME, Brunetto G, Muss H, et al. Whole abdominal radiotherapy versus combination doxorubicin-cisplatin chemotherapy in advanced endometrial carcinoma: A randomized phase III trial of the Gynecologic Oncology Group [abstract 3]. Proc Am Soc Clin Oncol 2003;22:2.

72. Mulder JE. Benefits and risks of hormone replacement therapy in young adult cancer survivors with gonadal failure. Med Pediatr Oncol 1999;33:46–52.

73. Castiel M. Management of menopausal symptoms in the cancer patient. Oncology (Huntingt) 1999;13:1363–72; discussion 1372, 1377–83.

74. Lin K, Runowicz CD. The wisdom of hormone-replacement therapy in survivors of ovarian and endometrial cancer. Surg Clin North Am 2001;81:987–93.

75. Writing Group for the Women's Health Initiative Investigators. Risks and benefits of estrogen plus progestin in healthy postmenopausal women: principal results from the Women's Health Initiative randomized controlled trial. JAMA 2002; 288(3):321–33.

76. Nathorst-Boos J, Fuchs T, von Schoultz B. Consumer's attitude to hysterectomy. The experience of 678 women. Acta Obstet Gynecol Scand 1992;71:230–4.

77. Alexander DA, Naji AA, Pinion SB, et al. Randomised trial comparing hysterectomy with endometrial ablation for dysfunctional uterine bleeding: psychiatric and psychosocial aspects. BMJ 1996;312:280–4.

78. Rhodes JC, Kjerulff KH, Langenberg PW, Guzinski GM. Hysterectomy and sexual functioning. JAMA 1999; 282(20):1934–41.

79. Bergmark K., Åvall-Lundqvist E, Dickman PW, et al. Vaginal changes and sexuality in women with a history of cervical cancer. N Engl J Med 1999;340:1383–9.

80. Crowther M, Corney R, Shepherd J. Psychosexual implications of gynaecological cancer: talk about it. BMJ 1994;308:869–70.

81. Klee M, Machin D. Health-related quality of life of patients with endometrial cancer who are disease-free following external irradiation. Acta Oncol 2001;40:816–24.

82. Robinson J W, Faris PD, Scott CB. Psychoeducational group increases vaginal dilation for younger women and reduces sexual fears for women of all ages with gynecological carcinoma treated with radiotherapy. Int J Radiat Oncol Biol Phys 1999;44:497–506.

83. Butler L, Banfield V, Sveinson T, Allen K. Conceptualizing sexual health in cancer care. West J Nurs Res 1998;20:683–99; discussion 700–5.

84. Kinsey AC, Pomeroy WB, Martin CE. Sexual behavior of the human male/female. Bloomington (IN): Indiana University Press; 1998.

85. Gagnon J. Sexual behavior in the human male, sexual behavior in the human female. The Kinsey Data: Marginal tabulations of the 1938–1963 interviews conducted by the Institute for Sex Research [Book review]. N Engl J Med 1999;340:571–2.

86. Penson RT, Gallagher J, Gioiella ME, et al. Sexuality and cancer: conversation comfort zone. Oncologist 2000;5:336–44.

87. Gallagher J. Chemotherapy-induced hair loss and quality of life. Quality of Life: A Nursing Challenge 1997;5:75–80.

88. Weisman A, Worden JW. Coping and vulnerability in cancer patients: research report. Boston: Project Omega, Harvard Medical School; 1977.

89. Masters WH, Johnson VE. Human sexual inadequacy. London: Churchill;1970.

90. Talcott JA, Rieker P, Clark JA, et al. Patient-reported symptoms after primary therapy for early prostate cancer: results of a prospective cohort study. J Clin Oncol 1998;16:275–83.

91. Leydon GM, Boulton M, Moynihan C, et al. Cancer patients' information needs and information seeking behaviour: in depth interview study. BMJ 2000;320:909–13.

92. Stead ML, Crocombe WD, Fallowfield LJ, et al. Sexual activity questionnaires in clinical trials: acceptability to patients with gynaecological disorders. Br J Obstet Gynaecol 1999;106:50–4.

93. Cull A, Howat S, Greimel E, et al. Development of a European Organization for Research and Treatment of Cancer questionnaire module to assess the quality of life of ovarian cancer patients in clinical trials: a progress report. Eur J Cancer. 2001;37:47–53.

94. Capone MA, Good RS, Westie KS, Jacobson AF. Psychosocial rehabilitation of gynaecologic oncology patients. Arch Phys Med Rehabil 1980;61:128–32.

95. Kauppila A. Progestin therapy of endometrial, breast and ovarian carcinoma. A review of clinical observations. Acta Obstet Gynecol Scand 1984;63:441–50.

8

Management of Recurrent or Metastatic Endometrial Carcinoma

MICHAEL V. SEIDEN, MD, PhD

Endometrial carcinoma is the most common gynecologic malignancy in the United States. Fortunately, the presenting symptom of blood per vagina in a postmenopausal woman is typically associated with early stage disease, and thus, less than 5% of women with a new diagnosis of endometrial carcinoma will present with stage IV disease.

The large majority of women with tumors of the endometrium have endometrioid tumors, and the focus of this chapter is on the management of women with recurrent or metastatic endometrioid endometrial cancer; management of serous and clear cell carcinomas are reviewed in Chapter 12.

It is anticipated that an additional 10 to 15% of women with a preexisting diagnosis of endometrial cancer will develop disease recurrence over their lifetime. Typical sites of recurrence include the vaginal cuff, pelvic sidewall, pelvic lymph nodes, and lung.[1] Peritoneal, liver, bone, and brain recurrence are also seen, although with lower frequency.

Risk factors for future recurrence and the pattern of these recurrences are partially dependent on histologic subtype, grade, and stage of tumor. Recently, physicians at the Mayo Clinic reviewed the patterns and risk factors for metastatic disease in a group of 610 women with epithelial endometrial cancer treated with hysterectomy and removal of the adnexa.[2] Table 8–1 reviews the factors associated with locoregional recurrence and/or hematogenous recurrence. After a median follow-up of 72 months, 23% of these women had tumor recurrence. In this series, 54% of the recurrences were local or regional, with 46% of recurrences consistent with hematogenous recurrences. Women with clear cell, papillary serous, and mixed müllerian tumors demonstrate different natural histories, with a higher relapse rate than the larger group of women with endometrioid carcinomas. The most common site of hematogenous dissemination is the lung followed by the liver. Other sites, such as adrenal, breast, heart, brain, bone, and skin, have also been reported predominantly in case reports.[2–10]

GENERAL MANAGEMENT ISSUES

The management of women with metastatic and/or recurrent disease begins with careful assessment of the patient. This includes a detailed physical examination, with a particular emphasis on the pelvis, with a vaginal Pap smear to evaluate the vaginal cuff. Examination of the inguinal, axillary, and supraclavicular areas for nodal metastases is also important, as are rectal and breast examinations to exclude a new primary malignancy. Computed tomographic (CT) scans of the chest, abdomen, and pelvis are necessary to evaluate the patient for potential pulmonary nodules or nodal metastases to the mediastinal, pelvic or para-aortic regions, as well as to evaluate the liver, peritoneal area, and/or pelvis for recurrent disease. Positron emission tomography (PET) may be useful for evaluating women for nodal recurrences. This may be particularly true for the high para-aortic or mediastinal regions in women with suspected nodal recurrences. Some of these women may be candidates for nodal resection.

Table 8–1. RISK FACTORS FOR LOCAL/REGIONAL OR METASTATIC DISEASE

Characteristic	Hematogenous Dissemination (%)	p Value	Local Regional Recurrence (%)	p Value
Stage I/II/III vs IV	6 vs 43	< .00001	5 vs 28	< .00001
Negative vs positive adnexa	7 vs 36	< .00001	5 vs 23	< .00001
Myometrial invasion: no vs yes	5 vs 23	< .00001	4 vs 16	< .00001
Peritoneal cytology: negative vs positive	6 vs 31	< .00001	4 vs 23	< .00001
LVI: no vs yes	4 vs 20	< .00001	3 vs 14	.00003
Grade I/II vs III	5 vs 19	< .00001	4 vs 11	.006
Endometroid vs nonendometroid	6 vs 15	.01	5 vs 8	.27

LVI = lymph-vascular invasion
Modified from Mariani A, et al.[2]

Because this cancer occurs in an elderly patient population, second primaries, particularly of the breast, colon, and lung, are possible, and this should be considered particularly when evaluating women with new metastatic lesions and a previous history of a low-stage endometrial carcinoma with favorable histologic features. Indeed, in the recent Portec study that studied the role of radiotherapy in women with early-stage disease, there were 45 second cancers and 19 deaths from second primary tumors.[11] Therefore, there should be a low threshold to obtain mammograms in all women with newly diagnosed metastatic disease. In addition, colonoscopy should be considered in the patient whose stool is guaiac positive. In smokers with a dominant lung lesion, an alternative diagnosis of a new primary lung cancer should be considered. In most circumstances, women with a new diagnosis of recurrent or metastatic disease should have either a biopsy of the metastatic lesion or, if clinically appropriate, have it resected for pathologic evaluation, including hormone receptors.

Despite the relative frequency of this cancer, the optimal approach to women with metastatic disease is complicated by the paucity of randomized studies in this clinical setting. This is explained, in part, by the limited number of women with metastatic or recurrent disease. In addition, this population of women are frequently obese, often diabetic, and frequently in their seventies. These populations have typically been under-represented in clinical studies. Therefore, in many circumstances, clinical practice is directed by clinical experience and the results from smaller phase II clinical trials evaluating numerous hormonal and chemotherapeutic agents.

HORMONAL THERAPY

The primary management of metastatic endometrial carcinoma remains as hormonal manipulation, particularly with progestin.[12]

In the normal endometrium, glandular proliferation is driven by estrogen, whereas cellular differentiation and apoptosis are driven by progestins. There are two estrogen receptors (ERs) and two progesterone receptors (PRs). These four hormone receptors are similar in structure and contain deoxyribonucleic acid (DNA) binding, hormone binding, and transcriptional activation domains (Figure 8–1). When the cytosolic receptors bind to the appropriate hormone, they dimerize with a second receptor-ligand complex and translocate to the nucleus. The dimerized hormone–hormone-receptor complex then binds to a consensus palindromic DNA sequence, either estrogen- or progesterone-response elements (ERE and PRE, respectively), driving transcription of a large collection of genes with ERE or PRE elements in their regulatory regions (Figure 8–2). Enhanced transcription through these upstream regulatory regions is mediated through two transcriptional domains, AF-1 and AF-2, located at the amino (NH_2) and carboxy (COOH) terminals of the hormone receptor (see Figure 8–1).[13,14] The family of estrogen-responsive genes is very large and includes the oncogenes *c-FOS, c-MYC, c-JUN,* as well as the progesterone receptor. There are two separate ERs (ERα and ERβ) as well as two PRs (PRA and PRB).[15,16] Well-differentiated tumors and some moderately differentiated tumors tend to retain functional receptors that continue to influence relevant biologically active hormone-dependent growth and apoptotic pathways.

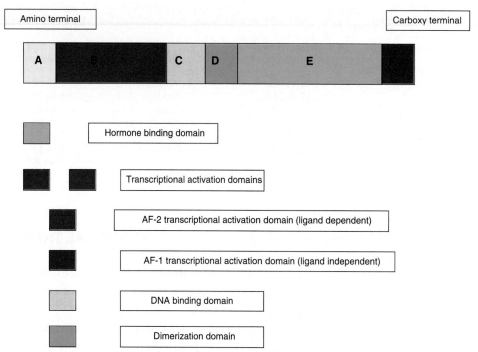

Figure 8–1. Schematic of the estrogen receptor. Color regions demonstrate principal regions involved in hormone binding, DNA binding, dimerization, and transcriptional activation. The AF-1 site is constitutively active and hence can drive some transcription even when the receptor is occupied with antagonists, such as tamoxifen. AF–2 directed transcription requires the natural ligand.

Poorly differentiated tumors typically do not have detectable ER and PR. The PRB progesterone receptor isoform has a longer amino terminal than the A isoform and may be preferentially upregulated by estrogens but may also be lost either first or preferentially in higher-grade tumors.[14,17] Experimental studies have suggested that reintroduction of PRA or PRB into receptor-negative cell lines may reinstate hormone sensitivity.[18] Most clinical studies have demonstrated that the clinical activity of hormonal manipulation in women with endometrial cancer is closely, albeit not perfectly, associated with hormone receptor status. Imperfect correlation may be due, in part, to variable techniques for evaluating hormone receptor status. In particular, few clinical laboratories use the ligand-binding assay, which is a more precise but also more cumbersome technique than immunohistochemistry. In other cases, tumors may have low receptor expression or may be lacking proteins that associate with the hormone–hormone-receptor complex and are necessary for activity. Several other technical and biologic issues potentially confound the evaluation of the tumor for the presence or absence of the hormone receptor, including the lack of perfect correlation between ER status in the primary tumor versus metastases. Other challenges in evaluating hormone status are reviewed in Table 8–2.

In the postmenopausal woman, estrogen is mainly derived from peripheral conversion of androstenedione to estrogens. Androstenedione, a product of the adrenal gland, is converted to estrone by aromatase present in adipose tissue, liver, and muscle and subsequently to estradiol by 17β-hydroxysteroid dehydrogenase.[19] Current endocrine-based therapies for the treatment of endometrial cancer are listed in Table 8–3. These include driving cells to terminal differentiation and subsequent apoptosis (progestins), blocking the ER (tamoxifen) or inhibiting estrogen synthesis (aromatase inhibitors), thus inhibiting estrogen-dependent growth and proliferation, and gonadotropin-releasing hormone (GnRH) receptor agonists also have activity in this disease, although the mechanism of inducing tumor response is not clearly defined.

Progestins

Progestins are the most extensively used hormonal agents in the treatment of recurrent or metastatic

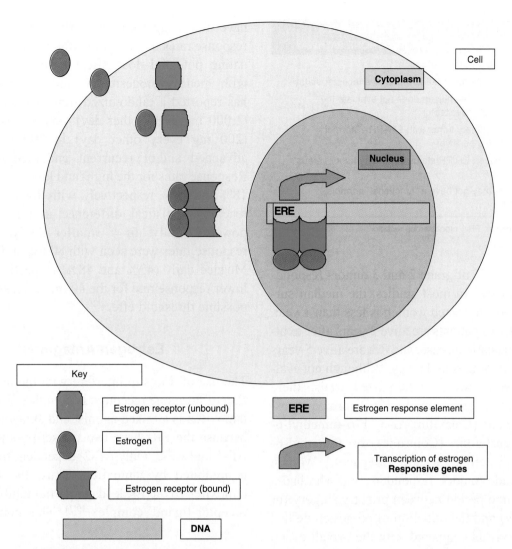

Figure 8–2. Schematic of estrogen-mediated gene transcription through the estrogen receptor. Estrogen diffuses passively through the cytoplasmic membrane and binds to the estrogen receptor leading to receptor dimerization and transport through the nuclear membrane. The bound receptor then binds to DNA at estrogen-responsive elements (ERE) with the subsequent transcription or enhanced transcription of a large family of genes. An identical model exists for the progesterone receptor.

endometrial cancer. Progestins antagonize estrogen-sensitive tumors through several mechanisms, including downregulation of estrogen receptors, conversion of estradiol to estrone, a weaker estrogen, and the direct triggering of apoptosis through the PR in the tumor tissue.[13,20] Studies performed on endometrioid tumors exposed to progestins demonstrate tumor differentiation and decreased proliferation.[21] Other effects include changes in BCL2 expression and suppression of vascular endothelial growth factor.[21,22] The use of progestins has included the intramuscular administration of medroxyprogesterone acetate (MPA) as well as the oral administra-

tion of MPA and megestrol acetate (Megace). Megace has a better pharmacokinetic profile and superior bioavailability than MPA. Therapy is generally well tolerated, with the most bothersome side effect typically being weight gain (Table 8–4).

Progestin therapy for endometrial cancer was first reported in 1951 by Kelley and Baker.[23] Although response rates to progestins were historically cited at 34%, contemporary trials using more stringent response definitions have reported response rates ranging from 9 to 16%.[1,24,25,26] Response rate is very dependent on tumor grade, with 30 to 40% of grade I tumors responding and

Table 8–2. CHALLENGES IN EVALUATING A FUNCTIONAL ESTROGEN/PROGESTRONE PATHWAY

Limited interlaboratory standardization

No consensus on what constitutes a "positive receptor status"

Immunohistochemistry technique does not evaluate the functional status of the receptor

Contamination of primary tumor with ER+PR + normal endometrium (false positive)

Discordance between ER/PR status of primary tumor versus metastasis

ER+/PR– tumors may not have a "functional" hormone receptor pathway

ER = estrogen receptor; PR = progesterone receptor.

only 17% and 2% of grade 2 and 3 tumors responding, respectively.[1] In most studies, the median survival of progestin-treated women is less than 1 year, although 19% of patients are alive 2 years after treatment for metastatic disease, and 8% are alive 5 years after initiating progestin therapy.[1] Although not evaluated by well-powered randomized trials, there appears to be no advantage to 17α-hydroxyprogesterone caproate (Delalutin), α-6, 17α-dimethyl-6-dehydroprogesterone (Colprone), or 6-methyl-6-dehydroprogesterone acetate (Megace).[1] Women with low-grade tumors, responders, and who had a prolonged time period between primary surgery (or radiotherapy) and the initiation of progesterone had superior survivals compared with the overall group that demonstrated a median survival of less than 1 year from the initiation of progesterone therapy (Table 8–5). High response rates have also been reported in individuals with single lesions, pulmonary nodules, and in nonirradiated versus irradiated lesions.[13] Other investigators have demonstrated a very durable response in a subset of low-grade ER-positive tumors.[25,27] The high response rate seen in well-differentiated tumors is due, at least in part, to the expression of the ER in this subset of endometrial carcinomas.

Current data suggest that oral and intramuscular administration of progestins has equivalent clinical activity and that there is no evidence to suggest a clinical superiority of one progestin to other members of this class of therapeutics.[24,26] This latter point has not been rigorously evaluated, although case-control studies evaluating hydroxyprogesterone versus medroxyprogesterone acetate (Depo-Provera)

have not suggested any difference in objective response rates or survival.[26] Randomized trials evaluating potential dose effect have been performed with medroxyprogesterone and Megace. Thigpen has reported a randomized trial of high-dose MPA (1,000 mg every other day) versus low-dose MPA (200 mg every other day) in 299 women with advanced and/or recurrent endometrial cancer.[28] Response rates for the high- and low-dose arms were 18% and 26%, respectively, with this difference not reaching statistical difference in this moderately powered study. In a smaller study, equivalent response rates were seen with 80 mg and 160 mg of Megace daily (43% and 48%, respectively) with a lower response rate for the 40 mg dose, suggesting a possible threshold effect.[29]

Estrogen Antagonist

The use of drugs to interfere with the normal function of hormone receptors is complex. For example, tamoxifen is a mixed agonist and antagonist. This is because the ERs have two transcriptional domains, AF-1 and AF-2. Only AF-2–dependent transcription is inhibited by tamoxifen. Thus, the binding of tamoxifen to the ER leads to partial inhibition of the receptor-ligand complex.[30,31] The tamoxifen-ER

Table 8–3. HORMONAL AGENTS WITH ACTIVITY IN ENDOMETRIAL CANCER

Progestins
  Delalutin
  Colprone
  Medroxyprogesterone acetate
  Megestrol acetate
Antiestrogens
  Tamoxifen
  Toremifene
Aromatase inhibitors
  Nonspecific
    Aminoglutethimide
  Selective steroidal inhibitors
    Formestane
    Exemestane
  Selective nonsteroidal inhibitors
    Anastrozole
    Letrozole
    Vorozole
Gonadotropinin-releasing hormone agonists
  Buserelin
  Goserelin
  Leuprolide
  Triptorelin

Table 8–4. SIDE EFFECTS OF PROGESTINS

Weight gain
Fluid retention
Muscle cramps
Liver function abnormalities
Thrombophlebitis
Hypertension
Hyperglycemia

complexes still dimerize and translocate to the nucleus and can still drive transcription of genes that rely on the AF-1 transcription domain. Thus, tamoxifen's actions on the normal endometrium are partially agonistic with increased uterine weight, endometrial proliferation, and an increased risk of carcinogenesis. Despite these effects, some antagonist activity persists, at least in the neoplastic endometrium, that can be used in the treatment of women with endometrioid tumors.

Tamoxifen is a triphenylethylene derivative that, when delivered orally, has a peak plasma level 2 to 6 hours after ingestion and has a long plasma half-life of 91 hours, with this half-life increasing with repeated administration. The potential antitumor activity of this drug includes its direct action on the hormone receptor (discussed above) and potentially secondary effects on epidermal growth factor (EGF), transforming growth factor-α (TGF-α) and insulin-like growth factors (IGFs).[32] Clinical response rates have been as high as 53% (average 23%) in women with untreated recurrent endometrial cancer and as low as 0% in women who have received prior progestin therapy.[33–35]

Toremifene is a tamoxifen analogue with a pharmacologic profile similar to that of tamoxifen and

has similar effects on the ER. It has similar efficacy to tamoxifen in the treatment of ER-positive breast cancer.[36] There are no obvious reasons why this drug should be superior or inferior to tamoxifen in the treatment of endometrial carcinoma, although trials evaluating its efficacy in endometrial cancer have not been reported.

Aromatase Inhibitors

The potential utility of aromatase inhibitors includes not only the inhibition of peripheral aromatization of androstenedione to estrone by peripheral tissues but also the potential for paracrine effects through the inhibition of aromatase found in the stroma of many endometrial tumors. The first aromatase inhibitor used in clinical practice was aminoglutethimide.[37] Although the agent is clinically active, it has numerous side effects, including reduction in cortisol levels, which required replacement of corticosteroids, as well as frequent lethargy, occasional ataxia, confusion, and even granulocytopenia. Aminoglutethimide is now primarily of historic interest, and aromatase inhibition is now accomplished with newer steroidal and nonsteroidal selective aromatase inhibitors (see Table 8–3). The nonsteroidal aromatase inhibitor, anastrozole (Arimidex) has been evaluated in women with metastatic endometrial cancer.[38] In a recent phase II trial of anastrozole, 2 of 23 women had partial responses for a response rate of 9%.[39] Although the response rate in this trial is modest, the majority of women had grade III tumors, and no attempt was made to select women with hormone receptor–positive tumors. It is note-

Table 8–5. RESPONSE AND SURVIVAL WITH HORMONAL THERAPY

Category	Characteristic	Response Rate (%)	Median Survival	5-Year Survival*(%)
Grade (Brorder)	1	40		20
	2	15		17
	3	2		0
	4	0		0
Response to therapy	Response		57 mo	
	Stable disease		13 mo	
	Progression		5 mo	
Time from primary therapy	< 12 mo			4.5
	12–36 mo			12.6
	> 36 mo			19

*From the time of progesterone therapy.

worthy that both responders had durable responses (13+ and 18+ months). Further study of this and other selective aromatase inhibitors in women with well-differentiated and hormone receptor–positive tumors is needed. There are no published reports of clinical activity with the other nonsteroidal aromatase inhibitors in gynecologic malignancies, but in light of the emerging breast cancer data, it is likely that these agents will be active.[40]

Steroidal aromatase inhibitors include exemestane and formestane.[41–44] Both drugs are suicide inhibitors and irreversibly inhibit aromatase and, thus, have a theoretic advantage over the nonsteroidal inhibitors anastrozole, letrozole, and vorozole, which bind reversibly to the active site of aromatase.[44,45] These agents are predicted to have activity in hormone-dependent tumors but formal studies are not yet available.

In addition, a selective pure antiestrogen agent, Faslodex, are now available and is a logical candidate for study in this clinical setting. This molecule inhibits receptor dimerization and leads to a shortened half-life of the estrogen receptors.[46] Lack of dimerization and induction of receptor degradation may lead to more effective inhibition of genes that are dependent on the ER–ligand complex for transcription. A trial evaluating Faslodex in endometrial cancer is under way in the Gynecologic Oncology Group in the US.

GnRH Analogues

Some endometrial carcinomas express luteinizing hormone (LH) and follicle stimulating hormone (FSH) receptors.[47–49] GnRH agonists are capable of effecting G_1-S arrest in vitro, and response rates of 25% have been reported in one clinical study, whereas other studies have showed essentially no activity.[50–52] Jeyarajah and colleagues reported on 32 consecutive women treated with monthly subcutaneous GnRH agonist with 9 responses.[51] Curiously, responses were seen more frequently in irradiated sites of disease, in women with grade 3 lesions, and women with prior exposure to progestin therapy. A second study involving 25 women had 8 women with stable disease but no formal responses, although many of these women had

received prior progestinal agents, chemotherapy, or even whole abdominal radiotherapy.[53] Further studies with these agents are needed.

Combination Hormonal Therapies

The correlation of hormone-receptor expression and the clinical activity of endocrine therapy have led to biologically based treatment programs designed to enhance hormone receptor expression or activity. For example, tamoxifen is known to increase PR levels, especially in grade 1/2 tumors that are ER positive but PR negative.[53] Carlson and colleagues treated 25 women with biopsy-documented endometrial cancer for 5 days prior to definitive hysterectomy.[53] Comparison of the initial endometrial biopsy with the hysterectomy specimen demonstrated an increase in the portion of PR-positive tumors from 52 to 84% ($p < .05$). Specifically, 100% of the grade 1 and 2 tumors were ER and PR positive, with 50% of high-grade tumors demonstrating PR expression.[53] Several groups have combined tamoxifen with progestins. Four trials involving 167 women have reported 46 responses (aggregate response rate 28%) in the same range as that expected for progestin therapy alone.[53,54] One study did suggest that in some cases, tamoxifen led to upregulation of PR content, yet in other specimens PR content might have decreased. Interferon in combination with either tamoxifen or medroxyprogesterone can result in enhanced antiproliferative activity in human tumor cell lines that express a functional ER.[55–57] Clinical studies have been performed with natural interferon (IFN)-β and recombinant (r)IFN-2β in women with primary endometrial cancer, with both studies demonstrating increased expression of both ER and PR in the malignant endometrium.[56,58] The potential utility of this approach in women with ER/PR-negative or marginally positive tumors has not been evaluated.

Summary of Hormonal Therapy

There is extensive clinical experience demonstrating the efficacy of hormonal therapies in the treatment of advanced or recurrent endometrial cancer (Table 8–6). Efficacy is limited to women whose tumors

Table 8–6. PHASE II TRIALS OF HORMONAL AGENTS IN ENDOMETRIAL CANCER				
Agent	N	RR (%)	CR (%)	Reference
Megace	63	24	11	25
Medroxyprogesterone	22	9		116
Medroxyprogesterone	331	18		117
Tamoxifen	49	20	12	33
Tamoxifen and Megace	25	33		53
Arimidex	23	9		39
Leuprolide	25	0		52
Leuprolide or goserelin	32	28	6	51

CR = complete risk; RR = relative risk.
*Response rate in grade 1 and 2 tumors.

express hormone receptors. A wide variety of hormonal agents demonstrate modest activity, with the greatest experience with progestins. Oral progestins are more convenient and as efficacious as intramuscular formulations. Limited data suggest there may be a threshold dose that should be exceeded, but that there are no data supporting very-high doses of progestins in the treatment of this disease. GnRH analogues and selective aromatase inhibitors may offer advantages in terms of side-effect profiles and are active, although they have not been formally proven to be as equally efficacious as progestins. New selective ER modulators (SERMs) and pure GnRH antagonists may provide additional therapeutic options in the future. Finally, more careful analysis of the expression of the hormone receptors in individual tumors may be important in selecting the most rational hormonal agent in the future.

CHEMOTHERAPY

Hormonal therapy is effective in providing palliation for many women with recurrent or metastatic ER/PR-positive tumors. This therapy typically provides disease control for 6 to 10 months. Once tumors are resistant to a primary hormonal therapy, secondary hormonal manipulations are unlikely to provide prolonged palliation. For women with progressive tumors after hormonal manipulation or for women with hormone receptor–negative tumors, chemotherapy is an option.

The high cure rate associated with primary therapy limits the number of women eligible for clinical trials involving chemotherapy. In addition, this is a tumor that typically occurs in elderly patients, often with significant comorbid diseases, such as diabetes. Thus, phase III studies evaluating chemotherapy strategies are limited and typically enroll a patient population that is a decade younger than the average woman afflicted with this cancer. Thus, it is difficult to make definitive conclusions regarding optimal chemotherapeutic strategies in women with recurrent disease.

Single-Agent Chemotherapy

Several agents have been evaluated in phase II clinical trials and Table 8–7 divides these agents into those with a predicted response of > 20% (active agents) versus those with lower response rates (less active agents). In reality, most of these agents have only been evaluated in modest-sized studies, and hence, the reported response rates may differ substantially from real response rates. With single-agent therapy, the large majority of responses are incomplete and have median durations of only 3 to 6 months. Currently, platinum compounds (cisplatin and carboplatin), anthracyclines (doxorubicin and epirubicin), and paclitaxel are among the most active

Table 8–7. CHEMOTHERAPY AGENTS USED TO TREAT ENDOMETRIAL CANCER			
More Active Agents		Less Active Agents	
Drug	References	Drug	References
Cisplatin	59–61, 118	Etoposide	92, 119
Carboplatin	120	Hexamethylmelamine	121
Doxorubicin	63, 68, 122, 123	Mitoxantrone	124
Paclitaxel	66	Methotrexate	125
Epirubicin	64	Vincristine	126
Methyl lomustine	127	Vinblastine	128
5-Fluorouracil	129	Cyclophosphamide	69
Ifosfamide	8, 129		

single agents, with 20 to 37% single-agent response rates (Table 8–8).[59-67] Complete responses are seen on occasion; however, median survival is less than 1 year. Randomized trials comparing single agents are limited to small randomized phase II studies. One such study suggests that doxorubicin is superior to cyclophosphamide, and the second suggests that ifosfamide is superior to cyclophosphamide.[68,69] Neither study demonstrated a survival advantage for either treatment arm, and indeed, both studies are too small to be conclusive. Trials that included women who had been treated with prior chemotherapy had lower response rates.

Combination Chemotherapy Regimens

A large number of combination regimens using two- or three-drug combinations have been evaluated in predominantly small phase II clinical trials (Table 8–9). Response rates for the reported trials tend to range between 30 and 65% and hence are higher than the single-agent trials, which, at most, have a 30% response rate.[34,62,70-76] In general, response rates in excess of 50% have included cisplatin, usually in combination with an anthracycline, most commonly doxorubicin (Adriamycin). The largest experience is with CAP chemotherapy (cisplatin, Adriamycin, and cyclophosphamide) with multiple phase II studies demonstrating a 40 to 60% response rate, including a 20 to 30% complete response rate.[70,71,72,77] Responses are usually brief, and overall survival is typically still less than 1 year. More recently, paclitaxel has been added into combination regimens. For example, paclitaxel and cisplatin (with granulocyte colony-stimulating factor [G-CSF] support) have a 67% response rate but a high rate of neuropathy, including severe peripheral neuropathy in 9% of patients. Progression-free survival and overall survival are 8 and 18 months, respectively.[78] The Gynecologic Oncology Group (GOG) has also recently reported a myelotoxic but active triplet regimen, using paclitaxel, doxorubicin, and cisplatin, to have a high response rate.[79]

Randomized trials comparing doublet therapy to single-agent therapy have demonstrated statistically superior response rates but not overall survival advantages (Figure 8–3 and Table 8–10).[62] GOG-107 compared doxorubicin as a single agent to doxorubicin and cisplatin. The response rate was superior for the doublet, with a marginal improvement in progression-free survival but apparently no advantage for overall survival. Higher response rates were seen in women with lung lesions, whereas women with a poor performance status, high-grade tumor, and liver or peritoneal disease were less likely to respond.[62]

Randomized trials comparing different doublet therapies have still not been reported in detail.[62,80] GOG-163 compares doxorubicin and cisplatin with doxorubicin and paclitaxel. Preliminary analysis of this randomized trial comprising 328 women demonstrates a complete response rate of 14% for doxorubicin and cisplatin versus 17% for doxorubicin and paclitaxel. To date, toxicity, overall response rate, and progression-free survival rates appear to be similar.[81] Preliminary reports have suggested that there will be no overall survival differences for women treated

Table 8–8. PHASE II SINGLE-AGENT CHEMOTHERAPY TRIALS IN ENDOMETRIAL CANCER					
Agent	Prior Therapy	Number Accrued	RR (%)	Median PFS	Reference
Carboplatin	No	27	30	2.7 mo	119
Cisplatin	Some	129	23	2.9–5 mo	59
					58, 90,116
Cyclophosphamide	No prior chemotherapy	14	14	7 wk	68
	Prior chemotherapy	15	0		
Doxorubicin	No	43	37	5 mo	62
Epirubicin	No	27	26	9.5 mo	63
Ifosfamide	No prior chemotherapy	37	24		129
Ifosfamide	No prior chemotherapy	16	25	7 wk	68
	Prior chemotherapy	16	0		
Ifosfamide	Some with prior chemotherapy	52	15	3.9 mo	89
Paclitaxel (24 h)		28	36	3.8 mo	65
Paclitaxel (3 h)	Previous CAP	19	36.5		64

CAP = cisplatin, Adriamycin, cyclophosphamide; PFS = progression-free survival; RR = response rate.

Agent	Prior Therapy	Number Accrued	RR (%)	Median PFS	Survival	Reference
Paclitaxel 175 mg/m² over 3 h Cisplatin 75 mg	None	24	67	8.4 mo	17.6 mo	78
MVAC	None	25	60			131
Cyclophosphamide Adriamycin	Hormones	13	46		10 mo	122
Cyclophosphamide Adriamycin Cisplatin	Hormones	17	45	6 mo		71
Cyclophosphamide Adriamycin Cisplatin	Hormones	18	56			77
Cyclophosphamide Adriamycin Cisplatin	Hormones	19	47			74
Cisplatin VM-26 Vincristine		44	52			132
Cyclophosphamide Adriamycin, 5-FU Vincristine		20	25		15 mo	73
Etoposide 5-FU, Adriamycin Cisplatin	4% prior chemotherapy	20	41	8 mo	17 mo	75
Paclitaxel Adriamycin Cisplatin	None	27	46	NA	NA	79
Adriamycin Platinum		19	36	5 mo	17 mo	133
Adriamycin Platinum (circadian dosing)		30	60	14 mo		134

Table 8–9. COMBINATION CHEMOTHERAPY TRIALS IN ENDOMETRIAL CANCER

5-FU = 5-Fluorouracil; MVAC = methotrexate, vinblastine, doxorubicin (Adriamycin), cisplatin; NA = not available; PFS = progression-free survival; RR = response rate; VM-26 = teniposide.

with the doxorubicin-cisplatin doublet compared with doxorubicin and (Cytoxan) or doxorubicin and paclitaxel doublets (Figure 8–4).

Recently, results of GOG-177 have suggested that the triplet regimen of Taxal, Adriamycin and cisplatin provides superior overall survival to Adriamycin and cisplatin with a hazard ratio of 0.79 (95% CI, 0.59–1.07).[82] Whether this reflects the synergy of the three drug regimen, or simply the addition of Taxal is unclear. A comparison of Taxal and carboplatin with the triplet is planned.[82]

In summary, multiagent chemotherapy probably offers a higher likelihood of tumor response than single-agent therapy. To date, none of the published multiagent chemotherapy trials demonstrates a survival advantage compared with single-agent ther-apy, although GOG-177 will likely challenge that paradigm.

In the absence of participation in clinical trials, single-agent carboplatin, paclitaxel, or doxorubicin is a reasonable choice. For patients with a significant burden of metastatic disease or in need of prompt cytoreduction, combination therapy offers a better chance of response but with greater toxicity. Currently, GOG-177 is the only trial that provides evidence that a multidrug regimen improves ultimate survival. For patients with good performance status after first-line chemotherapy, additional lines of therapy may offer further palliation. For patients with prolonged treat-ment-free intervals, a return to platinum-based therapy may once again generate a response, as seen in women with recurrent epithelial ovarian cancer.[83–85]

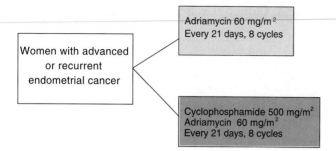

Figure 8–3. Schema of GOG-48 comparing doxorubicin (Adriamycin) to doxorubicin and cyclophosphamide.

Combination Chemotherapy with Hormonal Therapy

There have been only a few studies that have evaluated the potential benefit of delivering chemotherapy concurrently with hormonal therapy. In general, these studies have serious methodologic flaws, are underpowered, and do not include the most active chemotherapy agents.[86–89] There are only a few phase II trials that accrued more than 20 women. These trials demonstrate response rates of about 40 to 50%, which is in the range of that seen with combination chemotherapy without hormonal agents.[86,87] Randomized trials are limited and most compare two different chemotherapy regimens that contain progestins.[86,89] Only the study by Ayoub and colleagues compares CAF (cyclophosphamide, doxorubicin [Adriamycin], and 5-fluorouracil [5-FU]) with or without sequential medroxyprogesterone alternating with tamoxifen.[88] The study has only 43 patients and demonstrates that the hormone-containing arm has a response rate of 43% compared with 15% in the chemotherapy-alone arm. Median survival for the combination hormone-chemotherapy arm is 14 months compared with 11 months for the CAF-alone arm (not significant).[88] In summary, there is no evidence that simultaneous hormonal and chemotherapy is superior to the typical treatment strategy of hormonal therapy followed by chemotherapy at the time of disease progression.

Second-Line Chemotherapy Regimens

The treatment of women with recurrent or progressive disease after first-line chemotherapy is not exten-sively studied. Patients demonstrating a good and durable response to platinum and/or paclitaxel may respond again to the same agents.[84] Paclitaxel has demonstrated significant activity in women previously treated with cisplatin and Adriamycin, demonstrating that this agent has activity in platinum-resistant disease, thus paralleling the experience in epithelial ovarian cancer.[65] Ifosfamide, cisplatin, and docetaxel have also demonstrated activity as a second-line chemotherapy regimen, whereas etoposide has not demonstrated activity.[67,90,91,92]

SPECIAL SITUATIONS

Typically, recurrent endometrial cancer is amenable to palliative systemic therapies described above. Nevertheless, a few special situations deserve further discussion. In particular, certain patterns of pelvic recurrence represent regional and not systemic recurrence. In addition, in selected cases, oligometastatic disease may be amenable to long-term palliation with surgery.

Pelvic Recurrence

Prognosis and treatment planning is dependent on the extent of pelvic disease, prior treatment history, and the presence or absence of hematogenous or extrapelvic disease. In women with disease confined to the pelvis, the most important factors are whether the women have received prior pelvic radiotherapy and whether the site of recurrence within the pelvis. In particular, women who have not received prior pelvic radiotherapy and who have an isolated vaginal cuff recurrence have a relatively favorable outcome compared with all other women with recurrent or metastatic disease. In the recent Portec study, 2-year

Table 8–10. DOXORUBICIN VERSUS CYCLOPHOSPHAMIDE AND DOXORUBICIN		
	Doxorubicin	Doxorubicin + Cyclophosphamide
Patients	132	144
Complete responses	5%	13%
Partial responses	17%	17%
Overall response rate	22%	30%
Progression-free interval	3.2 mo	3.9 mo
Median survival	6.7 mo	7.3 mo

Adapted from Thigpen et al.[62]

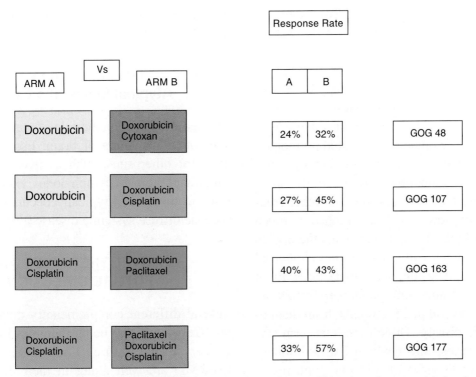

Figure 8–4. Evolution of randomized trials in endometrial cancer. This schematizes completed and ongoing randomized trials in women with advanced or recurrent endometrial cancer. To date, none of the trials has reported a statistically significant survival advantage for any of the arms in any of the studies.

survival after vaginal cuff recurrence was 79% compared with 21% for women with pelvic or distant disease.[11] Indeed, radiotherapy will provide long-term disease control and potentially cure 20 to 50% of women with isolated vaginal cuff recurrence (also reviewed in Chapter 7).[93–96] Long-term palliation is also possible but less likely in women with more extensive pelvic recurrences. Recurrent disease within the pelvic nodes typically indicates systemic disease, and very few of these women enjoy long-term disease control with pelvic radiotherapy.

Isolated Pelvic Recurrence in Women with Prior Radiotherapy

Women with high-risk stage I disease and surgical stage II/III disease typically receive radiotherapy. Randomized studies evaluating the role of radiotherapy in women with moderate- or high-risk local disease clearly demonstrates a lower local recurrence rate in the subgroup receiving postoperative radiation therapy compared with those treated with only surgery. For example, in a group of women with intermediate-

prognosis stage I disease, pelvic radiotherapy reduced pelvic recurrence rate to 4% at 5 years compared with 14% in the control group ($p < .0001$).[11] Even with more advanced pelvic disease at presentation, isolated pelvic recurrences at the time of relapse is uncommon and occurs in probably no more than 10 to 15% of cases (for a more detailed discussion, see Chapter 5). Isolated central pelvic recurrence after radiation therapy is rare. Carefully selected patients from large referral centers have demonstrated a modest long-term disease-free survival rate in women who have undergone exenterative surgery.[97] For example, the M.D. Anderson Cancer Center performed 20 such procedures over a 33-year period with a 45% 5-year disease-free survival.[97] These procedures are typically associated with a very high incidence of postoperative complications, including fistula, neovaginal flap necrosis, abscess, and vascular accidents.[97]

Isolated Pulmonary Nodules

Fuller and colleagues identified 100 women with pulmonary metastasis from a subset of 1,665 women with a diagnosis of uterine cancer.[27] Twenty-two of 100 women presented with pulmonary disease at the time of initial diagnosis, while the remainder had pulmonary metastasis identified at a mean of 29.4 months following primary therapy.[27] Median survival for the entire group was less then 1 year although 6% were alive 5 years after the diagnosis of metastatic disease. Women with isolated pulmonary nodules and response to progestin therapy comprised the most favorable group, with some responses lasting for > 5 years. As with other studies, women with low-grade tumors had a much higher chance of responding to hormonal therapy. In this series, 13 women had a history of endometrial carcinoma and solitary pulmonary metastases. Eight of these women underwent pulmonary resection, with a median survival of 25.6 months from diagnosis of metastatic disease. Three were long-term survivors in this series, all of whom had pulmonary resection. A second series of 6 women with resection of pulmonary nodule(s) demonstrated a median survival of 46 months.[98] Others have reported multi-year responses with progestin therapy.[99]

Brain Metastases

In reviews including 1,210 and 1,069 women with endometrial cancer, synchronous or, more commonly, metachronous brain metastases have been seen in 0.3 to 0.9% of women.[5,8] In a large Italian series, the median interval between diagnosis and documentation of brain involvement was 26 months, with most women presenting with headache (80%) or motor weakness (50%). In all series, a large subset of these patients have "brain-only" metastatic disease. In some cases, these metastases can even present prior or concurrently with discovery of the primary malignancy[3,8,100] Most women developing metastatic disease had high-grade primary tumors with evidence of deep myometrial invasion[100] While most patients have died of recurrent disease within months, there are reports of long-term survival (> 7 years) in individuals who underwent neurosurgical resection and brain radiotherapy.[5,8,9] Experience with this atypical presentation is too limited to make general recommendations, except to advocate that women with solitary brain metastasis and limited or

absent intra-abdominal/pulmonary disease should be considered potential neurosurgical candidates.

Metastasectomy for Atypical Metastatic Lesions

Limited data exist on the role of metastasectomy for sites other than lung or brain. Essentially no data exist for other sites, such as liver, skin, bone, or supradiaphragmatic lymph nodes, except that metastases to these sites typically occur with or shortly precede diffuse systemic disease.[6,7,10]

NOVEL THERAPIES AND FUTURE DIRECTIONS

Several different complementary areas of research are likely to provide better therapies for endometrial cancer in the future. First, pure antiestrogens (SERMs) are well along in their development as effective therapeutic agents in ER-positive breast cancer and will deserve careful evaluation in ER-positive endometrial cancer. Classic chemotherapeutic agents with novel mechanisms of actions are currently in phase I and early phase II trials. These drugs include new microtubule-specific agents (dolostatins and epothilones) as well as drugs that bind DNA (ET-743 and irofulven).[101–104] Biologic agents that target the tyrosine kinase of the EGF receptor family (Herceptin, CI-1033, C225, Iressa, EMD72,000, OSI774) have demonstrated activity in a broad range of tumors that express EGF receptors.[105] Pharmacologic agents that target proteins important in a broad range of cancers, such as RAS, other key cell cycle proteins, or even the proteosome machinery may deserve further evaluation in endometrial carcinoma. Preclinical experience suggests that many of these agents will be most active when combined with chemotherapeutic agents. Immunotherapeutic strategies continue to be evaluated in the treatment of carcinomas, including very limited studies in endometrial cancer, and will require further study.[106]

Technologies that replace absent tumor suppressor function may also be useful. Recently, PTEN, a dual-function phosphatase located on 10q23, has been found to be mutated or lost in a very large portion of malignant and premalignant endometrial lesions (see Chapter 2).[107,108] Interestingly, cells lacking PTEN may be selectively enriched in an estrogen-rich environment and attenuated by progestins.[109] Therapies that replace or restore PTEN function may provide therapeutic benefit or a preventive strategy in women with atypical hyperplasia.[107,110]

Additional therapies for endometrial carcinoma are likely to come from the improved understanding of the genetic alterations that define the malignant phenotype. First, evidence is mounting to suggest that endometrioid carcinoma may contain biologically distinct diseases within a single histologic phenotype; this is reviewed in Chapter 2.[111,112] These include estrogen-associated endometrioid carcinoma that is the most prevalent and associated with obesity, anovulation, nulliparity, diabetes, and the chronic unopposed use of estrogen or tamoxifen.[111–113] A second subtype is seen in younger women and probably does not have atypical hyperplasia as a precursor lesion.[111–113] These women are typically thin and do not have the classic risk factors for endometrial carcinoma. A third type may include women with the hereditary nonpolyposis colon carcinoma (HNPCC) syndrome (see Chapter 3). Finally, recent evidence has suggested that papillary serous carcinoma of the endometrium may be linked, in certain individuals, with the *BRCA1* germline mutation.[114] Currently, systemic therapies are not tailored to underlying mechanism of carcinogenesis, although distinguishing between these "molecular subtypes" of endometrial carcinoma will ultimately become logical when more rational therapeutics are available.

More global genome-wide surveys have been performed using comprehensive analysis of ribonucleic acid (RNA) transcripts through gene array technologies. Recently, Mutter and collaborators have evaluated the expression of 6,000 genes in malignant endometrial tumors compared with proliferative and secretory endometrium.[115] Evaluation of the general gene expression pattern in carcinomas was, in general, more similar to that of proliferative, compared with secretory, endometrium. Numerous changes in cell cycle, cytoskeletal extracellular matrix, hormone pathways, and oncogene/tumor-suppressor genes are worthy of further study in the hope that some of these will

be suitable targets for pharmacologic manipulation. Such efforts will require much more research.[115]

SUMMARY

The appropriate management of women with recurrent endometrial cancer depends on the localization of disease recurrence, hormone receptor status, and the general performance status of the patient. Isolated vaginal recurrences in women without prior radiation can be palliated and frequently cured with radiation therapy. Women with low-grade tumors that express PRs and ERs can often derive benefit for prolonged periods from progestin therapy and a growing list of alternative endocrine therapies. For women with hormone receptor–negative tumors or tumors that have progressed after hormonal therapy, a modest number of chemotherapy agents offer the chance of response. There is now data to suggest that multiagent chemotherapy may provide a survival advantage compared with sequential therapies. While some women with low-grade hormone receptor–positive tumors will live for many years, the median survival for women with metastatic disease is less than 1 year. New biologically targeted agents, either as single agents or in combination with chemotherapy, offer hope for women with recurrent or metastatic endometrial cancer in the future.

REFERENCES

1. Podratz KC, O'Brien PC, Malkasian GD Jr, et al. Effects of progestational agents in treatment of endometrial carcinoma. Obstet Gynecol 1985;66(1):106–10.
2. Mariani A, Webb MJ, Keeney GL, et al. Hematogenous dissemination in corpus cancer. Gynecol Oncol 2001;80(2):233–8.
3. Ruelle A, Zuccarello M, Andrioli G. Brain metastasis from endometrial carcinoma. Report of two cases. Neurosurg Rev 1994;17(1):83–7.
4. Arvold DS. Right ventricular metastasis of endometrial carcinoma: a case report. Gynecol Oncol 1988;29(2):231–3.
5. Cormio G, Lissoni A, Losa G, et al. Brain metastases from endometrial carcinoma. Gynecol Oncol 1996;61(1):40–3.
6. Dosoretz DE, Orr JW Jr, Salenius SA, Orr PF. Mandibular metastasis in a patient with endometrial cancer. Gynecol Oncol 1999;72(2):243–5.
7. Kushner DM, Lurain JR, Fu TS, Fishman DA. Endometrial adenocarcinoma metastatic to the scalp: case report and literature review. Gynecol Oncol 1997;65(3):530–3.
8. Petru E, Lax S, Kurschel S, et al. Long-term survival in a

patient with brain metastases preceding the diagnosis of endometrial cancer. Report of two cases and review of the literature. J Neurosurg 2001;94(5):846–8.

9. Sawada M, Inagaki M, Ozaki M, et al. Long-term survival after brain metastasis from endometrial cancer. Jpn J Clin Oncol 1990;20(3):312–5.

10. Siddiq MA, Bhudia SK, Gana P, Patel PJ. Metastatic endometrial carcinoma of the neck. J Laryngol Otol 2000; 114(3):229–30.

11. Creutzberg CL, van Putten WL, Koper PC, et al. Surgery and postoperative radiotherapy versus surgery alone for patients with stage-1 endometrial carcinoma: multicenter randomised trial. Lancet 2000;355:1404–11.

12. Emons G, Heyl W. Hormonal treatment of endometrial cancer. J Cancer Res Clin Oncol 2000;126(11):619–23.

13. Quinn MA. Hormonal treatment of endometrial cancer. Hematol Oncol Clin North Am 1999;13(1):163–87, ix.

14. Kumar NS, Richer J, Owen G, et al. Selective down-regulation of progesterone receptor isoform B in poorly differentiated human endometrial cancer cells: implications for unopposed estrogen action. Cancer Res 1998;58(9):1860–5.

15. Fujimoto J, Ichigo S, Hori M, et al. Expression of progesterone receptor form A and B mRNAs in gynecologic malignant tumors. Tumour Biol 1995;16(4):254–60.

16. Fujimoto J, Ichigo S, Hirose R, et al. Clinical implication of expression of progesterone receptor form A and B mRNAs in secondary spreading of gynecologic cancers. J Steroid Biochem Mol Biol 1997;62(5-6):449–54.

17. Ehrlich CE, Young PC, Stehman FB, et al. Steroid receptors and clinical outcome in patients with adenocarcinoma of the endometrium. Am J Obstet Gynecol 1988;158(4):796–807.

18. Dai D, Kumar NS, Wolf DM, Leslie KK. Molecular tools to reestablish progestin control of endometrial cancer cell proliferation. Am J Obstet Gynecol 2001;184(5):790–7.

19. Gadducci A, Genazzani AR. Endocrine therapy for gynecological cancer. Gynecol Endocrinol 1999;13(6):441–56.

20. Allegra JC, Kiefer SM. Mechanisms of action of progestational agents. Semin Oncol 1985;12 Suppl 1:3–5.

21. Saegusa M, Okayasu I. Progesterone therapy for endometrial carcinoma reduces cell proliferation but does not alter apoptosis. Cancer 1998;83(1):111–21.

22. Fujimoto J, Sakaguchi H, Hirose R, et al. Progestins suppress estrogen-induced expression of vascular endothelial growth factor (VEGF) subtypes in uterine endometrial cancer cells. Cancer Lett 1999;141(1-2):63–71.

23. Kelley RM, Baker WH. Progestational agents in the treatment of carcinoma of the endometrium. N Engl J Med 1961;264:216–22.

24. Kauppila A. Progestin therapy of endometrial, breast and ovarian carcinoma. A review of clinical observations. Acta Obstet Gynecol Scand 1984;63(5):441–50.

25. Lentz SS, Brady MF, Major FJ, et al. High dose megestrol acetate in advanced or recurrent endometrial carcinoma: a Gynecologic Oncology Group Study. J Clin Oncol 1996;14:357–61.

26. Piver MS, Barlow JJ, Lurain JR, Blumenson LE. Medroxyprogesterone acetate (Depo-Provera) vs. hydroxyprogesterone caproate (Delalutin) in women with metastatic endometrial adenocarcinoma. Cancer 1980;45(2):268–72.

27. Fuller AF Jr, Bouros D, Papadakis K, Siafakas N. Natural history of patients with pulmonary metastases from uterine cancer. Cancer 1996;78(3):441–7.

28. Thigpen JT, Homesley HD. A Randomized study of medroxyprogesterone acetate (MPA) 200 mg versus 1000 mg in the treatment of advanced, persistent or recurrent carcinoma of the endomtrium, In: Gynecologic Oncology Group Statistical Report-February 1990. Buffalo: Gynecologic Oncology Group, 1990;177.

29. Geisler H. The use of megestrol acetate in the treatment of advanced malignant lesions of the endometrium. Gynecol Oncol 1973;1:340.

30. Brzozowski AM, Pike AC, Dauter Z, et al. Molecular basis of agonism and antagonism in the oestrogen receptor. Nature 1997;389(6652):753–8.

31. Shiau AK, Barstad D, Loria PM, et al. The structural basis of estrogen receptor/coactivator recognition and the antagonism of this interaction by tamoxifen. Cell 1998;95(7): 927–37.

32. Jordan VC. Biochemical pharmacology of antiestrogen action. Pharmacol Rev 1984;36(4):245–76.

33. Quinn MA, Campbell JJ. Tamoxifen therapy in advanced/recurrent endometrial carcinoma. Gynecol Oncol 1989; 32(1):1–3.

34. Moore TD, Phillips PH, Nerenstone SR, Cheson BD. Systemic treatment of advanced and recurrent endometrial carcinoma: current status and future directions. J Clin Oncol 1991;9(6):1071–88.

35. Edmonson JH, Krook JE, Hilton JF, et al. Ineffectiveness of tamoxifen in advanced endometrial carcinoma after failure of progestin treatment. Cancer Treat Rep 1986;70(8): 1019–20.

36. Buzdar AU, Hortobagyi GN. Tamoxifen and toremifene in breast cancer: comparison of safety and efficacy. J Clin Oncol 1998;16(1):348–53.

37. Quinn MA, Campbell JJ, Murray R, Pepperell RJ. Tamoxifen and aminoglutethimide in the management of patients with advanced endometrial carcinoma not responsive to medroxyprogesterone. Aust N Z J Obstet Gynaecol 1981; 21(4):226–9.

38. Njar VC, Brodie AM. Comprehensive pharmacology and clinical efficacy of aromatase inhibitors. Drugs 1999; 58(2):233–55.

39. Rose PG, Brunetto VL, VanLe L, et al. A phase II trial of anastrozole in advanced recurrent or persistent endometrial carcinoma: a Gynecologic Oncology Group study. Gynecol Oncol 2000;78(2):212–6.

40. Dombernowsky P, Smith I, Falkson G, et al. Letrozole, a new oral aromatase inhibitor for advanced breast cancer: double-blind randomized trial showing a dose effect and improved efficacy and tolerability compared with megestrol acetate. J Clin Oncol 1998;16(2):453–61.

41. Venturino A, Comandini D, Granetto C, et al. Formestane is feasible and effective in elderly breast cancer patients with comorbidity and disability. Breast Cancer Res Treat 2000;62(3):217–22.

42. Kaufmann M, Bajetta E, Dirix LY, et al. Exemestane improves survival compared with megoestrol acetate in postmenopausal patients with advanced breast cancer who have failed on tamoxifen. Results of a double-blind randomised phase III trial. Eur J Cancer 2000;36 Suppl 4:S86–7.

43. Kaufmann M, Bajetta E, Dirix LY, et al. Exemestane is superior to megestrol acetate after tamoxifen failure in postmenopausal women with advanced breast cancer: results of a phase III randomized double-blind trial. The Exemestane Study Group. J Clin Oncol 2000;18(7):1399–411.

44. Hamilton A, Volm M. Nonsteroidal and steroidal aromatase inhibitors in breast cancer. Oncology (Huntingt) 2001;15(8):965–72; discussion 972, 977–9.

45. Buzdar A, Howell A. Advances in aromatase inhibition: clinical efficacy and tolerability in the treatment of breast cancer. Clin Cancer Res 2001;7(9):2620–35.

46. Fawell SE, White R, Hoare S, et al. Inhibition of estrogen receptor-DNA binding by the antiestrogen ICI 164,384 appears to be mediated by impaired receptor dimerization. Proc Natl Acad Sci U S A 1990;87(17):6883–7.

47. Srkalovic G, Wittliff JL, Schally AV. Detection and partial characterization of receptors for [D-Trp6]-luteinizing hormone-releasing hormone and epidermal growth factor in human endometrial carcinoma. Cancer Res 1990;50(6): 1841–6.

48. Noci I, Borri P, Taddei GL, et al. Human endometrial cancers contain follicle-stimulating hormone receptors: a preliminary study. Gynecol Endocrinol 1997;11(5):297–300.

49. Lamharzi N, Halmos G, Armatis P, Schally AV. Expression of mRNA for luteinizing hormone-releasing hormone receptors and epidermal growth factor receptors in human cancer cell lines. Int J Oncol 1998;12(3):671–5.

50. Kim JW, Lee YS, Kim BK, et al. Cell cycle arrest in endometrial carcinoma cells exposed to gonadotropin-releasing hormone analog. Gynecol Oncol 1999;73(3):368–71.

51. Jeyarajah AR, Gallagher CJ, Blake PR, et al. Long-term follow-up of gonadotrophin-releasing hormone analog treatment for recurrent endometrial cancer. Gynecol Oncol 1996;63(1):47–52.

52. Covens A, Thomas G, Shaw P, et al. A phase II study of leuprolide in advanced/recurrent endometrial cancer. Gynecol Oncol 1997;64(1):126–9.

53. Carlson JA Jr, Allegra JC, Day TG Jr, Wittliff JL. Tamoxifen and endometrial carcinoma: alterations in estrogen and progesterone receptors in untreated patients and combination hormonal therapy in advanced neoplasia. Am J Obstet Gynecol 1984;149(2):149–53.

54. Kline RC, Freedman RS, Jones LA, Atkinson EN. Treatment of recurrent or metastatic poorly differentiated adenocarcinoma of the endometrium with tamoxifen and medroxyprogesterone acetate. Cancer Treat Rep 1987;71(3):327–8.

55. van den Berg HW, Leahey WJ, Lynch M, et al. Recombinant human interferon alpha increases oestrogen receptor expression in human breast cancer cells (ZR-75-1) and sensitizes them to the anti-proliferative effects of tamoxifen. Br J Cancer 1987;55(3):255–7.

56. Sica G, Iacopino F, Recchia F. Interferon and hormone sensitivity of endocrine-related tumors. Anticancer Drugs 1996;7(2):150–60.

57. Goldstein D, Bushmeyer SM, Witt PL, et al. Effects of type I and II interferons on cultured human breast cells: interaction with estrogen receptors and with tamoxifen. Cancer Res 1989;49(10):2698–702.

58. Scambia G, Panici PB, Battaglia F, et al. Effect of recombinant human interferon-alpha 2b on receptors for steroid hormones and epidermal growth factor in patients with endometrial cancer. Eur J Cancer 1991;27(1):51–3.

59. Thigpen JT, Blessing JA, Homesley H, et al. Phase II trial of cisplatin as first-line chemotherapy in patients with advanced or recurrent endometrial carcinoma: a Gynecologic Oncology Group Study. Gynecol Oncol 1989;33(1): 68–70.

60. Seski JC, Edwards CL, Herson J, Rutledge FN. Cisplatin chemotherapy for disseminated endometrial cancer. Obstet Gynecol 1982;59(2):225–8.

61. Deppe G, Cohen CJ, Bruckner HW. Treatment of advanced endometrial adenocarcinoma with cis-dichlorodiammine platinum (II) after intensive prior therapy. Gynecol Oncol 1980;10(1):51–4.

62. Thigpen JT, Blessing JA, DiSaia PJ, et al. A randomized comparison of doxorubicin alone versus doxorubicin plus cyclophosphamide in the management of advanced or recurrent endometrial carcinoma: a Gynecologic Oncology Group study. J Clin Oncol 1994;12(7):1408–14.

63. Thigpen JT, Buchsbaum HJ, Mangan C, Blessing JA. Phase II trial of Adriamycin in the treatment of advanced or recurrent endometrial carcinoma: a Gynecologic Oncology Group study. Cancer Treat Rep 1979;63(1):21–7.

64. Calero F, Asins-Codoner E, Jimeno J, et al. Epirubicin in advanced endometrial adenocarcinoma: a phase II study of the Grupo Ginecologico Espanol para el Tratamiento Oncologico (GGETO). Eur J Cancer 1991;27(7):864–6.

65. Lissoni A, Zanetta G, Losa G, et al. Phase II study of paclitaxel as salvage treatment in advanced endometrial cancer. Ann Oncol 1996;7(8):861–3.

66. Ball HG, Blessing JA, Lentz SS, Mutch DG. A phase II trial of paclitaxel in patients with advanced or recurrent adenocarcinoma of the endometrium: a Gynecologic Oncology Group study. Gynecol Oncol 1996;62(2):278–81.

67. Gunthert AR, Pilz S, Kuhn W, et al. Docetaxel is effective in the treatment of metastatic endometrial cancer. Anticancer Res 1999;19(4C):3459–61.

68. Horton J, Begg CB, Arseneault J, et al. Comparison of Adriamycin with cyclophosphamide in patients with advanced endometrial cancer. Cancer Treat Rep 1978;2(1):159–61.

69. Pawinski A, Tumolo S, Hoesel G, et al. Cyclophosphamide or ifosfamide in patients with advanced and/or recurrent endometrial carcinoma: a randomized phase II study of the EORTC Gynecological Cancer Cooperative Group. Eur J Obstet Gynecol Reprod Biol 1999;86(2):179–83.

70. Dunton CJ, Pfeifer SM, Braitman LE, et al. Treatment of advanced and recurrent endometrial cancer with cisplatin, doxorubicin, and cyclophosphamide. Gynecol Oncol 1991;41(2):113–6.

71. Burke TW, Stringer CA, Morris M, et al. Prospective treatment of advanced or recurrent endometrial carcinoma with cisplatin, doxorubicin, and cyclophosphamide. Gynecol Oncol 1991;40(3):264–7.

72. Edmonson JH, Krook JE, Hilton JF, et al. Randomized phase II studies of cisplatin and a combination of cyclophosphamide-doxorubicin-cisplatin (CAP) in patients with progestin-refractory advanced endometrial carcinoma. Gynecol Oncol 1987;8(1):20–4.

73. Kauppila A, Janne O, Kujansuu E, Vihko R. Treatment of advanced endometrial adenocarcinoma with a combined

cytotoxic therapy. Predictive value of cytosol estrogen and progestin receptor levels. Cancer 1980;46(10):2162–7.

74. Kauppila A, Janne O, Kujansuu E, Vihko R. Cisplatin, doxorubicin, and cyclophosphamide chemotherapy for advanced endometrial carcinoma. Cancer Treat Rep 1985;69(5):465–7.

75. Pierga JY, Dieras V, Paraiso D, et al. Treatment of advanced or recurrent endometrial carcinoma with combination of etoposide, cisplatin, and 5-fluorouracil: a phase II study. Gynecol Oncol 1996;60(1):59–63.

76. Lissoni A, Gabriele A, Gorga G, et al. Cisplatin-, epirubicin- and paclitaxel-containing chemotherapy in uterine adenocarcinoma. Ann Oncol 1997;8(10):969–72.

77. Hancock KC, Freedman RS, Edwards CL, Rutledge FN. Use of cisplatin, doxorubicin, and cyclophosphamide to treat advanced and recurrent adenocarcinoma of the endometrium. Cancer Treat Rep 1986;70(6):789–91.

78. Dimopoulos MA, Papadimitriou CA, Georgoulias V, et al. Paclitaxel and cisplatin in advanced or recurrent carcinoma of the endometrium: long-term results of a phase II multicenter study. Gynecol Oncol 2000;78(1):52–7.

79. Fleming GF, Fowler JM, Waggoner SE, et al. Phase I trial of escalating doses of paclitaxel combined with fixed doses of cisplatin and doxorubicin in advanced endometrial cancer and other gynecologic malignancies: a Gynecologic Oncology Group study. J Clin Oncol 2001;19(4):1021–9.

80. Thigpen T, Blessing J, Homesley H, et al. Phase III trial of doxorubicin ± cisplatin in advanced or recurrent endometrial carcinoma: a Gynecologic Oncology Group (GOG) study. Proc Am J Clin Oncol 1993;12:261.

81. Fleming G. Randomized trial of doxorubicin plus cisplatin versus doxorubicin plus paclitaxel plus granulocyte colony-stimulating-factor (G-CSF) in patients with advanced or recurrent endometrial cancer: a report on Gynecologic Oncology Group (GOG) protocol #163. Proc Am Soc Clin Oncol 2000;9:379a.

82. Fleming GF, Brunetto VL, Mundt AJ, et al. Randomized trial of doxorubicin (DOX) plus cisplatin (CIS) versus DOX plus CIS plus paclitaxel (TAX) in patients with advances or recurrent endometrial carcinoma: A Gynecologic Oncology Group (GO) Study [abstract 807]. Proc Am Soc Clin Oncol 2002;22:202a.

83. Rose PG, Fusco N, Fluellen L, Rodriguez M. Second-line therapy with paclitaxel and carboplatin for recurrent disease following first-line therapy with paclitaxel and platinum in ovarian or peritoneal carcinoma. J Clin Oncol 1998;16:1494–7.

84. Markman M, Kennedy A, Webster K, et al. Persistent chemosensitivity to platinum and/or paclitaxel in metastatic endometrial cancer. Gynecol Oncol 1999;73(3):422–3.

85. Markman M, Rothman R, Hakes T, et al. Second-line platinum therapy in patients with ovarian cancer previously treated with cisplatin. J Clin Oncol 1991;9:389–93.

86. Horton J, Elson P, Gordon P, et al. Combination chemotherapy for advanced endometrial cancer. An evaluation of three regimens. Cancer 1982;49(15):2441–5.

87. Piver MS, Lele SB, Patsner B, Emrich LJ. Melphalan, 5-fluorouracil, and medroxyprogesterone acetate in metastatic endometrial carcinoma. Obstet Gynecol 1986;67:261–4.

88. Ayoub J, Audet-Lapointe P, Methot Y, et al. Efficacy of sequential cyclical hormonal therapy in endometrial cancer and its correlation with steroid hormone receptor status. Gynecol Oncol 1988;31(2):327–37.

89. Cohen CJ, Bruckner HW, Deppe G, et al. Multidrug treament of advanced and recurrent endometrial carcinoma: a Gynecologic Oncology Group study. Obstet Gynecol 1984;63:719–26.

90. Sutton GP, Blessing JA, Homesley HD, Malfetano JH. A phase II trial of ifosfamide and mesna in patients with advanced or recurrent mixed mesodermal tumors of the ovary previously treated with platinum-based chemotherapy: a Gynecologic Oncology Group study. Gynecol Oncol 1994;53(1):24–6.

91. Thigpen JT, Blessing JA, Lagasse LD, et al. Phase II trial of cisplatin as second-line chemotherapy in patients with advanced or recurrent endometrial carcinoma. A Gynecologic Oncology Group study. Am J Clin Oncol 1984;7(3):253–6.

92. Rose PG, Blessing JA, Lewandowski GS, et al. A phase II trial of prolonged oral etoposide (VP-16) as second-line therapy for advanced and recurrent endometrial carcinoma: a Gynecologic Oncology Group study. Gynecol Oncol 1996;63(1):101–4.

93. Mandell L, Nori D, Hilaris B. Recurrent Stage I endometrial carcinoma: results of treatment and prognosis factors. Int J Radiat Oncol Biol Phys 1985;11:1103–9.

94. Aalders J, Abeler V, Kolstad P. Recurrent adenocarcinoma of the endometrium: a clinical and histopathological study of 379 patients. Gynecol Oncol 1984;17:85–103.

95. Greven K, Olds W. Isolated vaginal recurrences of endometrial adenocarcinoma and their management. Cancer 1987;60(3):419–21.

96. Kuten A, Grigsby PW, Perez CA, et al. Results of radiotherapy in recurrent endometrial carcinoma. A retrospective analysis of 51 patients. Int J Radiat Oncol Biol Phys 1989;17:29–34.

97. Morris M, Alvarez RD, Kinney WK, Wilson TO. Treatment of recurrent adenocarcinoma of the endometrium with pelvic exenteration. Gynecol Oncol 1996;60(2):288–91.

98. Anderson TM, McMahon JJ, Nwogu CE, et al. Pulmonary resection in metastatic uterine and cervical malignancies. Gynecol Oncol 2001;83(3):472–6.

99. Crespo C, Gonzalez-Martin A, Lastra E, et al. Metastatic endometrial cancer in lung and liver: complete and prolonged response to hormonal therapy with progestins. Gynecol Oncol 1999;72:250–5.

100. Kottke-Marchant K, Estes ML, Nunez C. Early brain metastases in endometrial carcinoma. Gynecol Oncol 1991: 41(1):67–73.

101. Villalona-Calero MA, Baker SD, Hammond L, et al. Phase I and pharmacokinetic study of the water-soluble dolastatin 15 analog LU103793 in patients with advanced solid malignancies. J Clin Oncol 1998;16(8):2770–9.

102. Lee FY, Borzilleri R, Fairchild CR, et al. BMS-247550: a novel epothilone analog with a mode of action similar to paclitaxel but possessing superior antitumor efficacy. Clin Cancer Res 2001;7(5):1429–37.

103. Valoti G, Nicoletti MI, Pellegrino A, et al. Ecteinascidin-743, a new marine natural product with potent antitumor activity on human ovarian carcinoma xenografts. Clin Cancer Res 1998;4(8):1977–83.

104. Eckhardt SG, Baker SD, Britten CD, et al. Phase I and phar-

macokinetic study of irofulven, a novel mushroom-derived cytotoxin, administered for five consecutive days every four weeks in patients with advanced solid malignancies. J Clin Oncol 2000;18(24):4086–97.

105. Mendelsohn J, Baselga J. The EGF receptor family as targets for cancer therapy. Oncogene 2000;19(56):6550–65.

106. Santin AD, Hermonat PL, Ravaggi A, et al. Development and therapeutic effect of adoptively transferred T cells primed by tumor lysate-pulsed autologous dendritic cells in a patient with metastatic endometrial cancer. Gynecol Obstet Invest 2000;49(3):194–203.

107. Mutter GL, Lin MC, Fitzgerald JT, et al. Altered PTEN expression as a diagnostic marker for the earliest endometrial precancers. J Natl Cancer Inst 2000;92(11):924–30.

108. Maxwell GL, Risinger JI, Gumbs C, et al. Mutation of the PTEN tumor suppressor gene in endometrial hyperplasia. Cancer Res 1998;58(12):2500–3.

109. Mutter GL, Lin MC, Fitzgerald JT, et al. Changes in endometrial PTEN expression throughout the human menstrual cycle. J Clin Endocrinol Metab 2000;85(6):2334–8.

110. Levine RL, Cargile CB, Blazes MS, et al. PTEN mutations and microsatellite instability in complex atypical hyperplasia, a precursor lesion to uterine endometrioid carcinoma. Cancer Res 1998;58:3254–8.

111. Bokhman JV. Two pathogenetic types of endometrial carcinoma. Gynecol Oncol 1983;15:10–7.

112. Sherman ME. Theories of endometrial carcinogenesis: a multidisciplinary approach. Mol Pathol 2000;13:295–308.

113. Nyholm HCJ, Nielson AC, Norup P. Endometrial cancer in postmenopausal women with and without previous estrogen replacement treatment: comparison of clinical and histopathological characteristics. Gynecol Oncol 1993;49:229–35.

114. Geisler JP, Sorosky JI, Duong HL, et al. Papillary serous carcinoma of the uterus: increased risk of subsequent or concurrent development of breast carcinoma. Gynecol Oncol 2001;83:501–3.

115. Mutter GL, Baak JP, Fitzgerald JT, et al. Global expression changes of constitutive and hormonally regulated genes during endometrial neoplastic transformation. Gynecol Oncol 2001;83:177–85.

116. Quinn M, Cauchi M, Fortune D. Endometrial cancer: steroid receptors and response to medroxyprogesterone acetate. Gynecol Oncol 1985;21(3):314–9.

117. Thigpen J, Blessing J, Disaia P. Oral medroxyprogesterone acetate in advanced or recurrent endometrial carcinoma: results of therapy and correlation with estrogen and progesterone receptor levels. In: Balulieu E, Iacobilli S, McGuire W, editors. Proceedings of the First International Congress on Cancer and Hormones, Park Ridge, NJ: Parthenon;1986. p. 446.

118. Trope C, Grundsell H, Johnsson JE, Cavallin-Stahl E. A phase II study of Cis-platinum for recurrent corpus cancer. Eur J Cancer 1980;16(8):1025–6.

119. Poplin EA, Liu PY, Delmore JE, et al. Phase II trial of oral etoposide in recurrent or refractory endometrial adeno-

carcinoma: a Southwest Oncology Group Study. Gynecol Oncol 1999;74(3):432–5.

120. Burke TW, Munkarah A, Kavanagh JJ, et al. Prospective treatment of advanced or recurrent endometrial carcinoma with single-agent carboplatin. Gynecol Oncol 1993;51:397–400.

121. Seski JC, Edwards CL, Copeland LJ, Gershenson DM. Hexamethylmelamine chemotherapy for disseminated endometrial cancer. Obstet Gynecol 1981;58(3):361–3.

122. Campora E, Vidali A, Mammoliti S, et al. Treatment of advanced or recurrent adenocarcinoma of the endometrium with doxorubicin and cyclophosphamide. Eur J Gynaecol Oncol 1990;11(3):181–3.

123. Elit L, Hirte H. Novel strategies for systemic treatment of endometrial cancer. Expert Opin Invest Drugs 2000; 9(12):2831–53.

124. Hilgers RD, Legha SS, Johnston GA Jr, et al. Mitoxantrone in adenocarcinoma of the endometrium: a Southwest Oncology Group study. Invest New Drugs 1984;2(3):335–8.

125. Muss HB, Blessing JA, Hatch KD, et al. Methotrexate in advanced endometrial carcinoma. A phase II trial of the Gynecologic Oncology Group. Am J Clin Oncol 1990; 13(1):61–3.

126. Jackson DV Jr, Jobson VW, Homesley HD, et al. Vincristine infusion in refractory gynecologic malignancies. Gynecol Oncol 1986;25:212–6.

127. Omura GA, Shingleton HM, Creasman WT, et al. Chemotherapy of gynecologic cancer with nitrosourea: a randomized trial of CCNU and methyl CCNU in cancers of the cervix, corpus, vagina, and vulva. Cancer Treat Rep 1978;62:833–5.

128. Kavanagh JJ, Saul PB, Wharton JT, Rutledge FN. A trial of continuous-infusion vinblastine in refractory endometrial adenocarcinoma. Gynecol Oncol 1987;26(2):236–9.

129. Carbone P, Carter S. Endometrial cancer: approach to development of effective chemotherapy. Gynecol Oncol 1974; 2:348–53.

130. Sutton GP, Blessing JA, DeMars LR, et al. A phase II Gynecologic Oncology Group trial of ifosfamide and mesna in advanced or recurrent adenocarcinoma of the endometrium. Gynecol Oncol 1996;63(1):25–7.

131. Long H, Langdon R, Wieand H. Phase II trial of methotrexate, vinblastine, doxorubicin, and cisplatin (MVAC) in women with advanced endometrial cancer. Proc Am Soc Clin Oncol 1990;10:184.

132. Sorbe B, Wolmesjo E, Frankendal B. VM-26-vincristine-cisplatin combination chemotherapy in the treatment of primary advanced and recurrent endometrial carcinoma. Obstet Gynecol 1989;73:343–8.

133. Deppe G, Malviya VK, Malone JM, et al. Treatment of recurrent and metastatic endometrial carcinoma with cisplatin and doxorubicin. Eur J Gynaecol Oncol 1994;15(4):263–6.

134. Barrett RJ, Blessing JA, Homesley HD, et al. Circadian-timed combination doxorubicin-cisplatin chemotherapy for advanced endometrial carcinoma. A phase II study of the Gynecologic Oncology Group. Am J Clin Oncol 1993;16(6):494–6.

9

Primary Hormonal Therapy for Endometrial Carcinoma

LINDA R. DUSKA, MD
BO R. RUEDA, PhD

Endometrial cancer is the most common gynecologic malignancy. In the United States, the estimated number of new cases of endometrial cancer in 2003 is 40,100, and an estimated 6,800 women will die of this disease.[1] Endometrial cancer is statistically a tumor of postmenopause, with 75% of cases occurring after menopause and a mean age at diagnosis in 1990 to 1992 of 63.1 years.[2] However, previous studies suggest that between 2 and 14% of patients with endometrial cancer are 40 years of age or younger.[3–10] Endometrial cancer most often presents in early stages (confined to the corpus) and is typically curable with either surgery alone, consisting of total abdominal hysterectomy and bilateral salpingo-oophorectomy (TAH/BSO) with or without lymph node dissection, or with surgery plus radiation, if indicated by the extent of disease identified at surgical staging (see Chapter 7).

The most common histologic subtype of endometrial cancer, endometrioid adenocarcinoma, is believed to be associated with overexposure to estrogens without the differentiating effects of progesterone.[11–16] Endometrial hyperplasia and some endometrial cancers can be successfully treated with progesterone.[17–19] Progesterone treatment of endometrial cancer in early-stage, low-grade disease may preserve the uterus and future reproductive function. Currently, however, there is no way to identify those women with endometrial cancer for whom progesterone therapy may be successful, nor is there an adequate understanding of the action of steroid hormones on the malignant endometrium.

Our own study of patients at the Dana-Farber Partners Cancer Center included 95 patients under age 40 years with endometrial cancer; this number represented 4.5% of endometrial cancer cases over the period studied.[17] This series was one of the largest reported in the literature of young women with endometrial cancer. In an earlier study, the youngest patient with endometrial cancer reported in the English language literature was a 15-year-old female in a study of 10 patients who ranged up to 25 years. All but one of these women had grade 1 tumors.

From these studies, we can infer that in the United States, in 2002, between 780 and 5,500 women will present with endometrial cancer at age 40 years or less, that is, in their childbearing years. Thus, as more women in the United States postpone childbearing, the possibility of developing endometrial cancer or its premalignant precursor, complex atypical hyperplasia (CAH), increases. As this is a disease of the obese anovulatory young woman, and the incidence of obesity is increasing in the United States, so too will the incidence of low-grade endometrial carcinoma.

This chapter will focus on the primary hormonal treatment of young women with endometrioid adenocarcinoma of the endometrium who wish to preserve their uterus to maintain fertility options. All the data discussed will also apply to the older woman with endometrial cancer who is a nonsurgical candidate for medical reasons. However, many of these older women for whom fertility is not an issue may be better served by primary radiation therapy if they cannot undergo surgery.

ENDOMETRIAL CANCER PREMALIGNANT LESION

Kurman and Norris's classic paper in *Cancer* demonstrated the premalignant potential of CAH as well as the difficulties facing pathologists in making this diagnosis accurately and reliably, especially on the basis of preoperative dilatation and curettage (D & C).[20] In Kurman and Norris's *retrospective* study, 29% of patients with a preoperative diagnosis of CAH actually had grade 1 endometrioid adenocarcinoma on the final hysterectomy specimen (Figures 9–1 to 9–3). For that reason, many clinicians will counsel a woman who is peri- or postmenopausal and a good surgical candidate to undergo hysterectomy as definitive treatment for CAH. One must also understand from these statistics that in treating any young woman with CAH with progesterone, there is a significant chance that the clinician is actually treating an undiagnosed grade 1 adenocarcinoma.

A similar study to Kurman and Norris' is currently being conducted by the Gynecology Oncology Group (GOG) in a prospective fashion. This study (GOG-167) has two parts. In part A, the GOG is determining the accuracy of diagnosis of CAH by all pathologists by performing a central pathologic review of D & C specimens from both academic and community practices diagnosed as CAH. The preoperative diagnosis will then be compared with the final diagnosis on the hysterectomy specimen. Part A of the study, therefore, will provide information both on the accuracy of diagnosis of CAH across all practices and the predictive value of a preoperative diagnosis of CAH.

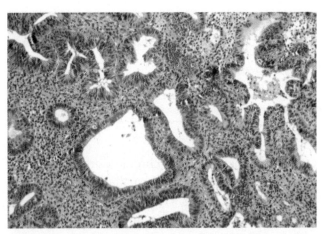

Figure 9–2.   Complex atypical hyperplasia (hematoxylin and eosin; ×10 magnification).

Because this study is being performed prospectively and because all women will undergo standard treatment with hysterectomy, this study should provide clinicians with better information regarding counseling patients with the diagnosis of CAH.

CHARACTERISTICS OF YOUNG WOMEN WITH ENDOMETRIAL CANCER

The anticipated characteristic of a patient with a hyperestrogenic state would be that of anovulation, commonly associated with the polycystic ovary syndrome (PCO) (Table 9–1). Most often, PCO is also associated with the findings of obesity, irregular menses, and excess endogenous estrogen, although women with PCO can also be of normal weight. The "classic" young woman with endometrial cancer is obese, nulliparous, and has irregular to no menstrual

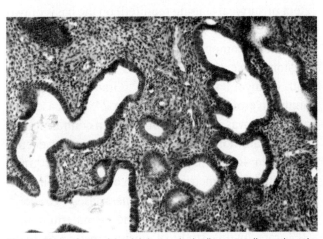

Figure 9–1.   Cystic (simple) hyperplasia (hematoxylin and eosin; ×10 magnification).

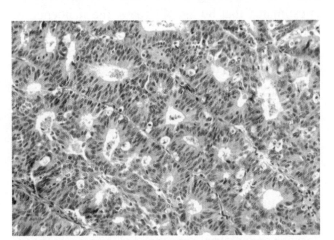

Figure 9–3.   Well-differentiated (grade 1) endometrioid adenocarcinoma (hematoxylin and eosin; ×10 magnification).

Table 9–1. CHARACTERISTICS OF YOUNG WOMEN WITH ENDOMETRIAL CANCER
Diagnosis made during infertility evaluation
Polycystic ovary syndrome
Genetic syndrome
Estrogen-producing ovarian tumors
Obesity and anovulation/increased sex hormone-binding globulin

cycles and, therefore, has chronic estrogen stimulation of her endometrium and usually grade 1 endometrial cancer as a result. Often, these women present with the primary complaint of infertility, and their endometrial cancer may be diagnosed by endometrial biopsy during infertility evaluation. Those women who present with infertility complaints are usually either amenorrheic or oligomenorrheic. The endometrium is often sampled as part of the infertility evaluation in the office or as part of a diagnostic laparoscopy done in the operating room. Once the diagnosis of endometrial cancer or CAH is made, the endometrial abnormality must be treated prior to proceeding with fertility treatment. These women are believed to have an excellent prognosis, with grade 1 tumors that often are confined to the endometrium and associated with adjacent CAH (see Chapter 6).

Alternatively, endometrial cancer in a young woman may represent part of a genetic syndrome (see Chapter 3). One such syndrome that includes endometrial cancer is the hereditary nonpolyposis cancer syndrome (HNPCC), or Lynch syndrome II, which includes colorectal cancer and endometrial cancer. Cancer of the endometrium is the second most common malignancy in Lynch syndrome II. It is estimated that by age 40 years, the incidence of endometrial malignancy for women with Lynch syndrome II is 1% annually, with a cumulative incidence by age 70 years of 60%.[21]

Finally, endometrial cancer can be associated with tumors of the ovary that produce estrogen. One such tumor is the granulosa cell tumor, which often produces high levels of estrogen. Young women may present with an ovarian mass, irregular menses, and/or infertility. Treatment involves removal of the ovarian tumor as well as D & C, which should always be performed in the setting of granulosa cell tumors because endometrial cancer or cancer precursors are so common in this setting.[22]

STANDARD OF CARE TREATMENT FOR ENDOMETRIAL CANCER

The primary use of hormonal therapy to manage low-risk endometrial cancer, by definition, omits surgical removal of the uterus as well as surgical staging, thus eliminating valuable prognostic information. The importance of surgical staging was first demonstrated by Lewis and colleagues, who documented the propensity of endometrial carcinoma to spread to the regional lymph nodes in the pelvis.[23] Subsequently, this observation was validated by the prospective GOG study of clinical stage I endometrial cancer reported by Creasman and colleagues.[24] This study defined a standard from which current practice was developed. The prognostic importance of lymph node status as well as the value of the depth of myometrial invasion in predicting the risk of nodal metastases (and adjuvant treatment recommendations) were demonstrated, and, as a result, surgical staging became the standard of care. The GOG defines surgical staging of endometrial cancer as including exploratory laparotomy (including exploration of the upper abdomen), pelvic washings, total abdominal hysterectomy, bilateral salpingo-oophorectomy, and sampling of pelvic and para-aortic lymph nodes (see Chapter 4). Adjuvant therapy (usually radiation) recommendations are made on the basis of tumor grade, depth of muscle invasion, and status of lymph nodes (see Chapter 7).

The results of the GOG staging study help clinicians to preoperatively and intraoperatively predict the surgical stage of disease (and thus, decide on the extent of surgical staging required) on the basis of two factors, neither of which can be 100% predicted preoperatively: tumor grade and depth of myometrial invasion. First, tumor grade can be correlated with depth of myometrial invasion.[24] Grade 1 tumors are noninvasive of the myometrium in 24% of cases but are deeply invasive in 10% of cases. In contrast, grade 3 tumors are noninvasive in 7% of cases but deeply invasive in 42% of cases. Second, both tumor grade and depth of myometrial invasion can be combined to predict risk of lymph node metastases. Grade 1 tumors that are noninvasive of the myometrium have a 0% rate in this study of positive pelvic or para-aortic nodes; in fact, the rate of lymph nodes metastases for *noninvasive* tumors of any grade is 3% or less. Grade 1 tumors that are deeply invasive, however, have an 11% rate of positive pelvic lymph nodes and a 6% rate of positive para-aortic nodes (indicating the need for adjuvant therapy). In contrast, grade 3 tumors that are deeply invasive are associated with positive pelvic nodes in 34% of cases and positive para-aortic nodes in 23% of cases.

The "standards" that help to determine the need for adjuvant therapy are only available if the complete surgery is performed. It has been demonstrated that preoperative tumor grade (determined on the basis of either office endometrial biopsy [EMB] or D & C) is not uniformly predictive of final tumor grade on hysterectomy. However, as the data presented below will demonstrate, a preoperative diagnosis of grade 1 cancer is more reliable than a diagnosis of grade 2 or 3 cancer.

PREDICTING GRADE

The 1985 study from Cowles and colleagues compared clinical staging with surgical staging in 62 consecutive patients.[25] In this study, 34% of patients had their preoperative grade changed on examination of the hysterectomy specimen. The study demonstrated that grade 1 tumors were upgraded as a result of surgery in 11% of cases. In contrast, grade 2 tumors were more likely to be upgraded (36%). Overall, although change of grade was 34%, rate of upgrading (more concerning when one is considering uterine preservation) was 19%. The paper did not detail whether the grade changed by more than one grade (either up or down).

A much larger study was reported by Daniel and Peters in 1988.[26] These authors reported their results from a retrospective review of 223 patients and looked at differences between EMB and D & C in preoperative grading. In this study, there was an overall upgrading rate of 15 to 20%. Table 9–2 was constructed from this study's results by combining data from both biopsy methods. (The "noresidual tumor" category was left out of Table 9–2, which is why the total number is not 223.)

In this study, only 1 case out of a total of 122 grade 1 tumors went up *more* than one grade. The two studies demonstrate that we do best predicting postopera-

tive grade correctly when the preoperative grade is 1 (and worst when the preoperative grade is 3).

Finally, a recent study is the multicentric Austrian study of Obermair and colleagues, who reviewed 137 consecutive patients with grade 1 adenocarcinoma of the endometrium and published the results in 1999. Of the 137 subjects, 78% had grade 1 tumors at hysterectomy, while 20.4% were upgraded.[27]

PREDICTING MYOMETRIAL INVASION AND LYMPH NODE STATUS

There is no completely reliable method to preoperatively determine depth of myometrial invasion, and there is no reliable way currently to predict lymph node status. Methods of assessing depth of myometrial invasion, including computed tomography (CT), ultrasonography, and magnetic resonance imaging (MRI), have all been suggested (see Chapter 4). None is completely reliable, and all are more accurate when detecting deep rather than superficial invasion. For determination of myometrial invasion, the accuracy of transabdominal ultrasonography has been reported to be 79% and for transvaginal ultrasonography, 60 to 77%.[28–31] Computed tomography is useful for identifying large volume extrauterine disease, but it fails to detect microscopic lymph node disease.[32] Accuracy of CT in predicting myometrial invasion has been reported to be 61 to 76%, increasing to 83% with deep invasion.[29,30,33] The accuracy of MRI ranges from 58 to 89% in determining myometrial invasion.[28,30] For both CT and MRI, the postmenopausal woman presents a special diagnostic difficulty because of the lack of a junctional zone (between the endometrium and the

Table 9–2. PREOPERATIVE COMPARED WITH POSTOPERATIVE GRADE OF TUMOR					
Preoperative Grade	n	Postoperative Grade			Total Upgraded
		1	2	3	
1	122	100 82%	21 17%	1 1%	22 18%
2	64	15 23%	43 67%	6 9%	6 9%
3	19	4 21%	4 11%	11 58%	None
Total					28/205 14%

myometrium). When dynamic contrast-enhanced MRI is used, accuracy rates increase to 85 to 93%.[33,34] Because MRI is the most accurate of the radiologic diagnostic techniques in assessing myometrial invasion, it is the one most frequently recommended to predict preoperatively the amount/presence of superficial myometrial invasion.[30,33,35] Like CT, MRI will not be able to accurately distinguish microscopically positive retroperitoneal lymph nodes.

CLINICAL DATA SUPPORTING PRIMARY HORMONAL THERAPY

Suggesting that a woman receive treatment less than the standard of care for a typically curable but potentially lethal disease, on the basis of tumor grade from a small biopsy and MRI prediction of myometrial invasion, therefore, is controversial at best. Nevertheless, multiple retrospective studies have suggested that uterine preservation in the setting of endometrial cancer may be safe under certain circumstances. One must keep in mind when reviewing this data that these studies are retrospective. Patients are not selected in a well-defined way nor are they treated in a standard fashion. In many of the studies, patients are gathered from pathology files and, often, are not treated primarily at the reporting institution.

One of the earliest reports was that of Bokhman and colleagues in 1985.[36] This study was reported prior to the surgical staging study of the GOG described above. In this report, 19 patients with endometrial cancer were treated with progesterone. Eleven had grade 1 tumors, and 8 had grade 2 tumors; all had *clinical* stage I disease. Seventeen patients had primary infertility and 14 were obese. All patients were treated with 500 mg/d of intramuscular oxyprogesterone caproate. After 3 months, all patients had their endometrium resampled to determine response. If the cancer persisted after 3 months, the patient was treated with hysterectomy. Of the 19 patients treated, 15 had complete resolution of their tumor. This study was the only one that included patients with grade 2 tumors.

In 1989, Lee and Scully reported on 10 young women with CAH and grade 1 adenocarcinoma ranging in age from 15 to 20 years.[37] There were 4 cases of adenocarcinoma and 6 cases of CAH. Four patients with CAH were treated with hormones, and, of these patients, 2 women had 3 successful pregnancies. Figure 9–4 demonstrates resolution of neoplactic epithelial changes with progestin. All 4 patients with cancer were treated with hormones, with one patient ultimately requiring hysterectomy. Pregnancy information was not provided for the patients with cancer.

Randall and Kurman reported their experience at Johns Hopkins Hospital in 1997.[38] They reviewed the treatment of 67 cases of atypical hyperplasia (32) and well-differentiated adenocarcinoma (35) over a 7-year period. Among the 33 women with adenocarcinoma considered eligible for the study, 12 were

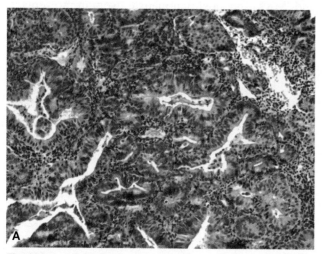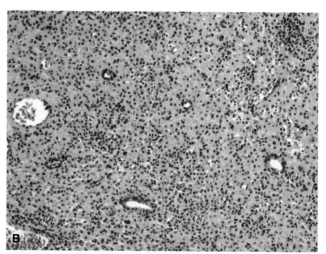

Figure 9–4.   *A,* Pretreatment appearance of grade 1 endometrioid adenocarcinoma. *B,* Post-treatment curettage from patient seen in *A* showing marked glandular atrophy and prominent stromal decidual change (hematoxylin and eosin; ×10 magnification).

treated with progestins, of whom 9 had regression of their lesions and 3 had progression. Most of the patients were treated with "high-dose progestins," although the treatment was not standardized. Most women were treated with megestrol acetate, ranging in dose from 80 mg/d to 400 mg/d. In this study, no woman had a tumor become more aggressive histologically, defined as a change from grade 1 to a higher-grade tumor on follow-up sampling. Two women were found to have coexistent ovarian carcinomas. Both of these were stage I endometrioid adenocarcinomas of the ovary thought to be second primaries. One patient who did have regression of her tumor was later found to have a recurrence and was successfully re-treated with hormonal therapy.

Kim and colleagues reported their experience at the University of California Los Angeles (UCLA) in the same year.[18] They reported 21 total patients with clinical stage IA grade 1 disease, 7 from their own institution and 14 from the literature. All data were combined in the report. Thirteen of 21 patients had an initial response to the progestin therapy (62% compared with 75% in Randall and Kurman's study). Three initial responders later developed recurrent disease, one of whom had extrauterine disease at laparotomy. Eight of 21 patients did not respond to progestins. Six infants were delivered by 3 patients. One patient had 1 delivery, one patient had 2 deliveries, and one patients had 3 deliveries.

Details were available for the 7 patients treated at the primary institution (UCLA). Seven premenopausal patients were treated with progestin alone, with an age range of 19 to 41 years. Four of the 7 were obese and were thought to have PCO, and 2 patients had a history of infertility. All 7 had grade 1 tumors and were treated with megestrol acetate at a dose of 160 mg/d. Four of the 7 had an initial response to therapy, and 2 of these later developed recurrent disease. Three patients did not have an initial response and were treated with hysterectomy. No pregnancies resulted from these 7 patients.

The other 14 patients reported in Kim's series were gathered from the literature. These patients ranged in age from 15 to 35 years, and all had grade 1 cancers. Obviously because of the retrospective nature of this collection, patients were treated with a variety of progestin regimens. Nine of

14 had an initial response to progestins, with 8 of 9 remaining free of recurrence at last follow-up. One patient subsequently developed a recurrent tumor and, when treated with surgical therapy, was found to have extrauterine disease. Three patients delivered viable infants.

The authors make the point that progestin therapy is not without risk. Three patients who were initial responders did later develop recurrence, and one of these was found to have extrauterine disease. In this particular patient, progestin therapy delayed definitive surgery and, therefore, may have adversely affected her prognosis. Like Randall and Kurman's study, all patients in Kim and colleagues' report had grade 1 tumors.

Our own study, reported in 2001, included 95 patients age 40 years and under with endometrial cancer.[17] Of these 95, 12 women were treated with progestins. Again, the study was retrospective, and, therefore, there was no standardization of therapy. The 12 women ranged in age from 24 to 40 years, and 8 presented with infertility as their primary complaint. All had grade 1 tumors. Two eventually required hysterectomy for persistent endometrial cancer, and one of these subsequently developed an endometrioid adenocarcinoma of the ovary. Four women achieved pregnancy, and 5 viable infants were delivered.

There are a large number of case reports, usually reporting one to four cases, of women with endometrial cancer who have achieved pregnancy (Table 9–3).[39–43] Most of the women described in these reports had grade 1 tumors that were extensively "clinically" staged with D & C, plus or minus hysteroscopy, CT, and/or MRI, and laparoscopy. One report is notable for a woman who achieved a successful triplet pregnancy but later was diagnosed with a tumor primary in the ovary. It is of note that many of these women reported were diagnosed during infertility evaluation, and many required artificial reproductive technology (ART) to achieve pregnancy. One must realize when considering these reports the phenomenon of selective recall bias. Because authors are more likely to report cases that are successes rather than failures, it is possible, if not likely, that the true pregnancy rate is lower, and, perhaps more importantly, that the risk of morbidity or death due to avoiding surgery may be higher.

Table 9–3. EXAMPLES OF CASE REPORTS				
Study	# of Patients	Grade of Tumor	Treatment	Pregnancy Outcome
Ogawa[39]	1	1	MPA 400 mg/d for 12 wk IVF	Singleton
Jobo[40]	2	1	MPA 600 mg/d Ovulation induction	Twins Singleton
Sardi[41]	4	Not stated	Not stated	2 patients had 3 babies
Shibahara[42]	1	1	Not stated IVF	Singleton
Kung[43]	1	1	Tamoxifen and megestrol acetate Doses not stated	

IVF = in vitro fertilization; MPA = medroxyprogesterone acetate.

To complicate matters further, there is no consensus among clinicians about (1) which progesterone formulation to use, (2) what schedule to use, (3) what dose to use, (4) how long to treat, and (5) how often to resample. Most clinicians agree that patients should be treated for at least 1 to 3 months prior to resampling to determine resolution. If carcinoma persists, some clinicians will then advise the patient to undergo hysterectomy, whereas others may continue with progesterone at a higher dosage. While many gynecologic oncologists use megestrol acetate as their first choice of progesterone, many also use medroxyprogesterone acetate (the GOG study uses this progesterone). Whether the drug is given cyclically, to allow a withdrawal bleed each month, or continuously is also debatable. The dose of megestrol acetate may vary by clinician from 40 mg qd to 40 mg qid to 200 mg qd (or higher). Although it is very unlikely that a prospective evaluation of progestin will be evaluated in this clinical scenario, it is notable that there is little evidence that progestin type or dose is important in the treatment of metastatic endometrial cancer (see Chapter 8). Finally, once regression of the endometrial neoplasia is achieved, there is no consensus on how often to resample, whether the patient with presumed unopposed estrogen should be maintained on progestins, or whether a patient should undergo completion hysterectomy once fertility is no longer an issue.

One institution, Johns Hopkins, has performed a study of the progesterone intrauterine device (IUD) in treating endometrial cancer.[44] Women with grade 1 endometrial cancer who were considered poor surgical candidates by virtue of American Society of Anesthesiologists statue were treated with progesterone IUD after radiologic findings confirmed noninvasive disease. Of the 12 women who completed the prospective trial, 6 had negative biopsies at the 12 month mark, indicating disease resolution.

Women with endometrial cancer treated with progesterone often then require ART to achieve pregnancy. Because ART generates very high serum estradiol levels (which, thereby, put the patient at high risk of recurrence of her endometrial cancer if pregnancy is not achieved), many community in vitro fertilization (IVF) programs may feel uncomfortable providing this essentially elective service. Moreover, from a reproductive standpoint, many of these women are older, which makes them more likely to have unsuccessful IVF attempts and more likely to require more than one attempt at ovulation induction to achieve pregnancy.

MECHANISMS OF HORMONE RECEPTOR ACTION IN ENDOMETRIAL CANCER

In order to make knowledgeable decisions about how and when a patient with endometrial cancer or CAH may be treated with progesterone, clinicians need a better understanding of the action of progesterone on the endometrium at the molecular and genetic levels. Although there is a plethora of *clinical* and *epidemiologic* data, as outlined above, with regard to the success of progesterone therapy both in preventing and reversing malignant change, there is a paucity of data related to the mechanism of action of this steroid hormone at the molecular or genetic level. Until recently, it was thought that there was a "generic" progesterone receptor (PR); currently, we have more information regarding the complexity of the receptor and the interactions between its two isoforms, progesterone receptor A and progesterone receptor B (PRA and PRB). Reportedly, the two isoforms have divergent responses, or alternatively, the ratio of the isoforms might be critical to the ultimate outcome. This could be further complicated by the number of cofactors and corepressors that can influence PR-mediated action.[45–50]

Despite improved understanding of the complexity of the PR receptor and PR-receptor signaling, we are still unable to use this information clinically. For example, in women with advanced endometrial cancer who are being treated with progesterone in the clinical setting, we are often unaware of the progesterone receptor status of the tumor, or we are only able to assess whether the PR is present and not answer more complex questions, such as: Is PRA or PRB present, and what is the ratio of these receptors? The answers to these questions might allow us to predict an individual patient's response to the steroid treatment being considered.

A better understanding of both the development and regression of endometrial cancer has become one of the focuses of the GOG and will be part B of the study of CAH described above. In part B of GOG-167, the GOG will be studying women with complex atypical hyperplasia who are first treated with progesterone for 3 months and then undergo hysterectomy. However, future studies may be needed to consider earlier time points to assess acute changes that result from progesterone therapy. The hysterectomy specimen will then be examined histologically to determine response to therapy. The choice of dose and schedule of progesterone (medroxyprogesterone acetate at 10 mg po qd versus Depo-Provera 150 mg IM q month, for 3 months) is based on the experience of the investigators. If the study demonstrates a high success rate for either of the doses, schedules, and types of progesterone, it might also then establish a new standard for treatment of CAH (and by extension, grade 1 endometrioid adenocarcinoma).

The majority of endometrioid endometrial cancers express PR, with PR levels and expression tending to vary with histologic grade of tumor.[51–53] The presence of PR has been correlated with well-differentiated tumors and better prognosis, as well as

response to progesterone treatment.[54–58] However, there is a variable response observed in patients with a tumor that has PR-positive and -negative areas.[59–62] Biologic effects may also be dependent on the ratio of PRA and PRB and the tissue in which the receptors are expressed.[63] Therefore, information about the generic PR receptor (usually provided by immunohistochemistry) may not be predictive of progesterone response.

An example of this problem is provided by the study of Arnett-Mansfield and colleagues.[63] The authors evaluated PR isoforms in archived human endometrial cancer tissue. They found that whereas 96% of tumors investigated expressed PR, 30% of tumors expressed PRA alone, 42% expressed both isoforms, and 28% expressed PRB alone. PRB-only tumors had low levels of PR. Those tumors that expressed both isoforms tended to express predominantly PRA, and those tumor expressing PRA alone or predominantly PRA represented over one-half of specimens. On the basis of these data, the authors hypothesized that loss of PRB resulted in development of endometrial cancer. Other authors have suggested that the *relative change* in isoform expression is as important as the total level of PR in the genesis of endometrial cancer.[64] Thus, it is likely that it is the ratio of PRA to PRB that is important both in the development of endometrial cancer and in predicting the ultimate success of progesterone therapy. Moreover, one could postulate that a progesterone agonist designed to target one or the other isoform might better achieve a clinical response than a "generic" progesterone that targets both isoforms.

Ultimately, to determine the safety of treating endometrial cancer with progesterone rather than surgery, we will need to perform prospective trials with standardized therapy for a large number of women. Rational prospective clinical trials will require a better understanding of the function/action of progesterones on the A and B receptors.

MONITORING WOMEN ON PROGESTERONE

Most clinicians agree that close surveillance of patients with endometrial cancer following progesterone treatment is necessary. There is not a consensus, however, on how to monitor either response to primary therapy or continued response. Most clinicians will resample between 1 and 3 months after initiating therapy, either via office endometrial biopsy or curettage (with or without hysteroscopy). Once reversal of the endometrial lesion is documented, the underlying condition (excess endogenous estrogen) must be addressed. A young patient can be placed on maintenance therapy with oral contraceptive pills. Older patients may continue a "maintenance" dose of progesterone or use cyclic progesterone to induce a withdrawal bleed at least every 3 to 6 months. A patient desiring pregnancy should actively pursue pregnancy (usually via ART). High progesterone levels during pregnancy should protect against recurrent disease (although endometrial cancer coexisting with pregnancy has been reported).[65–69] Patients should be resampled at least yearly and/or if any episodes of abnormal vaginal bleeding occur. Patients should also be monitored carefully for the possibility of a concurrent ovarian primary with careful pelvic examination, yearly ultrasonography, or both. Completion hysterectomy is usually recommended once childbearing is completed, if the patient is a good surgical candidate.

RISK IN CONSERVATIVE THERAPY

Data regarding the risk of later recurrence can only be gleaned by the large retrospective reviews detailed above; it is otherwise available only in the setting of case reports. In the study by Randall and Kurman, disease recurred in 1 of 35 (3%) women with adenocarcinoma, and, in the study by Kim and colleagues, 3 of 21 (14%) initial responders to progesterone experienced recurrent disease.[18,38] In Kim and colleagues' study, one patient who ultimately went to surgery had evidence of metastatic disease, and the authors raised the possibility of the progesterone therapy delaying definitive therapy, thereby possibly resulting in development of metastatic disease.[18] Certainly, this postponement of therapy is a significant concern. Although the risk of developing metastatic disease is probably low, given the slow growth rate of grade 1 tumors and the low rate of high-stage disease in endometrial cancer, the exact risk is unknown, making counseling of these women difficult.

There is a risk, although small, of endometrial cancer embolizing through the fallopian tube and metastasizing to the ovary. In the GOG staging study of clinical stage I endometrial cancer, the risk was 5%.[24] Gross ovarian metastases can be ruled out via pelvic examination and/or pelvic ultrasonography, but micrometastases cannot be easily demonstrated without histologic examination of the ovaries.

Several authors have demonstrated that women with endometrioid adenocarcinomas of the endometrium have a risk of concurrent primary in the ovary.[70–72] Coexistence of carcinoma in the ovary and endometrium occurs in slightly more than 5% of patients. In our own study, 10% of young women with endometrial cancer had a concurrent ovarian primary tumor.[17] Recently, the GOG performed a prospective trial of women with both ovarian and endometrial tumors.[73] Seventy-four patients were included in the study, and, in this study, most tumors were low grade and endometrioid in subtype. Most of these tumors are believed to be synchronous primaries, rather than a metastasis from one organ to the other.

FUTURE DIRECTIONS

As women in the United States continue to postpone childbearing, the risk of endometrial cancer during childbearing years will increase. Counseling of these women regarding uterine preservation is hampered by a lack of data and lack of standardized therapy. Prospective clinical trials will need to be performed to establish both the safety and efficacy of progesterone therapy as well as a standard drug, dose, and schedule of treatment and monitoring.

Prior to performing prospective trials, we will require a better understanding of the action of progesterone on the endometrium and its malignant lesions. Increased knowledge about the progesterone receptor and its isoforms will be needed before we can make clinical recommendations. Studies in cell lines are already reported, and studies of human tissue in the mouse model are ongoing and should provide valuable insights. GOG-167, once completed, will also provide information regarding the schedule of progesterone and its action on the endometrium.

For the present time, any young woman with endometrial cancer who wishes to preserve her fertility should be managed by a gynecologic oncologist or a clinician with the same experience/ knowledge about endometrial cancer. Only women with grade 1 tumors that appear to be confined to the endometrium should be considered for conservative therapy. Our own study failed to identify clinical factors other than grade that are predictive of stage IA disease and, thus, presumably predictive of successful conservative therapy. We support Kim and colleagues' conclusion that only women with grade 1 tumors should be considered for uterine conservation. The treating physician must also keep in mind the risk of concurrent ovarian malignancy in this population (range 11 to 29% reported in the literature).[5,9,10] Therefore, ultrasonography or MRI should be used as an imaging modality to aid in "staging" these patients.

Finally, patients who wish to proceed with progesterone therapy rather than surgery need to be counseled that this therapy represents a deviation from the standard of care for this disease. Treating with less than the standard of care could potentially result in a young woman dying of a surgically curable disease.

SUGGESTION FOR A MANAGEMENT SCHEMA

If a young woman diagnosed with endometrial cancer desires to maintain fertility:

- Confirm that the tumor is endometrioid and grade 1 via pathologic review. If the tumor is grade 2 or 3 or of high-risk histology, the patient should be counseled to undergo hysterectomy with bilateral salpingo-oophorectomy and surgical staging.
- Take a careful history and perform a physical examination, with particular attention to pelvic examination and any comorbid medical history (hypertension, diabetes) that might complicate pregnancy.
- Perform MRI (or ultrasonography, if MRI is not available) to rule out adnexal metastases and to assess myometrial invasion.
- If the tumor is well sampled, grade 1, and with no evidence of adnexal metastases or myometrial invasion, the patient should undergo careful informed counseling and then treatment with

progesterone and resampling in 3 months (preferably with D & C plus or minus hysteroscopy).

REFERENCES

1. Jemal A, Thomas A, Murray T, et al. Cancer statistics, 2002. CA Cancer J Clin 2002;52:23–47.
2. Creasman W, Odicino F, Maisonneuve P, et al. Carcinoma of the corpus uteri. J Epidemiol Biostat 2001;6:47–86.
3. Peterson EP. Endometrial carcinoma in young women. A clinical profile. Obstet Gynecol 1968;31:702–7.
4. Kempson RL, Pokorny GE. Adenocarcinoma of the endometrium in women aged forty and younger. Cancer 1968;21:650–62.
5. Crissman JD, Azoury RS, Barnes AE, et al. Endometrial carcinoma in women 40 years of age or younger. Obstet Gynecol 1981;57:699–704.
6. Gallup DG, Stock RJ. Adenocarcinoma of the endometrium in women 40 years of age or younger. Obstet Gynecol 1984;64:417–20.
7. Farhi DC, Nosanchuk J, Silverberg SG. Endometrial adenocarcinoma in women under 25 years of age. Obstet Gynecol 1986;68:741–5.
8. Jeffery JD, Taylor R, Robertson DI, et al. Endometrial carcinoma occurring in patients under the age of 45 years. Am J Obstet Gynecol 1987;156:366–70.
9. Gitsch G, Hanzal E, Jensen D, et al. Endometrial cancer in premenopausal women 45 years and younger. Obstet Gynecol 1995;85:504–8.
10. Evans-Metcalf ER, Brooks SE, Reale FR, et al. Profile of women 45 years of age and younger with endometrial cancer. Obstet Gynecol 1998;91:349–54.
11. Ziel HK, Finkle WD. Increased risk of endometrial carcinoma among users of conjugated estrogens. N Engl J Med 1975;293:1167–70.
12. Smith DC, Prentice R, Thompson DJ, et al. Association of exogenous estrogen and endometrial carcinoma. N Engl J Med 1975;293:1164–7.
13. Mack TM, Pike MC, Henderson BE, et al. Estrogens and endometrial cancer in a retirement community. N Engl J Med 1976;294:1262–7.
14. McDonald TW, Annegers JF, O'Fallon WM, et al. Exogenous estrogen and endometrial carcinoma: case-control and incidence study. Am J Obstet Gynecol 1977;127:572–80.
15. Greenwald P, Caputo TA, Wolfgang PE. Endometrial cancer after menopausal use of estrogens. Obstet Gynecol 1977;50:239–43.
16. Gray LA Sr, Christopherson WM, Hoover RN. Estrogens and endometrial carcinoma. Obstet Gynecol 1977;49:385–9.
17. Duska LR, Garrett A, Rueda BR, et al. Endometrial cancer in women 40 years old or younger. Gynecol Oncol 2001;83:388–93.
18. Kim YB, Holschneider CH, Ghosh K, et al. Progestin alone as primary treatment of endometrial carcinoma in premenopausal women. Report of seven cases and review of the literature. Cancer 1997;79:320–7.
19. Randall TC, Kurman RJ. Progestin treatment of atypical hyperplasia and well-differentiated carcinoma of the

endometrium in women under age 40. Obstet Gynecol 1997;90:434–40.

20. Kurman RJ, Norris HJ. Evaluation of criteria for distinguishing atypical endometrial hyperplasia from well-differentiated carcinoma. Cancer 1982;49:2547–59.

21. Fornasarig M, Viel A, Bidoli E, et al. Amsterdam criteria II and endometrial cancer index cases for an accurate selection of HNPCC families. Tumori 2002;88:18–20.

22. Gebhart JB, Roche PC, Keeney GL, et al. Assessment of inhibin and p53 in granulosa cell tumors of the ovary. Gynecol Oncol 2000;77:232–6.

23. Lewis BV, Stallworthy JA, Cowdell R. Adenocarcinoma of the body of the uterus. J Obstet Gynaecol Br Commonw 1970;77:343–8.

24. Creasman WT, Morrow CP, Bundy BN, et al. Surgical pathologic spread patterns of endometrial cancer. A Gynecologic Oncology Group Study. Cancer 1987;60:2035–41.

25. Cowles TA, Magrina JF, Masterson BJ, et al. Comparison of clinical and surgical-staging in patients with endometrial carcinoma. Obstet Gynecol 1985;66:413–6.

26. Daniel AG, Peters WA III. Accuracy of office and operating room curettage in the grading of endometrial carcinoma. Obstet Gynecol 1988;71:612–4.

27. Obermair A, Geramou M, Gucer F, et al. Endometrial cancer: accuracy of the finding of well-differentiated tumor at dilatation and curettage compared to the findings at subsequent hysterectomy. Int J Gynecol Cancer 1999;9:383–6.

28. DelMaschio A, Vanzulli A, Sironi S, et al. Estimating the depth of myometrial involvement by endometrial carcinoma: efficacy of transvaginal sonography vs MR imaging. AJR Am J Roentgenol 1993;160:533–8.

29. Gordon AN, Fleischer AC, Dudley BS, et al. Preoperative assessment of myometrial invasion of endometrial adenocarcinoma by sonography (US) and magnetic resonance imaging (MRI). Gynecol Oncol 1989;34:175–9.

30. Kim SH. Detection of deep myometrial invasion in endometrial carcinoma: comparison of transvaginal ultrasound, CT, and MRI. J Cell Biol 1995;130:1127–36.

31. Olaya FJ. Transvaginal sonography in endometrial carcinoma: preoperative assessment of the depth of myometrial invasion in 50 cases. Appl Environ Microbiol 2000;66:476–80.

32. Zerbe MJ, Bristow R, Grumbine FC, et al. Inability of preoperative computed tomography scans to accurately predict the extent of myometrial invasion and extracorporal spread in endometrial cancer. Gynecol Oncol 2000;78:67–70.

33. Hardesty LA, Sumkin JH, Hakim C, et al. The ability of helical CT to preoperatively stage endometrial carcinoma. AJR Am J Roentgenol 2001;176:603–6.

34. Seki H, Kimura M, Sakai K. Myometrial invasion of endometrial carcinoma: assessment with dynamic MR and contrast-enhanced T1-weighted images. Clin Radiol 1997;52:18–23.

35. Frei KA, Kinkel K. Staging endometrial cancer: role of magnetic resonance imaging. J Magn Reson Imaging 2001; 13:850–5.

36. Bokhman JV, Chepick OF, Volkova AT, et al. Can primary endometrial carcinoma stage I be cured without surgery and radiation therapy? Gynecol Oncol 1985;20:139–55.

37. Lee KR, Scully RE. Complex endometrial hyperplasia and

carcinoma in adolescents and young women 15 to 20 years of age. A report of 10 cases. Int J Gynecol Pathol 1989;8:201–13.

38. Randall TC, Kurman RJ. Progestin treatment of atypical hyperplasia and well-differentiated carcinoma of the endometrium in women under age 40. Obstet Gynecol 1997;90:434–40.

39. Ogawa S, Koike T, Shibahara H, et al. Assisted reproductive technologies in conjunction with conservatively treated endometrial adenocarcinoma. A case report. Gynecol Obstet Invest 2001;51:214–6.

40. Jobo T, Imai M, Kawaguchi M, et al. Successful conservative treatment of endometrial carcinoma permitting subsequent pregnancy: report of two cases. Eur J Gynaecol Oncol 2000;21:119–22.

41. Sardi J. Primary hormonal treatment for early endometrial carcinoma. Hum Reprod 1997;12:1649–53.

42. Shibahara H. Successful pregnancy in an infertile patient with conservatively treated endometrial adenocarcinoma after transfer of embryos obtained by intracytoplasmic sperm injection. Cancer Lett 2001;167:39–48.

43. Kung FT, Chen WJ, Chou HH, et al. Conservative management of early endometrial adenocarcinoma with repeat curettage and hormone therapy under assistance of hysteroscopy and laparoscopy. Hum Reprod 1997;12:1649–53.

44. Montz FJ, Bristow RE, Bovicelli A, et al. Intrauterine progesterone treatment of early endometrial cancer. Am J Obstet Gynecol 2002;186:651–7.

45. Conneely OM. Progesterone receptors in reproduction: functional impact of the A and B isoforms. Science 2000; 289:1751–4.

46. Conneely OM, Mulac-Jericevic B, Lydon JP, et al. Reproductive functions of the progesterone receptor isoforms: lessons from knock-out mice. Mol Cell Endocrinol 2001; 179:97–103.

47. Conneely OM. Perspective: female steroid hormone action. Arthritis Rheum 2001;44:782–93.

48. Rowan BG, Bai W. Progesterone receptor coactivators: differential phosphorylation of chicken progesterone receptor in hormone-dependent and ligand-independent activation. Steroids 2000;65:545–9.

49. Spitz IM. Progesterone receptor modulators at the start of a new millennium. Steroids 2000;65:817–23.

50. Bouchard P. Progesterone and the progesterone receptor. J Reprod Med 1999;44:153–7.

51. Ehrlich CE, Young PC, Cleary RE. Cytoplasmic progesterone and estradiol receptors in normal, hyperplastic, and carcinomatous endometria: therapeutic implications. Am J Obstet Gynecol 1981;141:539–46.

52. Ehrlich CE, Young PC, Stehman FB, et al. Steroid receptors and clinical outcome in patients with adenocarcinoma of the endometrium. Am J Obstet Gynecol 1988;158: 796–807.

53. Creasman WT, Soper JT, McCarty KS, et al. Influence of cytoplasmic steroid receptor content on prognosis of early stage endometrial carcinoma. Am J Obstet Gynecol 1985;151:922–32.

54. Nyholm HC, Nielsen AL, Lyndrup J, et al. Biochemical and immunohistochemical estrogen and progesterone receptors in adenomatous hyperplasia and endometrial carci-

noma: correlations with stage and other clinicopathologic features. Am J Obstet Gynecol 1992;167:1334–42.

55. Kleine W, Maier T, Geyer H, et al. Estrogen and progesterone receptors in endometrial cancer and their prognostic relevance. Gynecol Oncol 1990;38:59–65.

56. Sutton GP, Geisler HE, Stehman FB, et al. Features associated with survival and disease-free survival in early endometrial cancer. Am J Obstet Gynecol 1989;160:1385–91; discussion 1391–3.

57. Chambers JT, MacLusky N, Eisenfield A, et al. Estrogen and progestin receptor levels as prognosticators for survival in endometrial cancer. Gynecol Oncol 1988;31:65–81.

58. Fukuda K, Mori M, Uchiyama M, et al. Prognostic significance of progesterone receptor immunohistochemistry in endometrial carcinoma. Gynecol Oncol 1998;69:220–5.

59. Benraad TJ, Friberg LG, Koenders AJ, et al. Do estrogen and progesterone receptors (E2R and PR) in metastasizing endometrial cancers predict the response to gestagen therapy? Acta Obstet Gynecol Scand 1980;59:155–9.

60. Creasman WT, McCarty KS Sr, Barton TK, et al. Clinical correlates of estrogen- and progesterone-binding proteins in human endometrial adenocarcinoma. Obstet Gynecol 1980;55:363–70.

61. Martin PM, Rolland PH, Gammerre M, et al. Estradiol and progesterone receptors in normal and neoplastic endometrium: correlations between receptors, histopathological examinations and clinical responses under progestin therapy. Int J Cancer 1979;23:321–9.

62. Kauppila A, Kujansuu E, Vihko R. Cytosol estrogen and progestin receptors in endometrial carcinoma of patients treated with surgery, radiotherapy, and progestin. Clinical correlates. Cancer 1982;50:2157–62.

63. Arnett-Mansfield RL, deFazio A, Wain GV, et al. Relative expression of progesterone receptors A and B in endometrioid cancers of the endometrium. Cancer Res 2001;61:4576–82.

64. Dai D, Kumar NS, Wolf DM, et al. Molecular tools to reestablish progestin control of endometrial cancer cell proliferation. Am J Obstet Gynecol 2001;184:790–7.

65. Ayhan A, Gunalp S, Karaer C, et al. Endometrial adenocarcinoma in pregnancy. Gynecol Oncol 1999;75:298–9.

66. Mitsushita J, Toki T, Kato K, et al. Endometrial carcinoma remaining after term pregnancy following conservative treatment with medroxyprogesterone acetate. Gynecol Oncol 2000;79:129–32.

67. Vaccarello L. Endometrial carcinoma associated with pregnancy: a report of three cases and review of the literature. Br J Obstet Gynaecol 1994;101:547–9.

68. Hoffman MS, Cavanagh D, Walter TS, et al. Adenocarcinoma of the endometrium and endometrioid carcinoma of the ovary associated with pregnancy. Gynecol Oncol 1989; 32:82–5.

69. Schneller JA, Nicastri AD. Intrauterine pregnancy coincident with endometrial carcinoma: a case study and review of the literature. Gynecol Oncol 1994;54:87–90.

70. Zaino RJ, Unger ER, Whitney C. Synchronous carcinomas of the uterine corpus and ovary. Gynecol Oncol 1984;19: 329–35.

71. Piura B, Glezerman M. Synchronous carcinomas of endometrium and ovary. Gynecol Oncol 1989;33:261–4.

72. Falkenberry SS, Steinhoff MM, Gordinier M, et al. Synchronous endometrioid tumors of the ovary and endometrium. A clinicopathologic study of 22 cases. J Reprod Med 1996;41:713–8.

73. Zaino R, Whitney C, Brady MF, et al. Simultaneously detected endometrial and ovarian carcinomas—a prospective clinicopathologic study of 74 cases: a Gynecologic Oncology Group Study. Gynecol Oncol 2001;83:355–62.

10

Positive Peritoneal Cytology in Women with Endometrial Cancer

URSULA A. MATULONIS, MD
EDMUND S. CIBAS, MD

The goal of peritoneal cytology is to identify microscopic tumor deposits not visualized during surgery. The method was first applied to women with ovarian cancer and has been an established part of the surgical staging system for ovarian cancer for many years.[1,2] The significance of positive peritoneal cytology (PPC) in women with endometrial cancer, however, has been controversial ever since Creasman and Rutledge demonstrated an increased risk of recurrence of endometrial cancer in women with PPC.[3] Peritoneal cytology was incorporated into the revised International Federation of Gynecology and Obstetrics (FIGO) surgical staging system in 1988, and stage IIIA now includes tumors with invasion of the uterine serosa, adnexal involvement, and/or PPC.[4]

Since the work of Creasman and Rutledge over 30 years ago, many investigators have performed a similar investigation with conflicting results and conclusions. This chapter examines the method of cytologic evaluation and its accuracy, the biologic significance of malignant cells in the peritoneal cavity, the mechanisms whereby they enter the peritoneal cavity, the evidence for and against the predictive value of PPC in women with endometrial cancer, and the treatment strategies for women with PPC.

CYTOLOGY: SLIDE PREPARATION, EVALUATION, AND ACCURACY

Peritoneal washings are delivered to the cytology laboratory as a suspension of cells in a physiologic fluid.

An aliquot, typically 100 mL, is centrifuged to a cell pellet in a standard table-top centrifuge. The laboratory has a variety of options for preparing slides from this pellet. Slides can be prepared as direct smears by smearing the pellet onto a slide using a wooden applicator. In current practice, a liquid-based preparation method is more common. There are a variety of acceptable liquid-based methods, which include cytocentrifugation, a filter-transfer method (the ThinPrep technique), and a combined density and gravity sedimentation method (the SurePath technique). Slides prepared in this fashion are most commonly stained with a modified Papanicolaou stain. In many laboratories, the cell pellet, or a portion of it, is also fixed in formalin, embedded in paraffin, and sectioned and stained with hematoxylin and eosin (the "cell block" technique).

A normal peritoneal washing comprises sheets of mesothelial cells, histiocytes, and blood (Figure 10–1).[5] Fragments of skeletal muscle and fat, most likely from the incision site, are sometimes present. Benign mesothelial proliferations, such as those that occur in response to adhesions, can result in psammoma body formation. Psammoma bodies are concentric concretions of calcium, commonly associated with papillary serous tumors of the gynecologic tract. Because they are also occasionally induced by irritated, benign mesothelial cells, psammoma bodies per se are not diagnostic of malignancy. Malignant cells have enlarged nuclei, with coarsely textured chromatin and prominent nucleoli (Figure 10–2).[5] They are either isolated or arranged in clus-

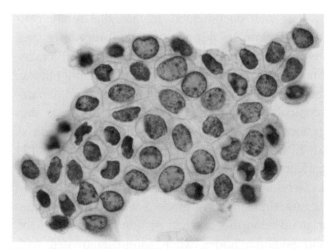

Figure 10–1. Negative peritoneal washing. A benign (ie, "negative") peritoneal washing contains sheets of benign mesothelial cells. The cells are similar to one another and evenly spaced (Papanicolaou stain).

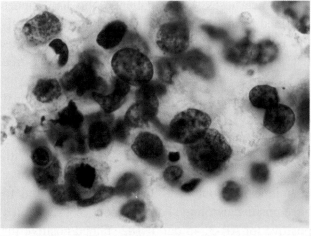

Figure 10–2. Positive peritoneal washing. This positive peritoneal washing is from a woman with an endometrial carcinoma, endometrioid type. The malignant cells are distinguished from benign mesothelial cells by their haphazard arrangement and larger and darker nuclei (Papanicolaou stain).

ters. The degree of nuclear atypia varies from mild to marked, depending on the grade of the tumor. Poor-prognosis types of endometrial cancer, such as papillary serous and clear cell carcinomas, are high-grade neoplasms whose cells are easily identified cytologically.

Results of peritoneal washing cytology are reported as "negative," "atypical," "suspicious," or "positive." "Atypical" and "suspicious" diagnoses should be avoided, whenever possible, because they are not helpful to a physician faced with making a treatment decision. In most medical centers, only an unequivocally positive diagnosis is considered "positive" for staging purposes; anything less in considered negative.

Cytologic examination has a false-negative rate that ranges from 23 to 52%.[5-8] The false-negatives are likely due primarily to sampling, meaning that the malignant cells are either not sampled during the washing procedure or do not make their way onto the slide preparations. Some of the false-negatives are due to the misinterpretation of malignant cells as benign. When peritoneal washings are examined as part of a second-look procedure, the false-negative rate is even higher, ranging from 31 to 86% of patients with biopsy-proven peritoneal metastases.[5] The high false-negative rate during second-look procedures is likely due to poor distribution of fluid because the abdominal cavity is altered by adhesions.

False-positive diagnoses occur in less than 5% of cases and have been attributed to reactive mesothelial proliferations with psammoma bodies[9] and endometriosis.[10] This false-positive rate may be underestimated, however, because PPC, even in the absence of histologic evidence of peritoneal disease, is generally considered a "true-positive." This stems from the original justification for peritoneal cytology as a more sensitive tool than visual inspection and directed histologic sampling. The specificity of PPC, however, has never been rigorously evaluated. Similarly, there have been no studies of the reproducibility of the cytologic diagnosis of malignancy in peritoneal washings. Some variability in the accuracy of cytologists may account for the controversy surrounding the significance of PPC in women with stage I and II endometrial cancer, discussed below.

Immunocytochemistry as an adjunct to conventional cytologic evaluation improves sensitivity but is not used routinely in the evaluation of peritoneal washings.[11] Luo and colleagues investigated the value of antibodies to the protein MOC-31, p53, cytokeratin 5/6, and leukocyte common antigen.[12] Using combined conventional and immunohistochemical (IHC) techniques, 18 out of 115 patients with endometrial cancer had positive cytology. PPC detected by the combination of conventional and IHC staining correlated with myometrial invasion, lymphovascular invasion, and the presence of peritoneal metastases. When patients who had cancer confined to the uterus were examined, having positive cytology performed by conventional as well as IHC means was correlated with poorer disease-free survival ($p < .0005$).[12]

Benevolo and colleagues used two monoclonal antibodies, AR-3 and B72.3, which in combination recognize more than 95% of endometrial cancers.[13] The authors examined washings in 182 patients with endometrial cancer. Using conventional cytology techniques, 27 out of 182 patients were found to have positive cytology. Forty-two out of 182 stained positive for AR-3, 45 out of 182 stained positive for B72.3, and 50 out of 182 stained for both. Disease-free survival was significantly lowered in the patients who had positive IHC readings compared with conventional cytology techniques.

Despite these results, immunocytochemistry is not used routinely for the evaluation of all peritoneal washings because there is no consensus that the increased sensitivity justifies the increased cost of the method. Conventional cytology remains the standard of care and is typically supplemented by immunocytochemistry only in difficult or borderline cases.

MECHANISMS OF ENTRY INTO THE PERITONEAL CAVITY AND BIOLOGY OF TUMOR CELLS IN THE PERITONEAL CAVITY

Malignant cells from an endometrial cancer can spread to the peritoneal cavity by direct extension through the myometrium and serosa, invasion of lymphatic or blood vessels, or retrograde migration through the fallopian tubes. Rarely, endometrial-type cancers arise as primary tumors in the peritoneum, often in association with endometriosis.

Many, if not most, women with PPC have other evidence of extrauterine disease, such as adnexal or lymph node involvement. Nevertheless, 2 to 15% of patients with disease limited to the uterus (and even to the endometrium) have PPC.[14,15] For this reason, it is believed that in some cases, endometrial cancer spreads to the peritoneum by retrograde migration through the fallopian tube. This may occur spontaneously or may be facilitated by diagnostic and/or therapeutic interventions.

It is well documented, in fact, that tumor cells can disseminate during surgical procedures that involve manipulation of the endometrial cavity. Endometrial contents are disturbed and spill out into the peritoneum during hysteroscopy and laparoscopic hysterectomy.[16–19] Some authors have suggested that these procedures confer an increased risk of PPC. Sonada and colleagues compared 131 patients with low-risk endometrial cancer (grade 1–2 endometrioid type cancer with no evidence of extrauterine spread or grade 3 with < 50% myometrial invasion, no cervical or adnexal involvement, and negative nodes when sampled) treated with laparoscopically assisted vaginal hysterectomy with 246 controls who underwent total abdominal hysterectomy (TAH).[17] Patients undergoing laparoscopy had the following interventions: placement of an inflatable intrauterine manipulator, laparoscopy, and vaginal hysterectomy. The cohorts were similar except that women treated with TAH had invasion into the myometrium; however, 10.3% of patients who underwent intrauterine manipulation had positive cytology compared with 2.8% of controls, a statistically significant result ($p = .003$).

Several case reports suggest that retrograde seeding of malignant cells occurs during hysteroscopy.[16,20,21] Romano and colleagues reported a case of woman with a stage IA, grade 2 endometrial cancer diagnosed via hysteroscopy. Surgical staging revealed PPC.[16] The patient underwent no further treatment, but 1 year later she developed a recurrence on the vaginal stump, suggesting that retrograde seeding had caused the recurrence.

Other investigators have not demonstrated an association between hysteroscopy and increased risk of PPC. Gu and colleagues retrospectively examined 284 women diagnosed with endometrial cancer either by endometrial biopsy or dilatation and curettage with or without hysteroscopy. Twenty-three underwent hysteroscopy, 177 did not, and no information was available for the remaining 84. There was no difference in the incidence of PPC among the three groups.[22]

To test the viability of hysteroscopy-disseminated tumor cells, Arikan and colleagues examined 24 women with endometrial cancer and collected run-off fluid through the fallopian tubes. A hysterectomy was performed, the uterus was flushed with saline in vitro, and the cells obtained were grown in culture. Tumor cells were found in 17 (71%) specimens, and in 10 (42%) cases, tumor cells were functionally viable.[23]

In summary, data suggest that endometrial carcinoma cells in peritoneal washings can be viable in vitro, but whether they progress to clinically significant disease in vivo has not been addressed in these studies.

SIGNIFICANCE OF POSITIVE PERITONEAL CYTOLOGY IN ENDOMETRIAL CANCER

Whether PPC is an independent prognostic indicator in women with endometrial cancer remains controversial. Many studies have been published on this subject (Table 10–1). It is fair to say that they have generated some light but certainly even more heat. A number of investigators have reported decreased survival and increased recurrence rates in women with PPC and have recommended postoperative treatment.[15,24–27] Others have shown that PPC correlates with other evidence of extrauterine spread and that PPC is not an independent prognostic indicator for women with endometrial cancer.[14,28–30] Still others have performed multivariate analyses, some of which confirm an independent prognostic value to PPC.[26,27,31,32]

Creasman and Rutledge published the first large experience of peritoneal cytology as a prognostic factor.[3] Between 1961 and 1968, 1,035 patients with gynecologic cancers underwent cytologic

examination of peritoneal washings. One hundred and ninety-four of them had uterine cancer, and 11.5% of patients had PPC. Staging information was not provided, and most patients received postoperative pelvic radiation therapy. These authors concluded that the survival of patients with negative peritoneal cytology was significantly better than that of patients with PPC.

Ten years later, Creasman and colleagues described 167 patients with clinical stage I endometrial cancer, 26 (16%) of whom had PPC.[24] PPC was correlated with increased depth of myometrial invasion. Postoperative therapy in the form of external beam irradiation was given to 46% with PPC and 18% with negative cytology. Recurrent cancer occurred in 10 (38%) of the patients with PPC and 14 (10%) of 141 with negative peritoneal cytology. Eighty-seven percent of patients with negative cytology were alive at 4 to 7 years whereas only 38% of those with PPC were alive. The authors concluded that PPC was an indicator of poor prognosis.

In a smaller study, the results of Imachi and colleagues contradicted those of Creasman.[33] Of the 35 clinical stage I patients, 5 (14.3%) had PPC and of 19 clinical stage II patients, 4 (21%) had PPC. There was no significant difference in survival between patients with and those without PPC, but there were few patients in this study, and they did not undergo surgical staging.

Many investigators have suggested that PPC is an indicator of poor prognosis only because it is associ-

Authors	Endometrial Cancers (N)	FIGO Stages Examined	% Positive Cytology	Independent Variable
Creasman[3]	194	Not known	12	Not done
Creasman[24]	167	Clinical I	16	Not done
Imachi[33]	54	Clinical I, II	Stage I: 14 Stage II: 21	Not done
Kadar[30]	269	Clinical I, II	13	No
Mariani[34]	51	Clinical IIIA	80	No
Konski[29]	134	Clinical I	14	No
Grimshaw[14]	322	Clinical I	5	No
Ebina[35]	114	Surgical I, II, III, IV	35	No
Takeshima[36]	534	Non-FIGO subgroups (see text)	22.	No
Turner[26]	567	Surgical I	5	Yes
Morrow[27]	895	Clinical I, II	11	Yes
Obermair[31]	369	Clinical I	4	Yes
Kashimura[32]	199	Clinical I, II, III, IV	15	Yes

TABLE 10–1. REVIEW OF STUDIES EXAMINING THE VALUE OF PERITONEAL WASHING CYTOLOGY IN ENDOMETRIAL CANCER, WITH EMPHASIS ON ITS VALUE AS AN INDEPENDENT PROGNOSTIC VARIABLE

FIGO = International Federation of Gynecology and Obstetrics.

ated with other evidence of extrauterine disease, such as adnexal or lymph node metastases. Kadar and colleagues reviewed 269 cases of clinical stage I and II endometrial cancer, all of which were surgically staged with selective pelvic and para-aortic lymphadenectomies.[30] Thirty-four patients (12.6%) had PPC. The authors found that PPC did not influence outcome if cancer was confined to the uterus. If disease had spread to the adnexae, lymph nodes, or peritoneum, however, PPC decreased overall survival at 5 years from 73 to 13%.

Mariani and colleagues retrospectively followed up 51 patients with stage IIIA endometrial cancer, 41 of whom had PPC.[34] Their hypothesis was that stage IIIA1 patients (PPC only) had better survival than stage IIIA2 (adnexal involvement or uterine serosal invasion or both). Of the 22 patients with stage IIIA1 disease and an endometrioid histology, without lymphatic and/or blood vessel invasion (LVI), none had a recurrence. Patients who had LVI, grade 3 histology, and/or nonendometrioid histology had a poorer prognosis and extra-abdominal sites of failure compared with the better prognostic group. Of the 22 patients with stage IIIA1 cancer with endometrioid histology and no LVI, no patients developed a recurrence. However, 17 had whole abdominal radiation therapy or intraperitoneal injection of ^{32}P and 2 had external beam radiation therapy.

Konski and colleagues reviewed 134 patients with clinical stage I endometrial cancer with washings obtained at surgery.[29] One hundred and fourteen of these patients had pathologic stage I cancers, and 19 out of 134 (14%) had PPC. Eleven out of 19 patients had pelvic radiation therapy, and 8 out of 19 underwent whole abdominal radiation therapy, some of whom also received intraperitoneal ^{32}P. Patients with negative cytology were treated with surgery alone or pelvic radiation therapy. There was no difference in the recurrence rate or survival of women with PPC and those with negative cytology.

Grimshaw and colleagues retrospectively reviewed 381 patients with endometrial cancer, and PPC was found in 24 out of 381 patients (6.3%).[14] In clinical stage I cancers, 16 of 322 (5.0%) had PPC. In women with surgical stage I cancers, there was no difference in 5-year survival between those with negative cytology and PPC (80% versus 86%, $p = .55$), and, importantly, no adjuvant treatment was given to patients with PPC alone.

Ebina and colleagues also found results similar to those of Grimshaw and colleagues. In women with surgical stage I cancers, there was no difference in survival between those who had negative peritoneal cytology and PPC.[35] None of the patients with surgical stage I endometrial cancers and PPC received any postoperative treatment.

Takeshima and colleagues retrospectively reviewed 534 patients with endometrial cancer and stratified them into three risk groups: (1) a low-risk group (disease limited to the uterus, grade 1, and depth of myometrial invasion less than or equal to 50%), (2) a moderate-risk group (disease limited to the uterus, grade 2 or 3, and/or depth of invasion > 50%), and (3) a high-risk group (extrauterine disease).[36] In each group, disease-free survival was compared in patients who had PPC versus those with negative cytology. The overall incidence of PPC was 22.3%. The 5-year disease-free survival of patients with PPC or negative cytology in the low-risk group was 98.1% versus 100% (n = 250), 77.5% versus 91.3% in the moderate-risk group (n = 211), and 42.9% versus 72.1% in the high-risk group (n = 73). The difference was statistically significant in the moderate- and high-risk groups but not in the low-risk group. They concluded that by itself, PPC is not an indicator of poor prognosis but that it impacts survival rates when associated with other poor prognostic indicators, such as higher grade of tumor and/or presence of extrauterine spread.

The data from other investigators, in contrast, support the original thesis of Creasman and Rutledge. Turner and colleagues retrospectively examined 567 patients and found that PPC indicated a poor prognosis in patients with stage I endometrial cancer.[26] PPC was found in 28 out of 567 patients (4.9%). Patients with negative cytology and those with PPC were treated similarly postoperatively. Forty-nine patients (8.5%) of the total group developed recurrent tumor; 7% with negative cytology and 32% with PPC ($p = .0002$). Sites of recurrence were similar between the two groups; 12.8% recurred in the pelvis and 87.2% developed distantly or in the upper pelvis.

Morrow and colleagues reviewed surgical and pathologic risk factors for clinical stage I and II endometrial cancer.[27] Patients were surgically staged, and a central review of the pathology was performed. Ninety-one patients out of 895 had PPC. Of those with PPC, 29.1% developed local or distant recurrences whereas 10.5% of patients with negative peritoneal cytology had a distant and/or local recurrence. Other poor prognostic predictors were grade 3 histology and outer one-third myometrial invasion. Of 36 cases whose only adverse pathologic factor was PPC, 32 had sufficient follow-up. Six (18.8%) of these 32 patients relapsed; 5 were abdominal recurrences. Twenty-two out of 32 had only superficial myometrial invasion, 5 of whom relapsed. These data suggest that PPC confers an independent increased risk of relapse and poorer outcome.

Obermair and colleagues examined 369 women with clinical stage I endometrial cancer, all of the endometrioid subtype.[31] The authors found that 3.5% of their cohort had PPC. PPC was not associated with depth of myometrial invasion or tumor grade. Women with negative washings had a disease-free survival of 96% at 36 months compared with 67% for women with PPC ($p < .001$).

Kashimura and colleagues came to a similar conclusion.[32] They examined 303 endometrial cancers, 199 of which were surgical stage I cancers. A multivariate analysis evaluated age, histologic type, grade, myometrial invasion, pelvic node metastasis, and peritoneal cytology. PPC was found to be an independent prognostic factor. These authors recommended that treatment protocols be established for patients with PPC because of their poorer outcome.

In conclusion, PPC is usually associated with other markers of poor prognosis, such as tumor grade and depth of myometrial invasion and is redundant as a prognostic marker when other accepted markers are present. In the case of low-stage and low-grade tumors, the significance of PPC is controversial, but data exist to suggest that women with surgical stage I or II cancers and PPC are at a higher risk of systemic recurrence. In time, pathologically staged patients entered into clinical trials, with adjudicated cytologic diagnoses, will help resolve this controversy.

TREATMENT OF WOMEN WITH POSITIVE PERITONEAL CYTOLOGY

Various local as well as systemic treatments have been attempted in women with a diagnosis of endometrial cancer and PPC, including pelvic radiotherapy, whole abdominal radiotherapy, intraperitoneal ^{32}P, and systemic chemotherapy. To date, there have been no randomized trials examining the relative efficacies of these therapies against each other or against clinical observation without adjuvant therapy to identify a standard of postoperative care for these patients.

Creasman and colleagues, after concluding that PPC was a marker of poor prognosis in women with stage I endometrial cancer, treated 23 patients with intraperitoneal ^{32}P following surgery.[24] Only 3 recurrences were seen, all at sites distant from the abdominal cavity.

Hormonal therapy has also been attempted in patients with PPC. Piver and colleagues prospectively treated 45 women with PPC and endometrial cancer confined to the uterus with progesterone for 1 year.[37] Patients with grade 1 or 2 cancers with < 50% myometrial invasion were treated with a total hysterectomy and bilateral oophorectomy followed by vaginal radium/cesium. Patients with grade 3 tumors or myometrial invasion > 50% had postoperative pelvic radiation therapy. Following 1 year of progesterone, patients then had second-look surgery. All 45 patients completed 1 year of progesterone, and 36 patients underwent second-look surgery. Thirty-four of the 36 had negative second-look surgery, and 2 had PPC and went on to receive another year of progesterone. One year later, at a third surgery, both of these women had negative cytology. The 5-year disease-free survival was 88.6%. Twenty patients did have hormonal receptors checked; 80% were estrogen receptor expressed and 90% were progesterone receptor expressed.

Other groups have examined the use of chemotherapy and radiation therapy, both pelvic and whole abdominal.[38–40] Obermair and colleagues recommend postoperative brachytherapy for women with low-stage endometrial cancer and PPC.[31] Unfortunately, there is no consensus on a standard of care, and prospective, randomized trials are needed to determine the optimal, if any, postoperative adjuvant therapy for stage IIIA endometrial cancer with PPC.

Schorge and colleagues examined postoperative treatment of 86 patients with pathologic stage III endometrial cancers, 48 of whom had stage IIIA disease with tumor invasion of uterine serosa and/or adnexae and/or PPC.[41] PPC was found not to be an important prognostic indicator. Stage IIIA tumors were grouped with stage IIIB tumors, making specific assessment of treatment on PPC impossible, but the authors concluded that no benefit from pelvic radiation therapy or chemotherapy was observed in stage IIIA/IIIB patients.

In conclusion, no standard of care following surgery has been identified for women with endometrial cancer and PPC. There appears to be little justification at the present time for adjuvant chemotherapy or hormonal therapy, except in the setting of investigational trials. Some investigators recommend some form of postoperative radiotherapy, including brachytherapy, limited pelvic radiotherapy, or even whole abdominal radiotherapy.[31] Randomized trials are clearly needed in this setting.

REFERENCES

1. Keetel WC, Elkins HB. Experience with radioactive colloidal gold in the treatment of ovarian cancer. Am J Obstet Gynecol 1956;71:553–68.
2. FIGO Cancer Committee. Staging announcement. Gynecol Oncol 1986;25:383–5.
3. Creasman WT, Rutledge F. The prognostic value of peritoneal cytology in gynecologic malignant disease. Am J Obstet Gynecol 1971;110:773–81.
4. FIGO Cancer Committee. Announcements. Gynecol Oncol 1989;35:125–7.
5. Cibas ES. Peritoneal washings. In: Cibas ES, Ducatman BS, editors. Cytology: diagnostic principles and clinical correlates. 2nd ed. London, UK: WB Saunders; 2003. p. 145–161.
6. Lowe E, McKenna H. Peritoneal washings cytology: a retrospective analysis of 175 gynecological patients. Aust N Z Obstet Gynecol 1989;29:55–61.
7. Ravinsky E. Cytology of peritoneal washings in gynecologic patients: diagnostic criteria and pitfalls. Acta Cytol 1986; 30:8–16.
8. Zuna RE, Mitchell ML, Mulick KA, Weijchert WM. Cyto-histologic correlation of peritoneal washing cytology in gynecologic disease. Acta Cytol 1989;33:327–36.
9. Sneige N, Fernandez T, Copeland LJ, Katz RL. Müllerian inclusions in peritoneal washings: potential source of error in cytologic diagnosis. Acta Cytol 1986;30:271–6.
10. Zuna RE, Mitcell ML. Cytologic findings in peritoneal wash-ings associated with benign gynecologic disease. Acta Cytol 1988;32:139–47.
11. Leong ASY. Immunostaining of cytologic specimens. Am J Clin Pathol 1996;105:139–40.
12. Luo ML, Sakuragi N, Shimizu M, et al. Prognostic significance of combined conventional and immunocytochemical cytology for peritoneal washings in endometrial cancer. Cancer 2001;93:115–23.
13. Benevolo M, Mariani L, Vocaturo G, et al. Independent prognostic value of peritoneal immunocytodiagnosis in endometrial carcinoma. Am J Surg Pathol 2000;24:241–7.
14. Grimshaw RN, Tupper WC, Fraser RC, et al. Prognostic value of peritoneal cytology in endometrial carcinoma. Gynecol Oncol 1990;36:97–100.
15. Harouny VR, Sutton GP, Clark SA, et al. The importance of peritoneal cytology in endometrial carcinoma. Obstet Gynecol 1988;72:394–8.
16. Romano S, Shimoni Y, Muralee D, Shalev E. Retrograde seeding of endometrial carcinoma during hysteroscopy. Gynecol Oncol 1992;44:116–8.
17. Sonada Y, Zerbe M, Smith A, et al. High incidence of positive peritoneal cytology in low-risk endometrial cancer treated by laparoscopically assisted vaginal hysterectomy. Gynecol Oncol 2001;80:378–82.
18. Beyth Y, Yaffe H, Levij S, Sadovsky E. Retrograde seeding of endometrium: a sequela of tubal flushing. Fertil Steril 1975;26:1094–7.
19. Obermair A, Geramou M, Gucer F, et al. Does hysteroscopy facilitate tumor cell dissemination? Incidence of peritoneal cytology from patients with early stage endometrial carcinoma following dilatation and curettage (D & C) versus hysteroscopy and D & C. Cancer 2000;88:139–43.
20. Schmitz MJ, Nahhas WA. Hysteroscopy may transport malignant cells into the peritoneal cavity. Case report. Eur J Gynaecol Oncol 1994;15:121–4.
21. Egarter C, Krestan C, Kurz C. Abdominal dissemination of maligant cells into the peritoneal cavity. Gynecol Oncol 1996;63:143–4.
22. Gu M, Shi W, Huang J, et al. Association between initial diagnostic procedure and hysteroscopy and abnormal peritoneal washings in patients with endometrial carcinoma. Cancer 2000;90:143–7.
23. Arikan G, Reich O, Weiss U, et al. Are endometrial carcinoma cells disseminated at hysteroscopy functionally viable? Gynecol Oncol 2001;83:221–6.
24. Creasman WT, DiSaia PJ, Blessing J, et al. Prognostic significance of peritoneal cytology in patients with endometrial cancer and preliminary data concerning therapy with intraperitoneal radiopharmaceuticals. Am J Obstet Gynecol 1981;141:921–7.
25. Mazurka JL, Krepart GV, Lotocki RJ. Prognostic significance of positive peritoneal cytology in endometrial carcinoma. Am J Obstet Gynecol 1988;158:303–6.
26. Turner DA, Gershenson DM, Atkinson N, et al. The prognostic significance of peritoneal cytology for stage I endometrial cancer. Obstet Gynecol 1989;74:775–80.
27. Morrow CP, Bundy BN, Kurman RJ, et al. Relationship between surgical-pathological risk factors and outcome in clinical stage I and II carcinoma of the endometrium: a Gynecologic Oncology Group Study. Gynecol Oncol 1991; 40:55–65.

28. Lurain JR, Rice BL, Rademaker AW, et al. Prognostic factors associated with recurrence in clinical stage I adenocarcinoma of the endometrium. Obstet Gynecol 1991;78:63–9.

29. Konski A, Poulter C, Keys H, et al. Absence of prognostic significance, peritoneal dissemination and treatment advantage in endometrial cancer patients with positive peritoneal cytology. Int J Radiat Oncol Biol Phys 1988;4:49–55.

30. Kadar N, Homesley HD, Malfetano JN. Positive peritoneal cytology is an adverse factor in endometrial carcinoma only if there is other evidence of extrauterine disease. Gynecol Oncol 1992;46:145–9.

31. Obermair A, Geramou M, Tripcony L, et al. Peritoneal cytology: impact on disease-free survival in clinical stage I endometrioid adenocarcinoma of the uterus. Cancer Lett 2001;164:105–10.

32. Kashimura M, Sugihara K, Toki N, et al. The significance of peritoneal cytology in uterine cervix and endometrial cancer. Gynecol Oncol 1997;67:285–90.

33 Imachi M, Tsukamoto N, Matsuyama T, Nakano H. Peritoneal cytology in patients with endometrial carcinoma. Gynecol Oncol 1988;30:76–86.

34. Mariani A, Webb MJ, Keeney GL, et al. Assessment of prognostic factors in stage IIIA endometrial cancer. Gynecol Oncol 2002;86:38–44.

35. Ebina Y, Hareyama H, Sakuragh N, et al. Peritoneal cytology and its prognostic value in endometrial carcinoma. Int Surg 1997;82:244–8.

36. Takeshima N, Nishida H, Tabata T, et al. Positive peritoneal cytology in endometrial cancer: enhancement of other prognostic indicators. Gynecol Oncol 2001;82:470–3.

37. Piver SM, Recio FO, Baker TR, Hempling RE. A prospective trial of progesterone therapy for malignant peritoneal cytology in patients with endometrial cancer. Gynecol Oncol 1992;47:373–6.

38. Mundt AJ, McBride R, Rotmensch J, et al. Significant pelvic recurrence in high-risk pathologic stage I-IV endometrial carcinoma patients after adjuvant chemotherapy alone: implications for adjuvant radiation therapy. Int J Radiat Oncol Biol Phys 2001;50:1145–53.

39. Burke TW, Gershenson DM. Chemotherapy as adjuvant and salvage treatment in women with endometrial cancer. Clin Obstet Gynecol 1996;39:716–27.

40. Potish RA, Twiggs LB, Adcock LL, Prem KA. Role of whole abdominal radiation therapy in the management of endometrial cancer: prognostic importance of factors indicating peritoneal metastases. Gynecol Oncol 1985;21:80–6.

41. Schorge JO, Molpus KL, Goodman A, et al. The effect of postsurgical therapy on stage III endometrial carcinoma. Gynecol Oncol 1996;63:34–9.

11

Papillary Serous, Clear Cell, and Small Cell Carcinomas of the Endometrium

NAJMOSAMA NIKRUI, MD
MICHAEL V. SEIDEN, MD, PhD

In 2003, the American Cancer Society (ACS) reported 40,000 new cases of endometrial cancer in the United States.[1] Although the large majority of these tumors have endometrioid histology, a wide variety of uncommon or rare subtypes make up approximately 5 to 13% of all cases. Annually, there are 4,700 deaths reported from endometrial cancer for an overall mortality of 12%. Women diagnosed with nonendometrioid histologies have, in general, a poorer prognosis, with up to a 50% mortality rate.[2] Although many studies have reported on the poor prognosis of nonendometrioid endometrial cancers, the rarity of these tumors limits systematic evaluation of different treatment approaches and clinical trials. Therefore, recommendations regarding best standards of care are typically based on expert consensus and not as a result of rigorous clinical study. Uterine papillary serous carcinoma (UPSC) and clear cell carcinoma (CCC) make up the large majority of these subtypes and will be the primary focus of this chapter with some additional comments on small cell tumors of the uterus. Additional information on rare subtypes can be found in Chapter 5.

INCIDENCE AND EPIDEMIOLOGY

There are several different types of endometrial carcinomas with nonendometrioid histology, with CCC and UPSC being the two most important. In addition, the endometrium is occasionally the site of metastatic disease from other gynecologic primary tumors (such as cancers of the ovary or fallopian tube) and, much less commonly, the site of metastatic tumors from primary tumors outside of the gynecologic organs. As serous carcinoma from the ovary and tube, in particular, can spread to the endometrium, care must be taken through careful combined clinical and pathologic evaluation to rule out such an explanation in bulky tumors that might involve the endometrium. Endometrioid carcinomas with squamous differentiation, secretory change, or mucinous components are variants of endometrioid endometrial carcinoma and carry similar prognostic and treatment recommendations.[2] A review of the pathology records from the Mayo Clinic between 1979 and 1983 demonstrated a 13% incidence of nonendometrioid tumors in a collection of 388 women with endometrial cancer.[2] Other series have reported a similar incidence (ranging from 5 to 13%). Younger women seem to have a somewhat lower incidence of nonendometrioid histologies, although Duska and colleagues' recent series of young women with endometrial carcinoma found that 10% of the younger cohort still had high-risk histologies.[3] Women with atypical histologies have slightly different epidemiologic factors from those with endometrioid histologies (Table 11–1). In some series, the age at diagnosis (63 years) has been comparable with endometrioid histologies whereas other studies have suggested that these atypical subtypes present in a slightly older age group. It does seem that these histologies are not associated with hyperestrogenic states (see Chapter 1). In addition, there does not seem to be a link between these atypical histologies and estrogen replacement therapy. African American women have a higher proportion of nonen-

Table 11-1. EPIDEMIOLOGY CHARACTERISTICS			
Characteristics or Race*	Endometrioid Histology	UPSC	CCC
White American	83%	66%	83
Black American	15	34%	17
Median age	62	65	68
Diabetes	22%	8%	17%
Estrogen use	48%	30%	33%

CCC = clear cell carconoma; UPSC = uterine papillary serous carcinoma.
*Numbers do not necessarily total 100 due to other race catagories.
Adapted from Cirisano FD Jr et al.[20]

dometrioid histologies (UPSC and CCC).[4,5] In a series of 401 women from New York, 40% of patients were identified as African American women; however, this subset of patients contained 88% UPSC and 77% of the CCC (*p* < .01).[4] A California study has suggested that nonendometrioid lesions may occur with identical frequency in both Black American and White American women, but that low-risk endometrioid lesions are much less common in Black American women. Thus, the high-risk lesion makes up a larger proportion of endometrial cancer in this group of women.[6]

Patients with pure nonendometrioid histologies or mixed histologies containing at least 25% of a poor histologic subtype, such as UPSC and CCC, tend to have advanced disease and a poor prognosis. Corn and colleagues have recently reviewed 394 women with International Federation of Gynecology and Obstetrics (FIGO) stage I to III endometrial cancer of which 13% demonstrated nonendometrioid histologies. Univariate analysis demonstrated a higher risk of local recurrence (21% versus 6%) and distant recurrence (36% versus 1%) for nonendometrioid histology. Although both these differences were highly significant on univariate analysis,

multivariate analysis identified stage, and not histology, as the primary prognostic factor.[7] Similarly, in a recent analysis of prognostic factors that predict peritoneal recurrence in women with stage I to III endometrial cancer, nonendometrioid histology was associated with a 28% incidence of peritoneal recurrence compared with 3% for women with endometrioid histology.[8]

Data are accumulating to suggest that the molecular phenotype of these unusual tumors will be important in defining prognosis and potentially defining therapeutic strategies in the future. Evaluation of dilatation and curettage (D & C) specimens from endometrioid and nonendometrioid histologies demonstrates that the nonendometrioid histologies have a higher likelihood of aneuploidy, high proliferative index, S-phase fraction, and P53 overexpression compared with the endometrioid histology.[9] P53 over-expression is particularly notable in UPSC.[10–13] The high proliferative thrust of these tumors may, in turn, be related to the loss of *P16*.[14] In contrast, nonendometrioid histologies have a lower frequency of microsatellite instability compared with endometrioid histology (Table 11–2).[15]

DIAGNOSIS AND PREOPERATIVE EVALUATION

Seventy-five percent of women present with postmenopausal bleeding, and ultrasonography demonstrates either endometrial thickening or a mass and an endometrial biopsy is usually diagnostic. Magnetic resonance imaging (MRI), although not part of formal staging strategies, can help define the extent of disease, including depth of myometrial invasion and status of pelvic and adnexal structures

Table 11-2. BIOLOGIC FACTORS AND PRESENTATION OF ENDOMETRIOID VERSUS NONENDOMETRIOID HISTOLOGIES				
Risk Factor	Endometrioid	Nonendometrioid	*p* Value	Reference
Median age	63	68	< .01	2
Exogenous estrogens	29%	17%		2
Body mass index	Typically high	Typically low		3
Diploid	74%	50%	.06	9
S-phase fraction ≥ 9%	36%	71%	.01	9
P16 loss	8%	45%	< .001	14
P53 abnormalities	10–30%	50–90%		10–13
Microsatellite instability	19%	8%	.03	15

(see Chapter 4). In a recent prospective study of 50 consecutive patients with clinical stage I endometrial carcinoma, MRI predicted the correct depth of myometrial invasion in 17 of 18 women with disease invading the myometrium and also correctly identified all of 3 women with cervical stromal invasion and all of 6 women with extrauterine involvement.[16] Although this test may be particularly useful in evaluating UPSC due to the tumor's proclivity for myometrial invasiveness, its usefulness is limited by the fact that most of these women should have aggressive surgical staging independent of radiologic findings.

STAGING

Since 1988, staging of all endometrial carcinoma is based on surgical staging. Extrauterine disease is very common in women with nonendometrioid histologies and is often found even with hysterectomy specimens that demonstrate only modest myometrial invasion. Indeed, there seems to be no correlation between depth of myometrial invasion and the evidence of extrauterine disease. Studies correlating the incidence of positive pelvic nodes with depth of myometrial invasion demonstrate that both UPSC and CCC have a propensity to metastasize to regional nodes with even modest invasion (Table 11–3). Similar data exist for peritoneal extension. For example, Geisler and colleagues found a 47.6% incidence of positive cytology in a series of 61 women with UPSC, including 26% of women who had > 2 cm tumor nodules in upper abdominal disease at the time of surgery.[17] Similar findings have been described by other investigators, including a recent series by Goff and colleagues, in which 72% were found to have extrauterine disease, including lymph node and upper abdominal disease.[18] The high propensity of extrauterine extension translates into a high inci-

dence of "upstaging" patients with UPSC and CCC with careful surgical staging (Table 11–4).

Although never studied in a rigorous prospective clinical trial, most experts have recommended that the evaluation of women with atypical histologies should include a full surgical staging similar to the staging of epithelial ovarian carcinoma.[17–20]

PAPILLARY SEROUS CARCINOMA

Uterine papillary serous carcinoma comprises between 3 and 10% of endometrial cancers. The range is, at least in part, probably due to variability in defining the histologic criteria required to make this diagnosis (see Chapter 5).[2,21–23] Despite the relatively low frequency of this subtype, up to 25% of endometrial cancer deaths are seen in the subpopulation of women with UPSC.[24] Although pure UPSC is the most common histologic pattern, a sizable minority of patients can have mixed histology, including admixtures of endometrioid and/or CCC. About 13% have a prior history of breast cancer, and, indeed, UPSC carcinoma has recently been found to be slightly over-represented in women harboring a *BRCA1* germ-line mutation.[25] In contrast, women with hereditary nonpolyposis colon cancer (HNPCC) syndrome are more likely to present with endometrioid histologies (see Chapter 3).

A clinicopathologic study of 30 women with UPSC demonstrated that this group of women were slightly older (67 years) with normal parity (2.4 births).[19] Most women presented with postmenopausal bleeding (80%). Pelvic pain was detected in 22%, and only 20% were classified as obese. Prior pelvic radiotherapy may increase the risk of subsequent UPSC.[26] A subset of patients will present initially with abnormal cervical cytology.[18,23,27–29] At the time of surgical

Table 11–3. FREQUENCY OF PELVIC NODAL METASTASES AS FUNCTION OF MYOMETRIAL INVASION

Invasion/ Histology (%)	Endometrioid (%) N = 493	UPSC (%) N = 49	CCC (%) N = 17
0 (noninvasive)	2	0	0
1–49	1	21	9
≥ 50	12	41	25

Table 11–4. FREQUENCY OF SURGICAL UPSTAGING IN WOMEN WITH CLINICAL STAGE I/II TUMORS

Tumor Grade/Histology	Frequency of Upstaging (%)
Endometrioid, grade 1	7
Endometrioid, grade 2	15
Endometrioid, grade 3	29
UPSC	47
CCC	39

CCC = clear cell carcinoma; UPSC = uterine papillary serous carcinoma. Adapted from Cirisano FD Jr et al.[20]

exploration, tumors are often bulky and exophytic and may fill the endometrial cavity (Figure 11–1). Massive extension into the adnexa can make it difficult or, in some cases, impossible to distinguish between primary ovarian, tubal, and endometrial carcinomas. In other cases, histopathologic evaluation will suggest multiple primary sites. Careful pathologic review of surgical specimens often demonstrates carcinoma in situ in other areas of the endometrium, fallopian tube, and cervix consistent with a more generalized field defect or potential transepithelial spread.[30] Hormone receptor studies demonstrate either weak or negative staining in essentially all tumors with this histologic variant.[31,32] Cancer antigen (CA) 125 is typically elevated at presentation and is useful in monitoring response to therapy.[33–36]

A group of 52 women with UPSC who were surgically staged at either the Massachusetts General Hospital or the University of Washington Medical Center demonstrated that metastases to the ovary,

pelvic/para-aortic lymph nodes, and omentum are common. For example, in the study by Kato and colleagues, 10 of 17 (58%) women with clinical stage I had their tumor upstaged by surgical staging.[19] This compares with a 20% chance of upstaging women with endometrioid histologies by surgical staging.[37] In Kato and colleagues' study, 66% of patients presented with surgical stage III/IV disease; other studies have reported even higher rates of advanced disease at primary presentation.[4,19] In contrast to the more common endometrioid histology, the risk of extrauterine extension is not correlated with depth of myometrial invasion and tumor grade; therefore, for prognostic reasons, complete surgical staging of women who present with these tumors, on curettage or biopsy, is important.[18,19]

Prognosis of Papillary Serous Carcinoma

Although earlier studies suggested that early-stage UPSC had a very poor prognosis, many of these other reports included patients with clinically staged tumor, which, in general, understages the majority of women with this disease. In a series of 320 women with stage IA or IB endometrioid tumors, the presence of a microscopic focus or foci of UPSC or CCC admixed in the tumor or found on diagnostic curettage did not seem to negatively influence prognosis.[38]

Treatment of Papillary Serous Carcinomas

The primary therapy for women with UPSC is surgery and because extrauterine disease is very common, it is recommended that all women should undergo total abdominal hysterectomy, bilateral salpingo-oophorectomy, pelvic and para-aortic lymphadenectomy, pelvic and peritoneal washing, peritoneal biopsy, and omentectomy. For patients with extensive upper abdominal disease, debulking is typically performed, although the clinical merit of such an approach has not been rigorously tested. Patients presenting with stage II, III, and IV disease are at very high risk of relapse and death. Relapses often resemble those of epithelial ovarian cancer with diffuse spread throughout the peritoneum including the upper abdomen.[19,27,39–41] Women with stage IC, II, or III disease have a high risk of recur-

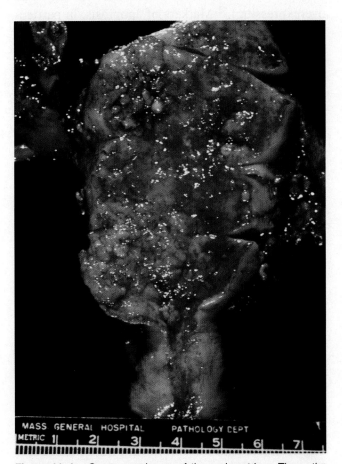

Figure 11–1. Serous carcinoma of the endometrium. The entire endometrial lining is covered by shaggy yellow-tan focally hemorrhagic tumor.

rence and many experts have advocated the use of postoperative adjuvant therapy. Both adjuvant chemotherapy and radiation have been proposed as useful modalities to reduce the recurrence rate.

The use of whole abdominal radiation has been reported in small retrospective series by a number of investigators. Some of these studies demonstrated low rates of upper abdominal recurrence whereas others have demonstrated high relapse rates.[39,42–45] A direct comparison of whole abdominal radiation therapy and chemotherapy (doxorubicin and cisplatin) was evaluated by the Gynecologic Oncology Group in Protocol 122.[46] The study includes about 80 women with UPSC (stage III/IV) that was successfully debulked to < 2 cm of residual disease. The trial demonstrates a progression free and overall survival advantage favoring chemotherapy.

Women who present with bulky abdominal disease, extra-abdominal systemic disease, or who develop recurrent disease are typically treated with palliative chemotherapy. There are only a limited number of small phase II clinical trials that focus on this uncommon tumor type.[34,47–49] Paclitaxel or the combination of paclitaxel with platinum are active with response rates in the 70% range.[34,47] In a recent study performed at the Cleveland Clinic, paclitaxel and carboplatin were used to treat 24 women with UPSC. Approximately half the women received this as adjuvant therapy, with the remaining women having persistent or recurrent tumor. A median progression-free interval of 30 months was reported for those women who received therapy in the adjuvant setting. Normalization of an elevated CA 125 to a pre-chemotherapy level was seen in 8 of 9 patients with residual disease, with a median progression-free interval of 13 months.[47] A regimen using single-agent paclitaxel at 200 mg/m^2 delivered over 24 hours demonstrated a complete response in 4 of 13 women who had measurable disease and received two or more cycles. Partial responses were seen in 6 of the remaining 9 women, for an overall response of 77% in this subgroup. Median survival is not typically meaningful in trials of this size but appears to be between 1 year and 18 months. Curiously, regimens that include platinum, but not paclitaxel, are less active, suggesting that paclitaxel may be the single most active agent in this disease.[34]

CLEAR CELL CARCINOMA

Clear cell carcinoma accounts for only 2 to 4% of endometrial carcinoma, and the histology is similar to those of clear cell tumors of the vagina, cervix, and ovary (Figure 11–2).[20,50] As with UPSC, the tumor tends to present in a population that is slightly older than those with endometrioid histology. There is no apparent epidemiologic link with in utero diethylstilbestrol (DES) exposure. Immunohistochemical studies of CCC demonstrate similar patterns of cytokeratin, carcinoembryonic antigen (CEA), vimentin, and CA 125 staining as clear cell tumors from other gynecologic sites.[51] Several investigators have suggested that these tumors are typically negative for progesterone receptor and have either low or absent estrogen receptor expression.[51,52] Studies at the Johns Hopkins Hospital have suggested that these tumors have a high proliferative thrust (high Ki-67) and tend not to overexpress P53 (compared with UPSCs, which are typically P53 overexpressing).[52] Markers of apoptosis, in particular, BAX (a proapoptotic) protein, have been found to be overexpressed in CCC compared with both endometrioid and UPSC tumors.[53] These data suggest that these tumors are genetically distinct from UPSC and endometrioid histologies.

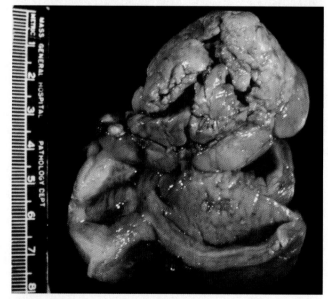

Figure 11–2. Clear cell carcinoma of the endometrium. A large polypoid yellow tumor that filled the endometrial cavity protrudes from the opened specimen.

Preoperative Evaluation and Surgical Staging of Clear Cell Carcinoma

Surgically staged patients with stage 1A/1B endometrioid tumors and evidence of small volumes of CCC in their initial D & C specimens seem to enjoy the same favorable prognosis as those women with pure endometrioid histology.[38] Indeed, several authors have described that preoperative histologies (typically from curettage or endometrial biopsies) are not always concordant with final histology. For patients with a preoperative diagnosis of CCC, plans should be made for thorough surgical staging, as described for UPSC. As with UPSC, women with CCC are frequently upstaged with careful surgical evaluation. Cirisano and colleagues reported upstaging at the time of surgery to surgical stage III/IV in 39% of CCC patients compared with 12% of women with endometrioid tumors.[20] Studies from Japan have shown similar trends with evidence of upstaging in 57% of nonendometrioid histologies (including CCC) compared with 22% of endometrioid histologies.[54] Upstaging occurred despite the fact that most patients with CCC had disease confined to the inner one-third of the myometrium.

Prognosis

As with UPSC, patients with CCC have an inferior survival compared with women with endometrioid histologies.[55] This is due, in part, to a more advanced stage at presentation. The largest series reviewed 181 patients from the Norwegian Radium Hospital spanning over 22 years and incorporated many different treatment modalities. In that study, 5- and 10-year actuarial disease-free survival as 43% and 39%, respectively, with two-thirds of relapses occurring outside the pelvis, including lung, liver, and brain metastases.[50,56] Prognosis for women with disease confined to the uterus is controversial, with some reports suggesting inferior survival and others reporting outcomes similar to those in women with endometrioid histologies. Precise estimates are lacking owing to the small number of women with CCC in each series. Series from North Carolina and the M.D. Anderson Cancer Center support the concept that those with low-stage CCC often do well, whereas

a study from Duke has suggested a worse prognosis.[57–59] In one series, patients with stage I/II disease had an estimated survival of 71% at 5 years compared with 39% for UPSC and 73% for endometrioid histologies, suggesting that CCC histologies may have a better prognosis than UPSC histologies. Similar findings are described in a relatively large collection of CCC patients seen at Yale University. Stage I and II CCC patients had 5-year survivals of 72% and 44%, respectively, as compared with a 5-year survival of 59% and 32%, respectively, for UPSC with stage I and II disease.[60] Review of the large Norwegian registry suggests that stage and age are important prognostic factors, with older women doing worse.[50] Women with surgically advanced stages did very poorly, with all patients with stage IV disease dying by 15 months (Figure 11–3).

Postsurgical Adjuvant Therapy

There are no specific studies designed to evaluate adjuvant radiotherapy or chemotherapy specifically targeted for CCC of the endometrium. As previously described, the Gynecologic Oncology Group (GOG) is comparing whole abdominal radiotherapy with anthracycline-based chemotherapy in women with high-risk endometrial carcinoma. This study included a modest number of CCC patients and demonstrated that patients treated with Adriamycin and cisplatin had a superior survival to those who received whole abdomen radiation therapy.[46] Although this study is important, the number of women with CCC was very small and thus it is difficult to make conclusions with confidence. Because of the high risk of extrapelvic disease, it may not be appropriate to consider pelvic radiation as a sole treatment modality in this patient population (see Figure 11–3).

Treatment for Advanced/Recurrent Disease

There are no specific chemotherapy trials designed to evaluate this patient population. Retrospective studies have demonstrated responses to platinum-based therapies.[50] In addition, there are anecdotal responses to tamoxifen and progestins.[50] In light of the pathologic similarities to CCC of the ovary, it would seem reasonable to consider agents that are typically used for that tumor.

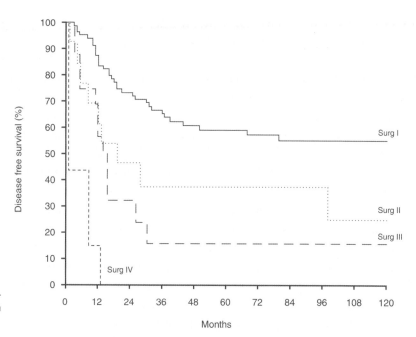

Figure 11–3. Survival of women with clear cell carcinoma by stage. Reproduced with permission from Abeler VM et al.[50]

SMALL CELL CARCINOMAS

Small cell carcinomas are typically found in the lungs of individuals with a history of tobacco smoking. In unusual cases, these tumors can be found in a wide variety of sites in the aerodigestive tracts and the gynecologic organs, including the ovary, cervix, and uterine corpus. Information on uterine small cell tumors is predominantly limited to case collections and one modest-size series reported from the Massachusetts General Hospital (MGH).[61–64] The median age of onset is typically 60 years, although patients as young as 30 years have been described. Most women have presented with vaginal bleeding, although a subset have presented with pain associated with metastatic disease. Vaginal involvement is often seen. In a few cases, bilateral diffuse uveal melanocytic proliferation with progressive visual loss has been described as a rare paraneoplastic disorder that accompanies this malignancy.[65]

The discovery of metastatic disease at the time of diagnosis or soon thereafter is the most common clinical scenario. In one series, metastatic disease was discovered in 8 of 13 women who had abdominal exploration.[1] In the MGH series, 8 of 16 cases presented with synchronous grade 1 or 2 endometrioid adenocarcinoma, and in an additional 2 cases, atypical endometrial hyperplasia was seen, suggest-

ing that early molecular events are shared between this rare tumor and the much more common endometrioid adenocarcinoma.

An overview of these cases and the single large series demonstrate a very high frequency of advanced-stage disease with many patients presenting with diffuse metastatic disease. Almost all patients die of metastatic disease soon after diagnosis, with a median survival of approximately 1 year.[1] Only anecdotal cases have survived for several years after surgery and adjuvant chemotherapy.[63] Due to the rarity of this tumor, there are no formal treatment recommendations that are grounded in prospective clinical trials. In our institution, we assume that essentially all patients have systemic disease and focus on the delivery of a chemotherapy regimen with activity for small cell carcinoma, typically extrapolating from information available from the small cell lung cancer literature. For example, such regimens as platinum and etoposide would be expected to be active in this disease.

CONCLUSION

Nonendometrioid endometrial tumors have a proclivity for extrapelvic dissemination when uterine tumors are still relatively small, and thus, a larger portion of patients presenting with these uncommon histologies have advanced stages of disease compared with women with endometrioid tumors. These tumors are not associated with chronic estrogen exposure. Immunohistochemical studies suggest molecular differences that distinguish the nonendometrioid tumors from the more common endometrioid histology. Secondary differences in *P53* and apoptotic regulatory molecules seem to distinguish UPSC from CCC variants.

Because of the tendency for upper abdominal and peritoneal dissemination, clinical consensus recommends that surgical treatment mimic that of ovarian cancer. Both radiation therapy and chemotherapy have activity, although the role of each modality remains undefined. Both CCC and UPSC are sensitive to platinum-based chemotherapy. UPSC also demonstrates clinical responses to paclitaxel.

REFERENCES

1. Jemal A, Murray T, Samuels A, et al. Cancer Statistics, 2003. CA Cancer J Clin 2003;53:5–26.
2. Wilson T, Podratz K, Gaffey T, et al. Evaluation of unfavorable histologic subtypes in endometrial adenocarcinoma. Am J Obstet Gynecol 1990;162:418–26.
3. Duska L, Garrett A, Rueda B, et al. Endometrial cancer in women 40 years old or younger. Gynecol Oncol 2001; 83:388–93.
4. Matthews RP, Hutchinson-Colas J, Maiman M, et al. Papillary serous and clear cell type lead to poor prognosis of endometrial carcinoma in black women. Gynecol Oncol 1997;65(2):206–12.
5. Liu JR, Conaway M, Rodriguez GC, et al. Relationship between race and interval to treatment in endometrial cancer. Obstet Gynecol 1995;86(4 Pt 1):486–90.
6. Plaxe SC, Saltzstein SL. Impact of ethnicity on the incidence of high-risk endometrial carcinoma. Gynecol Oncol 1997;65(1):8–12.
7. Corn BW, Lanciano RM, D'agostino R, et al. The relationship of local and distant failure from endometrial cancer: defining a clinical paradigm. Gynecol Oncol 1997;66(3):411–6.
8. Mariani A, Webb MJ, Aletti G, et al. Predictors of peritoneal failure in endometrial cancer. In: Annual Meeting of the Society of Gynecologic Oncology. Miami, FL: Society of Gynecologic Oncology; 2002.
9. Silverman M, Roche P, Kho R, et al. Molecular and cytokinetic pretreatment risk assessment in endometrial carcinoma. Gynecol Oncol 2000;77:1–7.
10. Berchuk A, Kohler M, Marks J, et al. The p53 tumor suppressor gene frequently altered in gynecologic cancers. Am J Obstet Gynecol 1994;170:246–52.
11. Boyd J. Molecular biology in the clinicopathologic assessment of endometrial carcinoma subtypes. Gynecol Oncol 1996;61:163–5.
12. Geisler J, Wiemann M, Zhou Z, et al. P53 as a prognostic indicator in endometrial cancer. Gynecol Oncol 1996; 61:245–8.
13. Zhen W, Cao P, Zheng M, et al. P53 overexpression and bcl-2 persistence in endometrial carcinoma: comparison of papillary serous and endometrioid subtypes. Gynecol Oncol 1996;61:167–74.
14. Salverson H, Das S, Akslen L. Loss of nuclear P16 protein expression is not associated with promoter methylation but defines a subgroup of aggressive endometrial carcinomas with poor prognosis. Clin Cancer Res 2000;6:153–9.
15. Basil JB, Goodfellow PJ, Rader JS, et al. Clinical significance of microsatellite instability in endometrial carcinoma. Cancer 2000;89(8):1758–64.
16. Chen S, Runamicik W, Spiegel G. Magnetic resonance imaging in stage I endometrial carcinoma. Obstet Gynecol 1990;75:274–7.
17. Geisler JP, Geisler HE, Melton ME, Wiemann MC. What staging surgery should be performed on patients with uterine papillary serous carcinoma? Gynecol Oncol 1999; 74:465–7.
18. Goff B, Kato D, Schmidt R, et al. Uterine papillary serous carcinoma: patterns of metastatic spread. Gynecol Oncol 1994;54:264–8.
19. Kato D, Ferry J, Goodman A, et al. Uterine papillary carcinoma (UPSC): clinicopathologic study of 30 cases. Gynecol Oncol 1995;59:384–9.
20. Cirisano FD Jr, Robboy SJ, Dodge RK, et al. Epidemiologic and surgicopathologic findings of papillary serous and clear cell endometrial cancers when compared to endometrioid carcinoma. Gynecol Oncol 1999;74:385–94.
21. Christopherson W, Alberhasky R, Connelly P. Carcinoma of the endometrium. II. Papillary adenocarcinoma: a clinical pathological study of 46 cases. Am J Clin Pathol 1982; 77:534–40.
22. Chamber J, Merino M, Kohorn E, et al. Uterine papillary serous carcinoma. Obstet Gynecol 1987;69:109–13.
23. Hendrickson M, Marinez A, Ross J, et al. Uterine papillary serous carcinoma: a highly malignant form of endometrial adenocarcinoma. Am J Surg Pathol 1982;6:93–108.
24. Rosenberg P, Boeryd B, Simonsen E. A new aggressive treatment approach to high-grade endometrial cancer of possible benefit to patients with stage I uterine papillary cancer. Gynecol Oncol 1993;48:32–7.
25. Geisler JP, Sorosky JI, Duong HL, et al. Papillary serous carcinoma of the uterus: increased risk of subsequent or concurrent development of breast carcinoma. Gynecol Oncol 2001;83:501–3.
26. Parkash V, Carcangiu ML. Uterine papillary serous carcinoma after radiation therapy for carcinoma of the cervix. Cancer 1992;69(2):496–501.
27. Nicklin JL, Copeland LJ. Endometrial papillary serous carcinoma: patterns of spread and treatment. Clin Obstet Gynecol 1996;39(3):686–95.
28. Sherman ME, Bitterman P, Rosenshein NB, et al. Uterine serous carcinoma. A morphologically diverse neoplasm with unifying clinicopathologic features. Am J Surg Pathol 1992;16(6):600–10.
29. Williams KE, Waters ED, Woolas RP, et al. Mixed serous-endometrioid carcinoma of the uterus: pathologic and

cytopathologic analysis of a high-risk endometrial carcinoma. Int J Gynecol Cancer 1994;4(1):7–18.

30. Jordan LB, Abdul-Kader M, Al-Nafussi A. Uterine serous papillary carcinoma: histopathologic changes within the female genital tract. Int J Gynecol Cancer 2001;11(4):283–9.

31. Carcangiu ML, Chambers JT, Voynick IM, et al. Immunohistochemical evaluation of estrogen and progesterone receptor content in 183 patients with endometrial carcinoma. Part I: clinical and histologic correlations. Am J Clin Pathol 1990;94(3):247–54.

32. Umpierre SA, Burke TW, Tornos C, et al. Immunocytochemical analysis of uterine papillary serous carcinomas for estrogen and progesterone receptors. Int J Gynecol Pathol 1994;13(2):127–30.

33. Abramovich D, Markman M, Kennedy A, et al. Serum CA-125 as a marker of disease activity in uterine papillary serous carcinoma. J Cancer Res Clin Oncol 1999;125(12):697–8.

34. Ramondetta L, Burke TW, Levenback C, et al. Treatment of uterine papillary serous carcinoma with paclitaxel. Gynecol Oncol 2001;82(1):156–61.

35. Rose PG, Sommers RM, Reale FR, et al. Serial serum CA 125 measurements for evaluation of recurrence in patients with endometrial carcinoma. Obstet Gynecol 1994;84(1):12–6.

36. Tseng PC, Sprance HE, Carcangiu ML, et al. CA 125, NB/70K, and lipid-associated sialic acid in monitoring uterine papillary serous carcinoma. Obstet Gynecol 1989;74(3 Pt 1):384–7.

37. Creasman WT, Morrow CP, Bundy BN, et al. Surgical pathologic spread patterns of endometrial cancer. A Gynecologic Oncology Group Study. Cancer 1987;60 8 Suppl: 2035–41.

38. Aquino-Parsons C, Lim P, Wong F, Mildenberger M. Papillary serous and clear cell carcinoma limited to endometrial curetting in FIGO 1a and 1b endometrial adenocarcinoma: treatment implication. Gynecol Oncol 1998;71:83–6.

39. Nguyen NP, Sallah S, Karlsson U, et al. Prognosis for papillary serous carcinoma of the endometrium after surgical staging. Int J Gynecol Cancer 2001;11(4):305–11.

40. Lee KR, Belinson JL. Papillary serous adenocarcinoma of the endometrium: a clinicopathologic study of 19 cases. Gynecol Oncol 1992;46:51–4.

41. Jeffrey J, Krepart G, Lotocki R. Papillary serous adenocarcinoma of the endometrium. Obstet Gynecol 1986;67:670–4.

42. Gibbons S, Martinez A, Schray M. Adjuvant whole abdominopelvic irradiation for high risk endometrial carcinoma. Int J Radiat Oncol Biol Phys 1991;21:1019–25.

43. Frank AH, Tseng PC, Haffty BG, et al. Adjuvant whole-abdominal radiation therapy in uterine papillary serous carcinoma. Cancer 1991;68:1516–9.

44. Mallipedi L, Dapp D, Teng N. Long-term survival with adjuvant whole abdominopelvic irradiation for uterine papillary serous carcinoma. Cancer 1993;71:385–94.

45. Smith R, Kapp DS, Chen Q, Teng N. Treatment of high-risk uterine cancer with whole abdominopelvic radiation therapy. Int J Radiat Oncol Biol Phys 2000;48:767–78.

46. Randall ME, Brunetto G, Muss H, et al. Whole abdominal radiotherapy versus combination doxorubicin-cisplatin chemotherapy in advanced endometrial carcinoma: A randomized phase III trial of the Gynecologic Oncology Group [abstract 3]. Proc Am Soc Clin Oncol 2003;22:2.

47. Zanotti KM, Belinson JL, Kennedy AW, et al. The use of paclitaxel and platinum-based chemotherapy in uterine papillary serous carcinoma. Gynecol Oncol 1999;74(2):272–7.

48. Levenback C, Burke TW, Silva E, et al. Uterine papillary serous carcinoma (UPSC) treated with cisplatin, doxorubicin, and cyclophosphamide (PAC). Gynecol Oncol 1992;46(3):317–21.

49. Price FV, Chambers SK, Carcangiu ML, et al. Intravenous cisplatin, doxorubicin, and cyclophosphamide in the treatment of uterine papillary serous carcinoma (UPSC). Gynecol Oncol 1993;51(3):383–9.

50. Abeler VM, Vergote IB, Kjorstad KE, Trope CG. Clear cell carcinoma of the endometrium. Prognosis and metastatic pattern. Cancer 1996;78(8):1740–7.

51. Vang R, Whitaker BP, Farhood AI, et al. Immunohistochemical analysis of clear cell carcinoma of the gynecologic tract. Int J Gynecol Pathol 2001;20:252–9.

52. Lax SF, Pizer ES, Ronnett BM, Kurman RJ. Clear cell carcinoma of the endometrium is characterized by a distinctive profile of p53, Ki-67, estrogen, and progesterone receptor expression. Hum Pathol 1998;29(6):551–8.

53. Kokawa K, Shikone T, Otani T, et al. Apoptosis and expression of Bcl-2 and Bax in patients with endometrioid, clear cell and serous carcinomas of the uterine endometrium. Gynecol Oncol 2001;81:178–83.

54. Sakuragi N, Hareyama H, Todo Y, et al. Prognostic significance of serous and clear cell adenocarcinoma in surgically staged endometrial carcinoma. Acta Obstet Gynecol Scand 2000;79:311–6.

55. Kurman RJ, Scully RE. Clear cell carcinoma of the endometrium: an analysis of 21 cases. Cancer 1976;37(2): 872–82.

56. Abeler V, Kjorstad K, Berle E. Carcinoma of the endometrium in Norway: a histopathological and prognostic survey of a total population. Int J Gynecol Cancer 1992; 2:9–22.

57. Malpica A, Tornos C, Burke TW, Silva EG. Low-stage clear-cell carcinoma of the endometrium. Am J Surg Pathol 1995;19(7):769–74.

58. Photopulos GJ, Carney CN, Edelman DA, et al. Clear cell carcinoma of the endometrium. Cancer 1979;43(4):448–56.

59. Cirisano FD Jr, Robboy SJ, Dodge RK, et al. The outcome of stage I-II clinically and surgically staged papillary serous and clear cell endometrial cancers when compared with endometrioid carcinoma. Gynecol Oncol 2000;77: 55–65.

60. Carcangi ML, Chambers JT. Early pathologic stage clear cell carcinoma and uterine papillary serous carcinoma of the endometrium: comparison of clinicopathologic features and survival. Int J Gynecol Pathol 1995;14(1):30–8.

61. Huntsman DG, Clement PB, Gilks CB, Scully RE. Small-cell carcinoma of the endometrium. A clinicopathological study of sixteen cases. Am J Surg Pathol 1994;18(4): 364–75.

62. Kumar NB. Small cell carcinoma of the endometrium in a 23-year-old woman: light microscopic and ultrastructural study. Am J Clin Pathol 1984;81:98–101.

63. Manivel C, Wick MR, Sibley RK. Neuroendocrine differentiation in müllerian neoplasms. An immunohistochemical study of a "pure" endometrial small-cell carcinoma and a

mixed müllerian tumor containing small-cell carcinoma. Am J Clin Pathol 1986:86:438–43.

64. Paz RA, Frigerio B, Sundblad AS, Eusebi V. Small cell (oat cell) carcinoma of the endometrium. Arch Pathol Lab Med 1985;109:270–2.

65. Chahud F, Young RH, Remulla JF, et al. Bilateral diffuse uveal melanocytic proliferation associated with extraocular cancers. Review of a process particularly associated with gynecologic cancers. Am J Surg Pathol 2001;25(2): 212–8.

12

Estrogen Replacement Therapy after Endometrial Cancer

ANNEKATHRYN GOODMAN, MD

Endometrial cancer is the most common pelvic malignancy and is the fourth most common cancer in women after breast, colon, and lung cancers. In the United States, 40,100 women are estimated to develop endometrial cancer in 2003, with 6,800 women dying from these cancers.[1] The average age of women who are treated for endometrial cancer is 65 years.[2] Less than 25% of women with this cancer are premenopausal, and 5% are less than 40 years old.[3] Risk factors for the development of endometrial cancer include unopposed estrogens, obesity, nulliparity, hypertension, diabetes, nutrition, family history, and the use of tamoxifen (also reviewed in Chapter 1).[4,5]

Surgical removal of the uterus, fallopian tubes, and ovaries is the mainstay of therapy for endometrial cancer.[6] As the majority of endometrial cancers are curable, the long-term consequences of therapy become important. The loss of estrogen can have far-reaching effects. Estrogen deficiency reduces quality of life and is an important etiologic reason for significant health problems in older women.[7,8] This chapter reviews the complex association of estrogen with endometrial cancer, the consequences of estrogen loss, and the possible solutions.

ESTROGEN AND THE DEVELOPMENT OF ENDOMETRIAL CANCER

To consider estrogen replacement therapy (ERT) after definitive treatment for endometrial cancer, the underlying etiology of the cancer must be understood. Theoretically, those women whose cancers may have been caused by excess estrogen would be at risk of recurrence with continued exposure to the inciting agent. Although the administration of estrogens is considered in women who have had their uterus and primary tumor removed, the risk of this therapy is associated with stimulation of occult disease. Therefore, prognostic factors, such as stage of cancer, grade, histologic subtype, and etiologic factors, will guide decisions about ERT (also see Chapter 6).[9]

Prolonged, noncyclic estrogen exposure has been a known element in the development of endometrial cancer.[10] Women with anovulatory cycles, such as those with polycystic ovarian syndrome, who lack the monthly stabilization of the endometrial lining by progesterone, have been noted to be at increased risk of the development of endometrial cancer. In addition, women with estrogen-secreting tumors have an increased risk of development of atypical endometrial hyperplasia, a precursor to cancer, and of cancer itself.[11] In the 1970s and 1980s, several case-control studies reported an association between unopposed estrogen use in the form of sequential birth control pills and postmenopausal estrogen therapy and the development of endometrial adenocarcinoma.[12,13] The relative risk of cancer with unopposed estrogen was increased 4-fold to 15-fold, and these cancers occurred with prolonged exposure of > 5 to 10 years.[14] While the current practice of prescribing combined estrogen-progesterone preparations has decreased the incidence of endometrial cancer, endometrial cancers continue to occur in women treated with less than the recommended 12 days of progesterone monthly.[15]

Two separate variants of endometrial cancer have been described on the basis of their histologic and clinical features.[16] Type 1, which has a generally good prognosis, is the more common variant. Associated with endogenous and/or exogenous estrogen exposure and usually diagnosed at an early stage, this variant is well differentiated, an endometrioid cell subtype, and associated with endometrial hyperplasia. Type 2 cancers do not appear to be associated with estrogen use or with hyperplasia and have adverse histologic features, including poorly differentiated tumors, papillary serous and clear cell subtypes, and commonly present with extrauterine disease.[2]

The underlying mechanism for estrogen-related carcinogenesis is not understood. Estrogen binds to and activates the nuclear estrogen receptor (ER), a deoxyribonucleic acid (DNA)-binding protein that is found in estrogen-responsive tissue. The activated ER binds to specific DNA sequences that lead to transcription of proliferative genes. In endometrial tissue, estrogen induces epithelial proliferation and increased concentrations of progesterone receptors (PRs).[17] In endometrial carcinomas, tumors often express ER, with expression more commonly seen in well-differentiated tumors. Progesterone-receptor concentrations also drop as the tumors become less differentiated.[18] Clear cell and serous tumors have significantly lower frequencies of ER and PR compared with the endometrioid variants.[19]

ESTROGEN DEFICIENCY SYNDROME

With the removal of the uterus and adnexa, a premenopausal woman will enter immediate surgical menopause. Postmenopausal women who have been treated for endometrial cancer are usually advised not to restart ERT if they had previously been on it. Estrogen deficiency has both immediate and long-range consequences (Table 12–1).[8,20] The vasomotor flush is experienced by most menopausal women. Fatigue, nervousness, insomnia, depression, irritability, joint and muscle pain, dizziness, and palpitations are frequent complaints, with varying degrees of intensity.[7,21] Epidemiologic studies have dispelled the notion of an increase in depression in naturally menopausal women.[22] In women facing cancer, the loss of autonomy in illness and decline in health can trigger depression.[23]

Genitourinary atrophy, accompanied by vaginitis, pruritus, dyspareunia, and vaginal and urethral stenosis, occurs and progresses over time after loss of estrogen.[24] Urethritis, recurrent urinary tract infections, urge incontinence, and urinary frequency can be debilitating symptoms of hypoestrogenism.[25,26]

Sexual dysfunction can occur from loss of libido and from anatomic changes secondary to hypoestrogenism.[27] There is a reduction in the production and volume of vaginal fluid, loss of vaginal wall elasticity, and thinning of the vaginal tissues.[28] Postmenopausal urogenital atrophy leads to vaginal dryness, burning, postcoital spotting, and a decreased ability to tolerate deep thrusting during intercourse.[29]

Osteoporosis, a direct effect of estrogen loss, leads to a significant incidence of bone fracture.[30] Osteoporosis-related fractures will occur in more than 40% of women over the age of 50 years. Twenty percent of women will die within 1 year of hip fracture.[31] One-fourth of survivors will be confined to long-term care facilities, and 50% will experience loss of mobility.[31] Associated risk factors in the development of osteoporosis and osteopenia include Caucasian or Asian descent, family history, and alcohol and tobacco use.[32]

Cardiovascular disease is the leading cause of death among women in the United States, and the death rate of women approaches that of men after menopause.[33] While estrogen increases high-density lipoprotein (HDL) cholesterol, the cardioprotective effect of estrogen has been recently challenged.[30]

Table 12–1. EFFECTS OF ESTROGEN DEFICIENCY

Vasomotor instability—hot flashes
Osteoporosis
Fatigue
Insomnia
Joint and muscle pains
Irritability
Palpitations
Vaginitis
Vulvar pruritus
Dyspareunia
Vaginal and urethral stenosis
Urinary incontinence
Recurrent urinary tract infection
Loss of libido

ESTROGEN REPLACEMENT THERAPY AFTER TREATMENT OF ENDOMETRIAL CANCER

Two major questions need to be addressed in deciding whether to offer ERT to women who have completed their therapy for endometrial cancer. First, does ERT cause recurrence of endometrial cancer? Second, does ERT increase the risk of second primaries in these women who may already be at heightened genetic risk of breast and colon cancers?

Currently, there are no conclusive data available to support specific recommendations regarding the use of ERT in women treated for endometrial cancer. The effect of ERT on the recurrence risk of endometrial cancer is unknown. There have been four retrospective reviews of this issue, which are discussed below.

The first study to address this question of ERT was a retrospective review of 221 patients with clinical stage I adenocarcinoma between the years 1975 and 1980. Forty-seven women received ERT, and 147 did not. Of those treated with estrogen, 34 took vaginal estrogen, 7 received oral estrogen, and 6 received both vaginal and oral preparations. One woman, who had used vaginal cream for 3 months, had a recurrence at 22 months compared with 26 recurrences (14.9%) in the nonuser group. The ERT users had better disease-free survival, even after controlling for other prognostic factors.[34]

Another retrospective review looked at 144 patients with clinical stage I adenocarcinoma who were treated between the years 1975 and 1985. Of the 44 patients who received ERT, there were no recurrences or deaths. Of the 99 nonusers, there were 8 recurrences and 8 deaths.[35]

One hundred and twenty-three women with surgical stages I and II adenocarcinoma of the endometrium between the years 1982 and 1994 were retrospectively analyzed. Sixty-two patients who received ERT were matched to 61 nonusers. Sixty percent of the patients started ERT within 1 year of surgery, 20% between 1 and 2 years, and 21% after 2 years. The overall recurrence rate was 6.5%. Of the 2 women taking estrogen who had a recurrence, 1 developed abdominal carcinomatosis 24 months after diagnosis, and 1 developed a vaginal cuff recurrence at 32 months. Six of the 61 nonusers had recurrences. Overall, there was no significant difference in recurrence rate or death from disease. When patients who started ERT within 1 year were compared with nonusers, ERT users did better ($p = .07$). However, ERT users were younger, more likely to have earlier-stage disease, less depth of invasion, and fewer intercurrent illnesses.[36]

The most recent study reviewed the cases of 249 women with surgical stages I, II, and III endometrial cancer who were treated between the years 1984 and 1998.[37] One hundred and thirty women received ERT after their primary cancers, and 49% of these women also received progesterone in addition to estrogen. Seventy-five matched treatment-control pairs were identified. The subjects were followed up for a mean of 83 months. Two recurrences (1%) occurred among ERT users compared with 11 recurrences (14%) in the controls. This was statistically significant favoring a longer disease-free interval among ERT users.[37]

There has been one recent case report of a groin and para-aortic node recurrence of a grade 1, stage IB adenocarcinoma 1 year after ERT was instituted. The patient had undergone a laparotomy, hysterectomy, and bilateral adnexectomy for a superficially invasive, well-differentiated adenocarcinoma of the endometrium. She was immediately started on oral estrogen after surgery.[38]

In general, all these reviews suggest that posttreatment ERT is safe. However, these retrospective reviews reflect the bias of practising oncologists who only select low-risk groups for the institution of ERT. One would expect these women to have a better survival from their cancers. Theoretically, one would assume that women with high-risk cancers that have a lower concentration of ER in the tumors would safely benefit from ERT as well. Presently, the Gynecologic Oncology Group (GOG) is conducting a prospective, double-blind, randomized trial of ERT versus placebo for women who have been treated for endometrial cancer.

The most significant genetic association of endometrial carcinoma is hereditary nonpolyposis colorectal cancer (HNPCC) syndrome.[39] Breast cancer is less associated with endometrial cancer genetically but has an epidemiologic association based on estrogen excess, obesity, and dietary risk factors.[40] A recent prospective randomized controlled trial of estrogen plus progesterone versus placebo looked at 16,608 healthy postmenopausal women who were followed up for a mean of 5.2 years. The hazard risk ratios for the development of breast, endometrial, and colon cancers were 1.26, 0.83, and 0.63, respectively.[30]

Endometrioid adenocarcinoma arising in endometriotic implants has been reported to occur after hysterectomy for endometriosis.[41] Unopposed estrogen replacement therapy has been implicated in the development of malignancy in the residual rests of peritoneal endometriosis.

PHYTOESTROGENS

Phytoestrogens are defined as naturally occurring compounds found in plants that may produce estrogenic effects.[42] Lignans and isoflavones have been the most extensively evaluated of the classes of phytoestrogens. Isoflavones are 500 to 1,000 times weaker than endogenous estrogens and may also act as antiestrogens by competing with estradiol at the ER.[43] Isoflavones predominantly express estrogenic activities in the central nervous system, blood vessels, bone, and skin and less so in the breast and uterus because of preferential binding to the beta form of ER.[44] This does raise the possibility that they are protective in hormone-related diseases, such as breast cancer.

Studies of the efficacy of isoflavones in alleviating vasomotor flashes have shown variable results. One study reported that only 27% of Thai women, who have a diet high in phytoestrogens, have hot flashes compared with 85% of Western women.[45] However, a randomized controlled trial of breast cancer survivors failed to elicit a difference between phytoestrogens and placebo.[46] The literature on the prevention of osteoporosis with phytoestrogen reports equally mixed results.[47]

At least four human studies have shown that a high isoflavone diet or isoflavone supplements in postmenopausal women does not increase endometrial thickness.[48–51] There have been no large studies of phytoestrogen use and endometrial cancer risk. Epidemiologic studies suggest a possible protective role of dietary phytoestrogen consumption in the prevention of endometrial cancer.[52] One case study reported the development of noninvasive grade 1 endometrial

cancer after excessive consumption of supplemental phytoestrogens. This patient also had a confounding history of infertility.[53] There is presently no literature evaluating the use of phytoestrogens after treatment of endometrial cancer.

ALTERNATIVE THERAPIES FOR ESTROGEN DEFICIENCY

Osteoporosis is the leading cause of morbidity and mortality from estrogen deficiency. There are several effective nonestrogen interventions, including raloxifene, bisphosphonates, and calcitonin (Table 12–2).[54] There are no effective alternatives to estrogen to treat urogenital atrophy and subsequent sexual dysfunction. Many water-soluble and oil-based lubricants have been advocated, with minor success. The estradiol vaginal ring has been recommended for breast cancer survivors. The relative potency is < 0.5% of serum level of oral conjugated estrogen. With continuous use, there are no detectable blood levels of estradiol or estrone.[15] Many herbal therapies have been suggested for the management of vasomotor symptoms, but these substances have not been rigorously evaluated.[55] Fluoxetine for the treatment of hot flashes showed promise in one randomized study.[56]

SUMMARY

The majority of women with endometrial carcinoma will survive their cancers and be faced with the lifelong consequences of estrogen deficiency. Although there are no conclusive data to support specific recommendations for ERT in women treated for endometrial cancer, the retrospective studies suggest that ERT in women with low-risk cancers is not

Table 12–2. NONHORMONAL ALTERNATIVES FOR ESTROGEN DEFICIENCY		
Symptom (Problem)	Treatment	Efficacy
Osteoporosis	Raloxifene	√√
	Bisphosphonates	√√
	Calcitonin	√
Vasomotor symptoms	Fluoxetine	√
	Clonidine	√
	Phytoestrogens	no data
	Various herbal remedies	no data
Urogenital atrophy	—	—

associated with an increased recurrence rate. The other long-term risks of ERT, such as increased breast cancer risk, must be kept in mind, but recent data suggest that for women at increased risk of colon cancer, ERT may be protective. For women who cannot take ERT, clinicians must be cognizant of the health risks and reduction in quality of life associated with estrogen deficiency. Active intervention with alternatives to estrogen should be part of the long-term care of these women.

REFERENCES

1. Jemal A, Thomas A, Murray T, Thun M. Cancer statistics, 2002. CA Cancer J Clin 2002;52:23–47.

2. Sividris E, Fox H, Buckley CH. Endometrial carcinoma: two or three entities? Int J Gynecol Cancer 1998;8:183–8.

3. Gallup DG, Stock RJ. Adenocarcinoma of the endometrium in women 40 years of age or younger. Obstet Gynecol 1984;64:417–20.

4. MacMahon B. Risk factors for endometrial cancer. Gynecol Oncol 1974;2:122–9.

5. Fornander T, Cedermark B, Mattsson A, et al. Adjuvant tamoxifen in early breast cancer: occurrence of new primary cancers. Lancet 1989;21:117–20.

6. International Federation of Gynecology and Obstetrics. Corpus Cancer Staging. Int J Gynecol Obstet 1989;28:190.

7. Sherwin BB. Effects of estrogen and/or androgen on somatic, affective, sexual, and cognitive functioning in hysterectomized and oophorectomized women. Diss Abstr Int B Sci Eng 1983;44:1275.

8. Yen SS. The biology of menopause. J Reprod Med 1977;18:287–96.

9. Creasman WT, Morrow CP, Bundy BN, et al. Surgical pathologic spread patterns of endometrial cancer: a Gynecologic Oncology Group study. Cancer 1987;60 Suppl:2035–41.

10. Gusberg SB. Classics in oncology—precursors of corpus carcinoma estrogens and adenomatous hyperplasia. CA Cancer J Clin 1989;39:179–92.

11. Bjorkholm E, Pettersson F. Granulosa cell and theca cell tumors: the clinical picture and long term outcome for the Radiumhemmet series. Acta Obstet Gynecol Scand 1980;59:361–5.

12. Antunes CM, Strolley PD, Rosenshein NB, et al. Endometrial cancer and estrogen use. N Engl J Med 1979;300:9–13.

13. Jelovsek FR, Hammond CB, Woodard BH, et al. Risk of exogenous estrogen therapy and endometrial cancer. Am J Obstet Gynecol 1980;137:85–91.

14. Rubin GL, Peterson HB, Lee NC, et al. Estrogen replacement therapy and the risk of endometrial cancer: remaining controversies. Am J Obstet Gynecol 1990;162:148–54.

15. American College of Obstetricians and Gynecologists. ACOG Educational Bulletin No. 247. Hormone replacement therapy. Washington, DC: The College; 1998:110.

16. Bokhman JV. Two pathogenetic types of endometrial carcinoma. Gynecol Oncol 1983;15:10–7.

17. Lessey BA, Killam AP, Metzger DA, et al. Immunohistochemical analysis of human uterine estrogen and progesterone receptors throughout the menstrual cycle. J Clin Metab 1988;67:334–40.

18. Erlich CE, Young PCM, Stehman FB, et al. Steroid receptors and clinical outcome in patients with adenocarcinoma of the endometrium. Am J Obstet Gynecol 1988;158:796–895.

19. Lax SF, Pizer ES, Ronnett BM, Kurman RJ. Clear cell carcinoma of the endometrium is characterized by a distinctive profile of p53, Ki-67, estrogen and progesterone receptor expression. Hum Pathol 1998;29:551–8.

20. Notman MT. Menopause and adult development. Ann N Y Acad Sci 1990;592:149–55.

21. Oldenhave A, Jaszmann LJB, Haspels AA, Everaerd WTAM. Impact of the climacteric on well-being. A survey based on 5213 women 39 to 60 years old. Am J Obstet Gynecol 1993;168:772–80.

22. Hunter MS. Emotional well-being, sexual behavior, and hormone replacement therapy. Maturitas 1990;12:299–314.

23. Derogatis LR, Morrow GR, Fetting J, et al. The prevalence of psychiatric disorders amongst cancer patients. JAMA 1983;249:751–7.

24. Bhatia NN, Bergman A, Karram MM. Effects of estrogen on urethral function in women with urinary incontinence. Am J Obstet Gynecol 1989;160:176–81.

25. Fantl JA, Wyman JF, Anderson RL, et al. Postmenopausal urinary incontinence: comparison between non-estrogen supplemented and estrogen-supplemented women. Obstet Gynecol 1988;71:823–8.

26. Staskin DR. Age-related physiologic and pathologic changes affecting lower urinary tract function. Clin Geriatr Med 1986;2:701–10.

27. Sarrel PM. Sexuality and menopause. Obstet Gynecol 1990; 74 4 Suppl:26S–30S.

28. Semmens JP, Tsai CC, Semmens EC, Loadholt CB. Effects of estrogen therapy on vaginal physiology during menopause. Obstet Gynecol 1985;66:15–23.

29. Masters WH, Johnson VE. Human sexual response. Boston, MA: Little Brown, and Co.;1966. p. 141–68.

30. Writing Group for the Women's Health Initiative Investigators. Risks and benefits of estrogen plus progestin in healthy postmenopausal women: principal results from the Women's Health Initiative randomized controlled trial. JAMA 2002;288:321–33.

31. Genant HK, Jergas M, Palermo L, et al. Comparison of semiquantitative visual and quantitative morphometric assessment of prevalent and incident vertebral fractures in osteoporosis. The study of osteoporotic Fractures Research Group. J Bone Miner Res 1996;11:984–96.

32. Hernandez-Avila M, Colditz GA, Stampfer MJ, et al. Caffeine, moderate alcohol intake, and risk of fractures of the hip and forearm in middle-aged women. Am J Clin Nutr 1991;54:157–63.

33. Wenger NK, Speroff L, Packard B. Cardiovascular health and disease in women. N Engl J Med 1993;329:247–56.

34. Creasman WT, Henderson D, Hinshaw W, Clarke-Pearson DL. Estrogen replacement therapy in the patient treated for endometrial cancer. Obstet Gynecol 1986;67:326–30.

35. Lee RB, Burke TW, Park RC. Estrogen replacement therapy

following treatment for stage I endometrial carcinoma. Gynecol Oncol 1990;36:189–91.

36. Chapman JA, DiSaia PJ, Osann K, et al. Estrogen replacement in surgical stage I and II endometrial cancer survivors. Am J Obstet Gynecol 1996;175:1195–200.

37. Suriano KA, McHale M, McLaren CE, et al. Estrogen replacement therapy in endometrial cancer patients: a matched control study. Obstet Gynecol 2001;97:555–60.

38. Carr JA, Schoon PA, Look KY. An atypical recurrence of endometrial carcinoma following estrogen replacement therapy. Gynecol Oncol 1996;60:498–9.

39. Lynch HT, Bardawil WA, Harris RE, et al. Multiple primary cancers and prolonged survival: familial colonic and endometrial cancers. Dis Colon Rectum 1978;21:165–8.

40. Lynch HT, Cavalieri RJ, Lynch JF, Casey MJ. Gynecologic cancer clues to Lynch syndrome II diagnosis: a family report. Gynecol Oncol 1992;44:198–203.

41. Jones KD, Owen E, Berresford A, Sutton C. Endometrial adenocarcinoma arising from endometriosis of the rectosigmoid colon. Gynecol Oncol 2002;86:220–2.

42. Nachtigall LE. Isoflavones in the management of the menopause. J Br Menopause Soc 2001;7 Suppl 1:8–12.

43. Jones KP. Menopause and cognitive function: estrogens and alternative therapies. Clin Obstet Gynecol 2000;43:198–206.

44. Kulper GG, Carlsson B, Grandien K, et al. Comparison of the ligand binding specificity and transcript tissue distribution of estrogen receptors alpha and beta. Endocrinology 1997;138:863–70.

45. Punyahotra S, Dennerstein L, Lehert P. Menopausal experiences of Thai women. Part I: symptoms and their correlates. Maturitas 1997;26:1–7.

46. Van Patten CL, Olivotto IA, Chambers K, et al. Effect of soy phytoestrogens on hot flashes in postmenopausal women with breast cancer: A randomized clinical trial. J Clin Oncol 2002;20:1449–55.

47. Ewies AAA. Phytoestrogens in the management of the menopause: up to date. Obstet Gynecol Surv 2002;57:306–13.

48. Duncan AM, Underhill KEW, XU X, et al. Modest hormonal effects of soy isoflavones in postmenopausal women. J Clin Endocrinol Metab 1999;84:3479–84.

49. Baber RJ, Templeman C, Morton T, et al. Randomized placebo-controlled trial of an isoflavone supplement and menopausal symptoms in women. Climacteric 1999;2:85–92.

50. Upmalis D, Lobo RA, Bradley L, et al. Vasomotor symptom relief by soy isoflavone extract tablets in postmenopausal women: a multicenter double blind, randomized, placebo-controlled study. Menopause 2000;7:236–42.

51. Scambia G, Mango D, Signorile PG, et al. Clinical effects of a standardized soy extract in postmenopausal women: a pilot study. Menopause 2000;7:105–11.

52. Goodman MT, Wilkens LR, Hankin JH, et al. Association of soy and fiber consumption with risk of endometrial cancer. Am J Epidemiol 1997;146:294–306.

53. Johnson EB, Muto MG, Yanushpolsky EH, Mutter GL. Phytoestrogen supplementation and endometrial cancer. Obstet Gynecol 2001;98:947–50.

54. American College of Obstetricians and Gynecologists. ACOG Educational Bulletin No 246. Osteoporosis. Washington, DC: The College; 1998:1–9.

55. Kass-Annese B. Alternative therapies for menopause. Clin Obstet Gynecol 2002;43:162–83.

56. Loprinzi CL, Sloan JA, Perez EA, et al. Phase III evaluation of fluoxetine for treatment of hot flashes. J Clin Oncol 2002;20:1578–83.

13

Endometrial Hyperplasia and Management of the Endometrium for Women on Tamoxifen

ANNEKATHRYN GOODMAN, MD

Tamoxifen has become the standard adjuvant therapy in women with breast cancer to reduce the risk of a second breast cancer and to reduce the recurrence rate of the primary breast cancer.[1] Tamoxifen has also been shown to reduce the risk of primary breast cancer in women with a high genetic risk.[2] Although it acts as an estrogen antagonist in the breast, tamoxifen's effect on the female genital tract is more complicated, acting both as an agonist and as an antagonist of estrogen.[3–5] Whereas many epidemiologic and genetic risk factors that predispose women to breast cancer can also increase the overall risk of endometrial cancer, tamoxifen use confers a two- to threefold increased risk of development of endometrial cancer.[2,6,7]

During the past decade, other endometrial pathologies ranging from polyps to endometrial hyperplasia to mixed müllerian tumors have been associated with tamoxifen use (Figures 13–1 to 13–5). This chapter reviews the literature on nonmalignant endometrial changes and strategies for intervention.

DEFINITIONS

In premenopausal women, the endometrium is in a state of dynamic change. After the completion of menses, the zona basalis of the endometrium regenerates with the estrogen stimulation of the proliferative phase. Following midcycle ovulation, the corpus luteum of the ovary produces progesterone. Progesterone stabilizes the endometrium during the secretory phase, which lasts for 14 days. In the absence of a pregnancy, the endometrium then sloughs. After menopause, the endometrial lining becomes atrophic. If estrogen replacement therapy is used, a mixed proliferative and secretory pattern results.

Endometrial polyps are proliferations of glandular endometrium within a fibrous stroma. The glandular component is usually altered with irregularly distributed glands, some of which are cystically dilated, associated with thick-walled or ecstatic vessels, and accompanied by unresponsiveness to progestational hormones.[8–11] Polyps are a common benign cause of postmenopausal bleeding. Recent cytogenetic studies

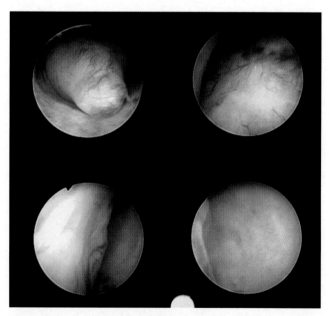

Figure 13–1. Hysteroscopic views of a tamoxifen-induced endometrial polyp. Note the atrophic background endometrium and the smooth, edematous nature of the polyp.

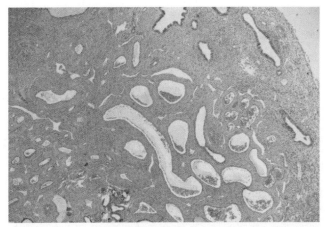

Figure 13–2. Histologic picture of tamoxifen-induced endometrial polyp. Note the prominent vessels and conspicuous fibrous stroma.

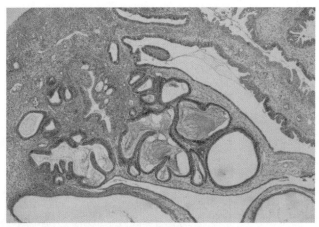

Figure 13–4. Histologic picture of tamoxifen-induced endometrial hyperplasia arising within an endometrial polyp.

have shown an inverted chromosome 6 at bands p21 and q22, consistently in all polyps tested suggesting that polyps may be neoplastic in nature.[12,13]

Endometrial hyperplasia is separated into categories on the basis of the complexity of the glandular architecture and atypia of the nuclei (Table 13–1). Simple hyperplasia refers to an excess of endometrial glands that are often cystic (cystic hyperplasia). It has minimal malignant potential. Complex hyperplasia refers to a more complex architectural proliferation with cytologic atypia, which, when severe, has been reported to have a 40% rate of malignant change.[11]

DIAGNOSIS

Abnormal bleeding is the most common symptom associated with endometrial lesions. Any staining,

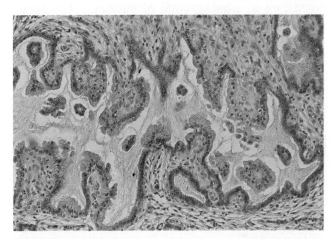

Figure 13–3. Histologic picture of papillary hyperplasia with mucinous metaplasia within a tamoxifen-induced endometrial polyp.

spotting, or bleeding after menopause should be considered abnormal and warrants an evaluation. A change in the quality of menses, such as heavier or longer bleeding or intermenstrual spotting in premenopausal women, can be due to endometrial pathology. Any abnormal bleeding needs to be evaluated with a pathologic evaluation of the endometrial cavity.

Women who have cervical stenosis will not have bleeding. A careful pelvic examination will reveal cervical stenosis. If a cytobrush or Q-tip cannot be passed through the external cervical os, stenosis is present. Asymptomatic women with cervical stenosis who have risk factors for endometrial pathology, such as strong family histories of pelvic malignancies, tamoxifen use, exogenous unopposed estrogen, and endogenous sources of excess estrogen, for example, obesity or chronic anovulation, should have an evaluation of the endometrial lining.

An office endometrial biopsy is the first procedure of choice to evaluate the lining (Table 13–2). However, this is not as sensitive and accurate as hysteroscopy and curettage.[14,15] The presence of cervical stenosis, vaginal stenosis, and extreme discomfort can preclude outpatient sampling and require dilatation and curettage under anesthesia. In one study,[16] 31% of 209 women with abnormal ultrasonographic findings of the endometrium had cervical stenosis that prevented outpatient endometrial sampling.

Ultrasonography has been used to evaluate the endometrial lining thickness. In general, an endometrial lining thickness > 8 mm on ultrasonography

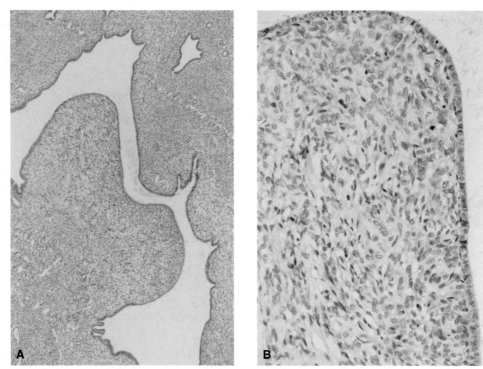

Figure 13–5. *A,* Histologic picture of tamoxifen-induced müllerian adenosarcoma. Typical intracystic polypoid fronds covered by epithelium are seen. *B,* On high power, the stroma has the features of low-grade malignant endometrial stroma. There is stromal cell atypia and a mitotic figure.

had a 100% positive predictive value for endometrial disease.[17] In women on tamoxifen, a duration-dependent increase in the stromal component of the endometrial lining caused an increased false-positive rate for ultrasonographic evaluation of endometrial pathology.[18–23] One study found a 46% false-negative rate of transvaginal ultrasonography.[24] In a review of 48 studies evaluating the accuracy of ultrasonography in diagnosing endometrial cancers in women with postmenopausal bleeding, the detection rate was inadequate, with a high false-positive rate.[25] These data reinforce the need for invasive diagnostic testing in symptomatic women.

Sonohysterography (SHG), a technique that involves the sterile instillation of saline into the endometrial cavity followed by ultrasonography, can better delineate the endometrial thickness and con-

tour.[26–30] It has been suggested that SHG is the best diagnostic imaging study to evaluate the endometrial lining. However, as no differentiation between benign and malignant lesions can be made by this technique, SHG cannot replace evaluating histopathology of the endometrium,

Recent studies have found that endometrial abnormalities occurring in the setting of tamoxifen use seem to be more heterogeneous than in the absence of tamoxifen, with focal hyperplastic lesions coexisting in a background of atrophy.[31] The false-negative rate by office biopsy may be higher, arguing in favor of a dilation and curettage with hysteroscopy as the best method to target an abnormal area within the cavity for histologic evaluation (see Figure 13–1).

Table 13–1. CLASSIFICATION OF ENDOMETRIAL HYPERPLASIA

Simple hyperplasia
Complex hyperplasia (adenomatous)
Simple atypical hyperplasia
Complex atypical hyperplasia (adenomatous with atypia)

Table 13–2. ENDOMETRIAL HYPERPLASIA: DIAGNOSTIC TOOLS

Pelvic examination (look for cervical stenosis)
Office endometrial biopsy
Office hysteroscopy
Transvaginal ultrasonography
Sonohysterography
Dilation and curettage (D & C) and hysteroscopy

TAMOXIFEN-INDUCED ENDOME TRIAL CHANGES

About 40% of postmenopausal women receiving tamoxifen have some type of endometrial abnormality (Table 13–3).[17] However, only 2 to 3 per 1,000 per year develop symptomatic endometrial cancer. Laboratory and clinical data have demonstrated the potential for tamoxifen to have proliferative effects on the endometrium and to act as a tumor promoter. Tamoxifen binds to the estrogen receptor and initially exerts an estrogen-like effect. The tamoxifen-receptor complex shows long-term nuclear retention so that prolonged estrogen antagonism follows early estrogenic manifestations.[32] The ratio of proliferative to atrophic uterine mucosa in postmenopausal women taking tamoxifen is much higher than seen in comparable controls.[33] Although epidemiologic evidence indicates that unopposed estrogens act at a late stage of promotion in the development of endometrial cancer,[34] tamoxifen has been shown in animal studies to act as an initiating agent by producing deoxyribonucleic acid (DNA)-covalent adducts.[35] DNA flow cytometry evaluated endometrial biopsy specimens from 33 women receiving 20 mg/d of tamoxifen compared with 37 women without breast cancer.[23] Although there were no findings of malignancy during the 36-month follow-up, there was a time-dependent proliferative effect on the endometrium. This effect appeared to be mediated by the stromal component.

Reviews of the gynecologic side effects of tamoxifen have not clearly separated out the differences in effects and neoplastic risks between pre- and post-menopausal women.[36–40] The menstrual cycle becomes irregular or amenorrheic in about 50% of premenopausal tamoxifen users.[41] Although follow-up is short, only those premenopausal women with low serum estradiol levels seem to be at increased risk

---

Table 13–3. TAMOXIFEN-INDUCED ENDOMETRIAL PATHOLOGY: LIST OF LESIONS ENCOUNTERED IN DESCENDING ORDER OF FREQUENCY

Endometrial polyps (often showing metaplasia and sometimes showing hyperplasia)
Endometrial hyperplasia
Endometrial adenocarcinoma
Mixed müllerian tumors

---

of tamoxifen-associated endometrial pathology.[42,43] Sixty-seven breast cancer patients on tamoxifen who had abnormal vaginal bleeding were compared with 48 equally symptomatic breast cancer patients who were not taking tamoxifen.[44] Twenty-three percent of the premenopausal tamoxifen-treated women had abnormal endometrial histopathology compared with 12% of the nontamoxifen group. In contrast, 66.7% of tamoxifen-treated postmenopausal women had abnormal findings compared with 30.4% of the nontamoxifen-treated postmenopausal women. These cohort analyses suggest that postmenopausal women are at highest risk of tamoxifen-induced endometrial lesions.

A retrospective histologic review of the endometrium from 700 patients who had received tamoxifen 20 mg/d for 1 to 16 years (mean 4 years) showed 46% with inactive endometrium, 15% with proliferative or secretory endometrium, 23% with benign polyps, 12.9% with polyps with atypical hyperplasia, 8% with hyperplasia, and 4.7% with endometrial cancer.[45] Tamoxifen may exert its variable and inconsistent effects on the endometrium because the epithelial elements respond variably. Different parts of the same endometrium in an individual patient may manifest atrophy, proliferation, hyperplasia, and cancer with tamoxifen exposure.[46,47]

Overall, endometrial polyps have been the most common endometrial pathology described in association with tamoxifen (see Figures 13–1 to 13–3).[48,49] Polyps are found in 13.4% of asymptomatic and 35.7% of symptomatic patients with breast cancer. Three to 10% of endometrial polyps resected from tamoxifen-treated postmenopausal patients have malignant changes.[48,50] Endometrial polyps from tamoxifen-treated patients are grossly different from those seen in patients not exposed to tamoxifen. They are more translucent, edematous, and microscopically more fibrotic and more often associated with metaplasia of the epithelial component (see Figure 13–3).[45] Risk factors for tamoxifen-induced polyps include obesity, older menopausal age, and longer duration of breast disease than similar patients without endometrial pathology.[51, 52] Long-term tamoxifen therapy of > 48 months increases the frequency of endometrial lesions, especially polyps.[53] Starting with an empty endometrial cavity, 3 years of tamoxifen stimulates the growth of endometrial polyps in 29% of women and an atrophic appearance in the remainder.[54] Histopathologic studies of tamoxifen-induced polyps suggest a possible neoplastic potential; in one study, 15 of 33 cancers arose directly in the endometrial polyps.[45] Tamoxifen-induced polyps also seem to be more likely to harbor cancers than those in controls.[4,55]

Ectopic endometrium, even when it is inactive, can respond to tamoxifen. Tamoxifen may induce or unmask endometriosis in both pre- and postmenopausal patients with no prior history. Polypoid, hyperplastic, and neoplastic changes may arise within endometriotic foci.[56] Adenomyosis—ectopic endometrial tissue located in the myometrium—was found three to four times more frequently in hysterectomy specimens from women receiving tamoxifen compared with those who have not been exposed to this drug.[57]

Endometrial hyperplasia in both polyps (see Figure 13–4) and the endometrial lining in tamoxifen-exposed women is consistent with a tissue response to estrogenic stimulation. A preliminary report of endometrial hyperplasia in an oophorectomized woman receiving tamoxifen suggested a direct etiologic role for tamoxifen in endometrial lesions.[58] A prospective evaluation of 111 women on tamoxifen revealed 2 (2%) with simple hyperplasia and 1 with atypical complex hyperplasia.[59] A retrospective review of symptomatic women demonstrated a 20% incidence of hyperplasia.[45] There are no prospective studies evaluating the malignant potential of tamoxifen-associated endometrial hyperplasia. However, the background hyperplasia and the polyps showing atypical hyperplasia raise the possibility that these lesions are intermediate between simple hyperplasia and endometrial carcinoma.[4] The estrogen model of progression from endometrial proliferation to hyperplasia and cancer does not seem to apply for tamoxifen. Tamoxifen-induced lesions seem to originate from the endometrial stroma and progress via polypoid growth, whereas the overlying endometrium remains atrophic.[54]

TREATMENT

Estrogen-induced hyperplasia is frequently responsive to high-dose progestagens.[60] Endometrial

malignancies in patients on tamoxifen are often morphologically different from those usually arising from unopposed estrogen.[61] The concomitant use of progesterone does not seem to prevent or reverse tamoxifen-associated endometrial changes.[62] Cyclic progestagens during tamoxifen use failed to reverse endometrial abnormalities identified by ultrasonography.[14] Moreover progestagens may blunt the antitumor action of tamoxifen on breast tissue.[63,64] A recent randomized controlled trial of postmenopausal women on at least 1 year of tamoxifen evaluated them with a levonorgestrel intrauterine device (IUD) versus those undergoing routine surveillance only. No new endometrial polyps were seen in the IUD group after 12 months.[65] Longer follow-up will be needed to assess the efficacy of this IUD, as tamoxifen-induced effects are duration dependent and no short term differences in the endometrial lining have been reported with tamoxifen use up to 26 months.[66]

For those lesions that are premalignant by Silverberg and Kurman's criteria,[11] a hysterectomy should be strongly considered. Women who have gene mutations, such as *BRCA1* and *BRCA2* that place them at high risk of breast and ovarian cancers should be counseled about prophylactic removal of the ovaries and fallopian tubes. For women in this group who then develop tamoxifen-induced endometrial lesions, the uterus should be removed along with the adnexa. For women with breast cancer, a family history of hereditary nonpolyposis colon cancer gives a lifetime risk of endometrial cancer of 50 to 60%, and prophylactic hysterectomy is a reasonable intervention (also see Chapter 3).[67]

RECOMMENDATIONS

Prior to the institution of tamoxifen, patients should undergo a careful gynecologic history, pelvic examination, and Papanicolaou smear. Consideration should be given to obtaining a baseline transvaginal ultrasonogram to identify occult preexisting benign and malignant abnormalities in the endometrium. Routine monitoring with endometrial biopsy and ultrasonography in asymptomatic women who are taking tamoxifen is not recommended. However, transvaginal ultrasonography should be considered in women who are difficult to examine because of obesity, cervical stenosis, or vaginismus. Annual endometrial biopsy is recommended for women with familial cancer syndromes, such as hereditary nonpolyposis colon cancer.[68]

Asymptomatic women with an abnormal transvaginal ultrasonogram should undergo a sonohysterography. Women with abnormal bleeding or vaginal biopsy must have an endometrial biopsy. If the biopsy is negative, a dilation and curettage with hysteroscopy is necessary. A Papanicolaou smear showing atypical glandular cells or the finding of benign endometrial cells indicates the need for endometrial sampling (Table 13–4).

SUMMARY

Women who take tamoxifen as adjuvant therapy for breast cancer have a cumulative risk of developing endometrial pathology. Most significant endometrial lesions cause abnormal vaginal bleeding, and these women must be evaluated by endometrial biopsy. All women on tamoxifen need annual pelvic examinations. Women who have cervical stenosis will not develop bleeding in the setting of an endometrial lesion, and pelvic ultrasonography to evaluate the endometrial lining is important. Most tamoxifen-induced endometrial pathology is benign. However, severely atypical hyperplasia is a significant premalignant lesion and should be treated by

hysterectomy. Careful monitoring will also enable detection of the occasional patient who develops carcinoma or, rarely, other malignant lesions, such as müllerian adenosarcoma or even malignant mixed mullerian tumor.[69–71]

REFERENCES

1. Early Breast Cancer Trialists Collaborative Group. Systematic treatment of early breast cancer by hormonal, cytotoxic, or immune therapy: 133 randomized trials involving 31,000 recurrences and 2400 deaths among 75,000 women. Lancet 1992;339:71–85.
2. Fisher B, Constantino JP, Wickerham DL, et al. Tamoxifen for the prevention of breast cancer: Report of the national Surgical Adjuvant Breast and Bowel Project P-1 Study. J Natl Cancer Inst 1998;90:1371–88.
3. Gottardis MM, Robinson SP, Satyaswaroop PG. Contrasting actions of tamoxifen on endometrial and breast tumor growth in the athymic mouse. Cancer Res 1988;48:812–5.
4. Ismail S. Pathology of endometrium treated with tamoxifen. J Clin Pathol 1994;47:827–33.
5. Daniel Y, Inbar M, Bar-am A, et al. The effects of tamoxifen treatment on the endometrium. Fertil Steril 1996;65:1083–9.
6. Curtis RE, Boice JD, Shriner DA, et al. Second cancers after adjuvant therapy for breast cancer [brief communication]. J Natl Cancer Inst 1996;88:332–4.
7. Fornander T, Cedermark B, Mattson A, et al. Adjuvant tamoxifen in early breast cancer: occurrences of new primary cancers. Lancet 1989;ii:117–9.
8. Gompel C, Silverberg SG, editors. The corpus uteri. In: Pathology in gynecology and obstetrics. Philadelphia, PA: Lippincott; 1994. p. 163–283.
9. Kurman RJ, Mazur MT. Benign disease of the endometrium. In: Kurman RJ, editor. Blaustein's pathology of the female genital tract. 4th ed. New York, NY: Springer-Verlag; 1994. p. 367–409.
10. Zaino RJ, editor. Abnormal proliferations, hyperplasia, and polyps: the non-neoplastic proliferations. In: Interpretation of endometrial biopsies and curettings. New York, N Y: Lippincott-Raven. 1996. pp. 203–40.
11. Silverberg SG, Kurman RJ, editors. Endometrial polyps and hyperplasias. In: Tumors of the cervix and gestational trophoblastic disease: atlas of tumor pathology – fascicle 3. Washington D.C.: Armed Forces Institute of Pathology; 1992. p. 15–22.
12. Dal Cin P, De Wolf F, Klerckx P, van den Berghe H. The 6p21 chromosome region is nonrandomly involved in endometrial polyps. Gynecol Oncol 1992;46:393–6.
13. Speleman F, Dal Cin P, Van Roy N, et al. Is t(6;20) (p21q13) a characteristic change in endometrial polyps? Genes Chromosomes Cancer 1991;3:318–9.
14. Powles TJ, Bourne T, Athanasiou S, et al. The effect of noresthisterone on endometrial abnormalities identified by transvaginal ultrasound screening of healthy postmenopausal women on tamoxifen or placebo. Br J Cancer 1998;78:272–5.

Table 13–4. WORK-UP OF ENDOMETRIAL PATHOLOGY IN WOMEN ON TAMOXIFEN

Indication for a transvaginal ultrasound in asymptomatic women
  Compromised examination
  Cervical stenosis
  Genetic risk factors
    Family history of ovarian cancer
    Family history of endometrial cancer
    Hereditary nonpolyposis colon cancer syndrome
Indication for endometrial biopsy or dilation and curettage
  Abnormal premenopausal vaginal bleeding
  Any postmenopausal bleeding
  Abnormal vaginal discharge
  Papanicolau smear showing:
    Atypical glandular cells
    Benign endometrial cells out of phase with menstrual cycle
    Benign endometrial cells in a postmenopausal woman
  Abnormal transvaginal ultrasonogram
    Fluid in the uterus
    Endometrial stripe > 5 mm
  Abnormal sonohysterogram

15. Neven P, Vernaeve H. Guidelines for monitoring patients taking tamoxifen treatment. Drug Saf 2000;22:1–11.

16. Cecchini S, Ciatto S, Bonardi R, et al. Screening by ultrasonography for endometrial carcinoma in postmenopausal breast cancer patients under adjuvant tamoxifen. Gynecol Oncol 1996;60:409–11.

17. Kedar RP, Bourne TH, Powles TJ, et al. Effects of tamoxifen on the uterus and ovaries of postmenopausal women in a randomized breast cancer prevention trial. Lancet 1994;343:1318–21.

18. Bertelli G, Venturini M, Del Mastro L, et al. Tamoxifen and the endometrium: findings of pelvic ultrasound examination and endometrial biopsy in asymptomatic breast cancer patients. Breast Cancer Res Treat 1998;47:41–6.

19. Hann Le, Giess CS, Bach AM, et al. Endometrial thickness in tamoxifen-treated patients: correlation with clinical and pathologic findings. AJR Am J Roentgenol 1997; 168:657–61.

20. Achiron R, Lipitz S, Sivan E, et al. Changes mimicking endometrial neoplasia in postmenopausal, tamoxifen-treated women with breast cancer: a transvaginal Doppler study. Ultrasound Obstet Gynecol 1995;6:116–20.

21. Goldstein SR. Unusual ultrasonographic appearance of the uterus in patients receiving tamoxifen. Am J Obstet Gynecol 1994;170:447–51.

22. Bornstein J, Auslender R, Pascal B, et al. Diagnostic pitfalls of ultrasonographic uterine screening in women treated with tamoxifen. J Reprod Med 1994;39:674–8.

23. Decensi A, Fontana V, Bruno S, et al. Effect of tamoxifen on endometrial proliferation. J Clin Oncol 1996;14:434–40.

24. Love CDB, Muir BB, Scrimgeour JB, et al. Investigation of endometrial abnormalities in asymptomatic women treated with tamoxifen and an evaluation of the role of endometrial screening. J Clin Oncol 1999;17:2050–4.

25. Tabor A, Watt HC, Wald NJ. Endometrial thickness as a test for endometrial cancer in women with postmenopausal vaginal bleeding. Obstet Gynecol 2002;99:663–70.

26. Achiron R, Lipitz S, Sivan E, et al. Sonohysterography for ultrasonographic evaluation of tamoxifen-associated cystic thickened endometrium. J Ultrasound Med 1995;14: 685–8.

27. Schwartz LB, Snyder J, Horan C, et al. The use of transvaginal ultrasound and saline infusion sonohysterography for the evaluation of asymptomatic postmenopausal breast cancer patients on tamoxifen. Ultrasound Obstet Gynecol 1998;11:48–53.

28. Tepper R, Beyth Y, Altaras MM, et al. Value of sonohysterography in asymptomatic postmenopausal tamoxifen-treated patients. Gynecol Oncol 1997;64:386–91.

29. Bonilla-Musoles F, Raga F, Osborne NG, et al. Three-dimensional hysterosonography for the study of endometrial tumors: comparison with conventional transvaginal sonography, hysterosalpingography, and hysteroscopy. Gynecol Oncol 1997;65:245–52.

30. Valenzano M, Bertelle GF, Costantini S, et al. Transvaginal ultrasonography and hysterosonography to monitor endometrial effects in tamoxifen-treated patients. Eur J Gynaecol Oncol 2001;22:441–4.

31. Cohen I, Altaras MM, Shapira J, et al. Different coexisting endometrial histological features in asymptomatic postmenopausal breast cancer patients treated with tamoxifen. Gynecol Obstet Invest 1997;43:60–3.

32. Neumannova M, Kauppila A, Kivinen S, Vinko R. Short-term effects of tamoxifen, medroxyprogesterone acetate, and their combination on receptor kinetics and 17 beta-hydroxysteroid dehydrogenase in human endometrium. Obstet Gynecol 1985;66:695–700.

33. Neven P, De Muylder X, Van Belle Y, et al. Tamoxifen and the uterus and endometrium [letter]. Lancet 1989;i:375.

34. Van Leeuwen FE, Rookus MA. The role of exogenous hormones in the epidemiology of breast, ovarian, and endometrial cancer. Eur J Cancer Clin Oncol 1989;25: 1961–72.

35. Han X, Liehr JG. Induction of covalent DNA adducts in rodents by tamoxifen. Cancer Res 1992;52:1360–3.

36. Wolf DM, Jordan VC. Gynecologic complications associated with long term adjuvant tamoxifen therapy for breast cancer. Gynecol Oncol 1992;45:118–28.

37. Neven P, Shepherd JH, Lowe DG. Tamoxifen and the gynaecologist. Br J Obstet Gynaecol 1993;100:893–7.

38. Cohen CJ. Tamoxifen and endometrial cancer: Tamoxifen effects on the human female genital tract. Semin Oncol 1997;24 Suppl 1:55–64.

39. Ugwumadu AHN, Carmichael PL, Neven P. Tamoxifen and the female genital tract. Int J Gynaecol Cancer 1998;8:6–15.

40. Benshushan A, Brzezinski A. Tamoxifen effects on menopause-associated risk factors and symptoms. Obstet Gynecol Surv 1999;54:272–8.

41. Sunderland MC, Osborne CK. Tamoxifen in premenopausal patients with metastatic breast cancer. A review. J Clin Oncol 1991;9:1283–97.

42. Chang J, Powles TJ, Ashley SE, et al. Variation in endometrial thickening in women with amenorrhea on tamoxifen. Breast Cancer Res Treat 1998;48:81–5.

43. Hulka CA, Hall DA. Endometrial abnormalities associated with tamoxifen therapy for breast cancer: Sonographic and pathologic correlation. AJR Am J Roentgenol 1993; 160:809–12.

44. Cheng W-F, Lin H-H, Torng P-L, Huang S-C. Comparison of endometrial changes among symptomatic tamoxifen-treated and nontreated premenopausal and postmenopausal breast cancer patients. Gynecol Oncol 1997; 66:233–7.

45. Deligdisch L, Kalir T, Cohen CJ, et al. Endometrial histopathology in 700 patients treated with tamoxifen for breast cancer. Gynecol Oncol 2000;78:181–6.

46. Ugwumadu AHN, Bower D, Ho PKH. Tamoxifen induced adenomyosis and adenomyomatous endometrial polyp. Br J Obstet Gynaecol 1993;100:386–8.

47. Corley D, Rowe J, Curtis MT, et al. Postmenopausal bleeding from unusual endometrial polyps in women on chronic tamoxifen therapy. Obstet Gynecol 1992;79:111–6.

48. Gibson LE, Barakat RR, Venkarraman ES. Endometrial pathology at dilation and curettage in breast cancer patients: comparison of tamoxifen users and nonusers. Cancer J 1996;2:35–8.

49. Schlesinger C, Kamoi S, Ascher S, et al. Endometrial polyps: a comparison study of patients receiving tamoxifen with two control groups. Int J Gynecol Pathol 1998; 17:302–11.

50. Cohen I, Perel E, Flex D, et al. Endometrial pathology in postmenopausal tamoxifen treatment: comparison between gynecologically symptomatic and asymptomatic breast cancer patients. J Clin Pathol 1999;52:278–82.

51. Cohen I , Bernheim J, Azaria R, et al. Malignant endometrial polyps in postmenopausal breast cancer tamoxifen-treated patients. Gynecol Oncol 1999;75:136–41.

52. Cohen I, Azaria R, Bernham J, et al. Risk factors of endometrial polyps resected from postmenopausal patients with breast carcinoma treated with tamoxifen. Cancer 2001; 92:1151–5.

53. Cohen I, Altaras MM, Shapira J, et al. Time-dependent effect of tamoxifen therapy on endometrial pathologies in asymptomatic, postmenopausal breast cancer patients. Int J Gynecol Pathol 1996;15:152–7.

54. Neven P. Local levonorgestrel to prevent tamoxifen-related endometrial lesions. Lancet 2000;356:1698–9.

55. Neven P, De Muylder X, Van Belle Y. Tamoxifen-induced endometrial polyp. N Engl J Med 1997;336:1389.

56. Schlesinger C, Silverberg SG. Tamoxifen-associated polyps (basalomas) arising in multiple endometriotic foci: a case report and review of the literature. Gynecol Oncol 1999; 73:305–11.

57. Cohen I, Beyth Y, Tepper R, et al. Adenomyosis in postmenopausal breast cancer patients treated with tamoxifen: a new entity? Gynecol Oncol 1995;58:86–91.

58. Cross SS, Ismail SM. Endometrial hyperplasia in an oophorectomized woman receiving tamoxifen therapy. Case report. Br J Obstet Gynaecol 1990;97:190–2.

59. Barakat RR, Gilewski TA, Almadrones L, et al. Effect of adjuvant tamoxifen on the endometrium in women with breast cancer: a prospective study using office endometrial biopsy. J Clin Oncol 2000;18:3459–63.

60. Randall TC, Kurman RJ. Progestin treatment of atypical hyperplasia and well-differentiated carcinoma of the endometrium in women under age 40. Obstet Gynecol 1997;90:434–40.

61. Dallenbach-Hellweg G, Hahn U. Mucinous and clear cell adenocarcinomas of the endometrium in patients receiving antiestrogens (tamoxifen) and gestagens. Int J Gynecol Pathol 1995;14:7–15.

62. De Muylder X, Neven P, De Somer M, et al. Endometrial lesions in patients undergoing tamoxifen therapy. Int J Gynaecol Obstet 1991;36:127–30.

63. Robinson SP, Jordan VC. Reversal of the antitumor effect of tamoxifen by progesterone in the 7, 12-dimethylbenzanthracene rat mammary carcinoma model. Cancer Res 1987;47:5386–90.

64. Mourisden HT, Ellemann K, Mattson W, et al. Therapeutic effect of tamoxifen vs. tamoxifen and medroxyprogesterone acetate in advanced breast cancer in postmenopausal women. Cancer Treat Rep 1979;63:171–5.

65. Gardner FJE, Konje JC, Abrams KR, et al. Endometrial protection from tamoxifen-stimulated changes by a levonorgestrel-releasing intrauterine system: a randomized controlled trial. Lancet 2000;356:1711–7.

66. Gibson LE, Barakat RR, Venkatraman ES, Hoskins WJ. Endometrial pathology at dilatation and curettage in breast cancer patients: comparison of tamoxifen users and nonusers. Cancer J Sci Am 1996;2:35–8.

67. Emery J, Lucassen A, Murphy M. Common hereditary cancers and implications for primary care. Lancet 2001; 358:56–63.

68. Watson P, Vasen HF, Mecklin JP, et al. The risk of endometrial cancer in hereditary nonpolyposis colon cancer. Am J Med 1994;96:516–20.

69. Carcangiu ML. Uterine pathology in tamoxifen-treated patients with breast cancer. In: Rosai J, Carcangiu ML, Delellis RA, editors. Anatomic pathology. Vol. 2. Chicago, IL: ASCP Press; 1997. p. 53–70.

70. Clement PB, Oliva E, Young R. Müllerian adenosarcoma of the uterine corpus associated with tamoxifen therapy: a report of six cases and a review of tamoxifen-associated endometrial lesions. Int J Gynecol Pathol 1996;15: 222–9.

71. McCluggage WG, Abdulkader M, Price JH, et al. Uterine carcinosarcoma in patients receiving tamoxifen. A report of 19 cases. Int J Gynecol Cancer 2000;10:280–4.

14

Evaluation of Uterine Smooth Muscle, Stromal, and Malignant Mixed Müllerian Neoplasms: Symptoms, Radiologic Evaluation, and Diagnostic Techniques

SUSANNA I. LEE, MD, PHD

B. HANNAH ORTIZ, MD

ROSS S. BERKOWITZ, MD

EPIDEMIOLOGY

Uterine sarcomas represent fewer than 5% of all uterine corpus cancers and have an incidence of approximately 17.1 per million.[1,2] This chapter reviews the presentation and evaluation of women with sarcomas of the uterus. Included within the section is a review of malignant mixed müllerian tumors (MMMTs), despite the current thinking that these may be epithelial in origin. In most series, MMMT or carcinosarcoma is the most common type of uterine sarcoma (8.2 cases per million), typically followed by leiomyosarcoma (LMS, 6.4 cases per million), and endometrial stromal sarcoma (ESS, 1.8 cases per million).[2] In addition, some tumors are examples of the rare adenosarcoma. Some series have reported a higher incidence of LMS, as high as 53.4% of uterine sarcomas in one study.[3–5]

The average age of diagnosis of uterine sarcoma differs among the subtypes. MMMT is relatively uncommon through middle age, after which it rises sharply with age, with a peak incidence occurring in the 60- to 70-year age range, 10 years later than for ESS or LMS.[5–7] The incidence of LMS has been noted to rise gradually throughout the reproductive years with a peak in the later reproductive years.[2] The mean age is 45 years for LMS, 53 years for MMMT, and 35 years for ESS

in one series.[4] Black women are at greater risk than White women of developing uterine LMS and MMMT. The increased risk of uterine sarcoma in Black American women is opposite to that of endometrial cancer in which the rate among White American women is two to three times higher than among Black American women.[2]

RISK FACTORS

There is much speculation in the literature about the differences in incidence rates between the most common uterine sarcomas: MMMT and LMS. The patient age difference between MMMT and LMS suggests an association between estrogen levels and LMS. The age-specific incidence of uterine LMS and ESS more closely resembles that of tumors of the endometrium, ovary, and breast, which arise in a younger age group.[2,5] This suggests a possible role for sex hormones in the development of these tumors.[5] Small case series have suggested that LMS and ESS may be associated with unopposed estrogen in the etiology of certain histologic types of uterine sarcoma.[8] Conditions associated with uterine sarcomas include obesity (40%), hypertension (33%), and heart disease (30%). However, as many as 30% of patients have no associated comorbid conditions at diagnosis.[6]

Other potential risk factors have been sought. In one classic paper, 5% of patients presenting with uterine sarcomas had received prior pelvic radiation (though not all of those diagnosed were treated for cancer).[6] Similarly, another group reported a 2.4% prior irradiation rate, with a particular association with MMMT.[9,10] Although prior pelvic irradiation has been reported in some patients with uterine sarcoma, there is insufficient evidence to conclude that there is a clear causal relationship.

There is some debate about the potential role for tamoxifen in the etiology of uterine sarcomas. There are case reports and one small series of müllerian adenosarcomas arising in patients after variable periods of tamoxifen use.[11–13] Finally, a single case of pleomorphic rhabdomyosarcoma has also been reported in the setting of tamoxifen use.[14]

The use of oral contraceptives has been positively correlated with the risk of leiomyosarcoma, primarily in patients who have used oral contraceptives for 15 or more years.[8] The use of noncontraceptive estrogens was directly associated with the risk of MMMT but only among recent and long-term users.[8] Women who never smoked cigarettes were at a reduced risk of LMS and ESS but not MMMT, but this risk reduction did not increase with increased smoking.[8]

Even in the presence of risk factors loosely associated with uterine sarcomas, no effective screening is currently available, and the relative rarity of these tumors makes it unlikely that even targeted screening will be useful in reducing mortality from these diseases.

CLINICAL DIAGNOSIS

Clinical presentation patterns differ for the histologic subtypes. Leiomyosarcomas and endometrial stromal sarcomas tend to present earlier and at earlier stages.[7]

The most common symptom, occurring in approximately 80 to 90% of patients, is postmenopausal vaginal bleeding or abnormal uterine bleeding in a pre- or perimenopausal woman.[6,14–16] Occasionally, LMS may present with rapid uterine growth in a pre- or postmenopausal woman with symptoms related to an enlarging pelvic mass. Because LMS is typically an intramural process, abnormal vaginal bleeding may not be associated with this tumor. Although benign leiomyomata can be large and are much more common, there are no validated clinical or radiologic criteria that can accurately distinguish benign from malignant tumors. Any woman presenting with rapid uterine growth can be imaged conservatively with ultrasonography, computed tomography (CT), or magnetic resonance imaging (MRI) (see below) or undergo exploration and possible hysterectomy. However, there is little way to distinguish benign from malignant rapid uterine growth in the vast majority of women with a rapidly enlarging uterine corpus. Indeed, not infrequently, LMS is an incidental finding after myomectomy or hysterectomy for uterine leiomyomata. Other less common symptoms include abdominal or pelvic pain (19%), abdominal mass (15%), weight loss (7%), and vaginal discharge (4%).[6] Other symptoms, such as increasing pelvic pressure, hematuria, constipation, and back pain, may also be seen in association with a large or invasive pelvic mass.

Evaluation of abnormal uterine bleeding is the most important step in making the diagnosis and includes sampling of the endometrium. The simplest method is an outpatient endometrial biopsy, performed easily in an office setting. The most common symptom during and after this procedure is uterine cramping, which resolves in a few hours and can be controlled with nonsteroidal anti-inflammatory drugs.

Operative hysteroscopy may be an effective alternative to endometrial sampling or curettage. There are reports of endometrial stromal sarcoma being diagnosed at operative hysteroscopy, although distinguishing this from an endometrial stromal nodule is difficult on limited sampling (see Chapter 15).[17] In one case, a 26-year-old woman underwent operative hysteroscopy for a polypoid lesion, a 4 cm polyp with long, smooth, dilated vessels, which turned out to be a low-grade endometrial stromal sarcoma. Complete resection of all intracavitary lesions has been recommended by some authors.[18] However, in essentially all cases, surgical resection of the uterus is required, unless extensive metastatic disease is confirmed.

Although endometrial sampling is the gold standard for preoperative evaluation, its sensitivity is limited in stromal tumors because uterine sarcomas may be limited to the myometrium and not involve the endometrium. One study has suggested that endometrial sampling may miss more than 50% of sarcomas. Endometrial sampling is only about 30% sensitive for the diagnosis of uterine leiomyosarcoma and endometrial stromal sarcomas.[19,20]

Preoperative evaluation for extrauterine disease should be thorough and include abdominal and pelvic CT and chest CT. Metastatic disease includes lung metastasis and, less commonly, peritoneal or nodal disease. Occasionally, bizarre sites of metastases, such as the scalp and soft tissue, may be seen. The development of highly sensitive spiral CT scans has complicated evaluation because it is typical to identify very small pulmonary nodules of uncertain etiology. Lesions are often too small for transthoracic needle biopsy or evaluation by positron emission tomography (PET). Central nervous system disease is extremely rare, and evaluation should be limited to women with neurologic symptoms. Complete blood work is seldom useful in staging or establishing diagnosis, although evaluation of renal function is useful in women with large pelvic masses as hydronephrosis results from uterine enlargement or retroperitoneal lymphadenopathy that may compress the ureters.

RADIOLOGIC EVALUATION OF PRIMARY TUMOR

Diagnostic imaging is limited in its ability to differentiate between benign and malignant uterine masses. The most specific feature for distinguishing benign from malignant masses is documented rapid interval growth of a mass on imaging studies in the absence of exogenous estrogen or evidence of extrauterine disease, for example, lymphadenopathy, hepatic metastases, or intraperitoneal tumor implants.[21] Figures 14–1 to 14–3 demonstrate a leiomyosarcoma presenting as a large pelvic mass with central necrosis. This malignant tumor can be distinguished from a benign leiomyoma because of the lymphadenopathy seen in the upper abdomen (see Figure 14–3).

Imaging studies have been used most successfully in preoperative staging of uterine malignancies and to assess the extent of pelvic or extrapelvic disease.[22] MMMT on MRI (Figure 14–4) is seen as a large mass replacing the uterus with heterogeneous signal intensity. It demonstrates irregular borders and frond-like contrast enhancement typical of many malignant uterine masses. The presence of an enlarged pelvic node confirms the extrauterine extension of the tumor.

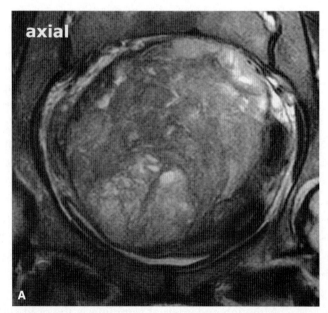
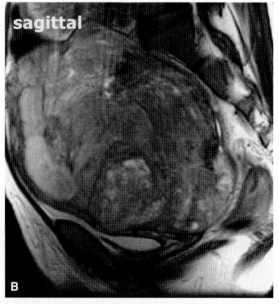

Figure 14–1.   Leiomyosarcoma. Magnetic resonance imaging of the uterus on T_2-weighted axial (A) and sagittal images (B) demonstrates an irregular mass of mixed signal intensity replacing the uterus.

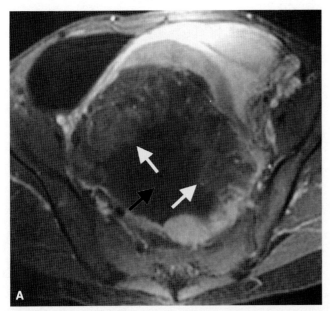
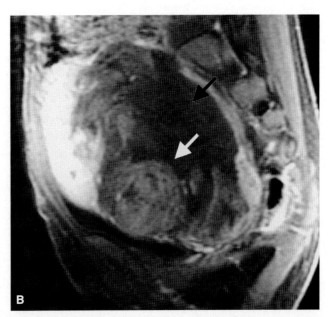

Figure 14–2. On gadolinium administration, the mass demonstrates patchy peripheral enhancement (*white arrows*) with central areas of nonenhancement (*black arrows*) corresponding to tumor necrosis. Right side (*A*), left side (*B*).

Ultrasonography of uterine sarcoma demonstrates an enlarged irregularly shaped uterus with a heterogeneous echotexture. A disordered echotexture, with a mixture of hyperechoic and cystic areas irregularly scattered in the myometrium, was the most predictive pattern (Figure 14–5). This echo pattern appeared to be highly associated with uterine sarcomas.

Positron emission tomography with fluorodeoxyglucose (FDG) imaging is based on metabolic activity in tissues, and its diagnostic usefulness for various malignant tissues has been reported. In contrast to imaging in the head and neck or chest, where PET imaging has proven to be highly sensitive and specific, PET imaging in the abdomen and pelvis has limited use due to signal from the normal uptake and excretion of FDG by the bowel, kidney, and bladder. Thus, even though the specificity of PET remains high (100%), sensitivity is lower (80%).[23]

FIGO STAGING

In 1988, the FIGO (International Federation of Gynecology and Obstetrics) adopted surgical staging as the standard of care for patients presenting with uterine malignancies. Although uterine sarcomas that originate in the endometrium (eg, ESS,

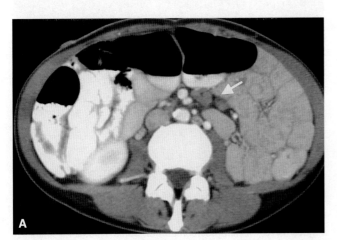
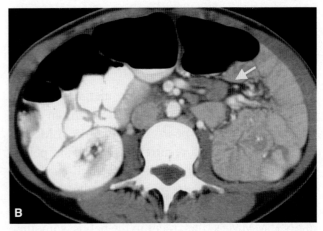

Figure 14–3. An axial computed tomographic image through the upper abdomen of the same patient as in Figure 14–2 shows abnormally enlarged intra-abdominal lymph nodes (*arrows*). Right side (*A*), left side (*B*).

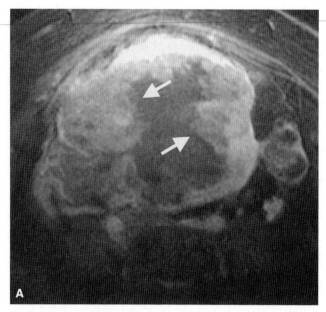
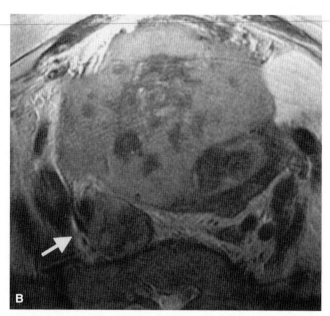

Figure 14–4. MMMT. *A*, Gadolinium-enhanced axial MRI image of the uterus shows a large mass replacing the uterus with frond-like irregular enhancement (*arrows*) typical of many malignant uterine tumors. *B*, Axial-weighted, T$_2$-weighted image shows a uterine mass of mixed signal intensity. An enlarged right obdurator node (*arrow*) confirms extrauterine extension of the tumor.

MMMT) can be staged surgically according to the FIGO staging system for endometrial adenocarcinoma, this is impossible with a sarcoma arising from the myometrium (eg, LMS) because stage I cannot be divided into substages. The FIGO surgical staging for endometrial adenocarcinomas has been adapted to uterine sarcomas as follows:

Stage I: tumor confined to the uterine body
Stage II: tumor confined to the uterine body and cervix
Stage III: tumor spread outside the uterus but confined to the true pelvis
Stage IV: tumor spread outside the true pelvis.[24,25]

EVALUATION OF RECURRENT OR PERSISTENT DISEASE

The overall recurrence rate for uterine sarcomas varies, depending on stage and patient mix in a particular study, but may be in excess of 50%.[7] LMS has demonstrated a 14% recurrence rate in the pelvis. There is a high rate of distant recurrent disease, with initial recurrences in the lungs reportedly as high as 41%.[7] MMMT demonstrates a higher recurrence rate of 56%. MMMTs often recur in the pelvis, sometime very rapidly after primary surgical debulking.[7] One

author reported a 37% recurrence rate in the lungs.[15] For all histologies, among women with tumor diameters < 5 cm, 45% had recurrences at 3 years compared with a 57% recurrence rate in patients who presented with a tumor diameter of 6 to 10 cm. Patients with an initial tumor diameter > 10 cm had a recurrence rate of 69%.[7]

Another prognostic indicator is lymph node metastasis, which was a significant prognostic factor for MMMT in one study. In addition, adnexal

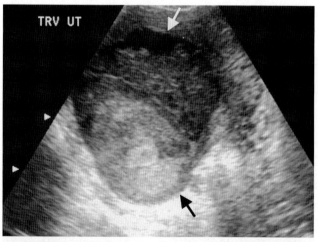

Figure 14–5. Leiomyosarcoma. Transverse ultrasound image of the uterus demonstrates a predominantly solid mass with mixed hypo- (*white arrow*) and hyperechoic (*black arrow*) features.

spread, tumor size, lymph-vascular space invasion, histologic grade, cell type, peritoneal cytology, cervical or isthmic involvement, and depth of myometrial invasions are important prognostic factors.[7]

Surgery remains the mainstay of treatment to achieve local control and has a role in recurrent disease (see Chapter 16). Because most recurrences occur distantly, improved survival will depend on the development of more effective systemic treatment.

In summary, the preoperative diagnosis and evaluation of uterine sarcomas is limited by the relative rarity of this tumor and the lack of specific imaging features to distinguish this from other benign entities of the uterine corpus. Guided biopsies, PET, CT, and MRI may provide useful staging information, but their availability is unlikely to aid in earlier diagnosis and, thus, affect survival.

REFERENCES

1. Curtin, JP, Kavanagh, JJ, Fox, H, Spanos, WJ. Corpus: mesenchymal tumors. In: Hoskins WJ, Perex CA, Young RC, editors. Principles and practice of gynecologic oncology. Philadelphia (PA): Lippincott Williams & Wilkins; 2002. p. 919.
2. Harlow BL, Weiss NS, Lofton S. The epidemiology of sarcomas of the uterus. J Natl Cancer Inst 1986;76:399–402.
3. Gonzalez-Bosquet E, Martinez-Palones JM, Gonzalez-Bosquet J, et al. Uterine sarcoma: a clinicopathological study of 93 cases. Eur J Gynaecol Oncol 1997;18:192–5.
4. Ayhan A, Tuncer ZS, Tanir M, et al. Uterine sarcoma: the Hacettepe hospital experience of 88 consecutive patients. Eur J Gynaecol Oncol 1997;18:146–8.
5. Nordal RR, Thoresen SO. Uterine sarcomas in Norway 1956–1992: incidence, survival and mortality. Eur J Cancer 1977;33:907–11.
6. Salazar OM, Bonfiglio TA, Patten SF, et al. Uterine sarcomas: natural history, treatment and prognosis. Cancer 1978;42:1152–60.
7. Major FJ, Blessing JA, Silverberg SG, et al. Prognostic factors in early-stage uterine sarcoma: a Gynecologic Oncology Group Study. Cancer 1993;71:1702–9.
8. Schwarz SM, Weiss NS, Daling JR, et al. Exogenous sex hormone use, correlates of endogenous hormone levels, and the incidence of histologic types of sarcoma of the uterus. Cancer 1996;15:717–24.
9. George M, Pejovic MH, Kramar A. Uterine sarcomas: prognostic factors and treatment modalities—study on 209 patients. Gynecol Oncol 1987;24:58–67.
10. Norris HJ, Taylor HB. Postirradiation sarcomas of the uterus. Obstet Gynecol 1965;26:689–94.
11. Clement PB, Oliva E, Young RH. Müllerian adenosarcoma of the uterine corpus associated with tamoxifen therapy: a report of six cases and a review of tamoxifen-associated endometrial lesions. Int J Gynecol Pathol 1996;15(3): 222–9.
12. Arici DS, Aker H, Yildiz E, Tasyurt A. Müllerian adenosarcoma of the uterus associated with tamoxifen therapy. Arch Gynecol Obstet 2000;264:105–7.
13. Carvalho FM, Carvalho JP, Motta EV, Souen J. Müllerian adenosarcoma of the uterus with sarcomatous overgrowth following tamoxifen treatment for breast cancer. Rev Hosp Clin Fac Med Sao Paulo 2000;55:17–20.
14. Okado DH Rowland JB, Petrovic LM. Uterine pleomorphic rhabdomyosarcoma in a patient receiving tamoxifen therapy. Gynecol Oncol 1999;75:509–13.
15. Salazar OM, Bonfiglio TA, Patten SF, et al. Uterine sarcomas: analysis of failures with special emphasis on the use of adjuvant radiation therapy. Cancer 1978;42:1161–70.
16. Olah KS, Gee GH, Blunt S, et al. Retrospective analysis of 318 cases of uterine sarcoma. Eur J Cancer 1991;27: 1095–99.
17. Flam F, Radestad A. Endometrial stromal sarcoma diagnosed by operative hysteroscopy. Hum Reprod 1996;11:2797–8.
18. Marabini A, Gubbini G, De Jaco P, et al. A case of unsuspected endometrial stromal sarcoma removed by operative hysteroscopy. Gynecol Oncol 1995;59:409–11.
19. Schwartz SM, Thomas DB. A case control study on risk factors for sarcomas of the uterus. Cancer 1989;64: 2487–92.
20. Umesaki N, Tanaka T, Masato M, et al. Positron emission tomography with ^{18}F-Fluorodeoxyglucose of uterine sarcoma: a comparison with magnetic resonance imaging and power doppler imaging. Gynecol Oncol 2001;80:372–7.
21. Walsh JW. Computed tomography of gynecological neoplasms. Radiol Clin North Am 1992;30:817–30.
22. Bragg DG, Hricak H. Imaging in gynecological malignancies. Cancer 1993;71:1648–51.
23. Torizuka T, Nobezawa S, Kanno T, et al. Ovarian cancer recurrence: role of whole-body positron emission tomography using 2-[fluorine-18]-fluoro-2-deoxy-D-glucose. Eur J Nucl Med Mol Imag 2002;29:797–803.
24. Lewis JL, Berchuck A, Rubin SC, et al. Uterine sarcomas. In: Shiu MH, Brennan M, editors. Surgical management of soft tissue sarcoma. Philadelphia (PA): Lea & Febiger; 1989. p. 213.
25. Piura B, Rabinovich A, Yanai-Inbar I, et al. Uterine sarcoma in the south of Israel: study of 36 cases. J Surg Oncol 1997;64:55–62.

15

Pathology of Sarcomas and Mixed Müllerian Tumors of the Uterine Corpus

ESTHER OLIVA, MD
PHILIP B. CLEMENT, MD
ROBERT H. YOUNG, MD, FRCPath

Mesenchymal neoplasms of the uterus are uncommon when benign smooth muscle tumors are excluded. Among uterine malignancies, sarcomas account for approximately 3%, leiomyosarcoma being the most common of them. In this chapter, the most frequently encountered sarcomas of the uterine corpus are discussed in detail, with special emphasis on their gross and microscopic features and their differential diagnosis with benign or other malignant tumors. The correct pathologic diagnosis of these tumors has major therapeutic and prognostic implications for the patient. Rarer sarcomas are also briefly considered, as their recognition is also important, mainly from the prognostic viewpoint. Tumors with both epithelial and stromal components that may be clinically malignant (müllerian adenosarcoma) or are notoriously aggressive (malignant müllerian mixed tumor [MMMT], carcinosarcoma) are reviewed, even though they are thought to be of endometrioid epithelial cell lineage. From the clinical viewpoint, particularly in the case of the MMMT, they have traditionally been grouped with the sarcomas. Finally, two tumors not fundamentally considered sarcomatous, intravenous leiomyomatosis and the uterine tumor resembling ovarian sex cord tumor, are considered for the reasons noted in the footnotes to Table 15–1.

LEIOMYOSARCOMA

Leiomyosarcoma of the uterus accounts for approximately 80% of uterine sarcomas when MMMTs are

excluded. They are typically large solitary masses.[1–4] Although rapid enlargement of a myometrial tumor suggests leiomyosarcoma, a similar phenomenon may be seen with leiomyomas, particularly in pregnant women or those taking oral contraceptives, but occasionally with neither association. Approximately two-thirds of uterine leiomyosarcomas are intramural, one-fifth submucosal, one-tenth subserosal, and one-twentieth arise in the cervix. They are

Table 15–1. CLASSIFICATION OF UTERINE SARCOMAS AND RELATED NEOPLASMS

Leiomyosarcoma
 Spindled
 Myxoid
 Epithelioid
 Others
Intravenous leiomyomatosis*
Low-grade endometrial stromal sarcoma
High-grade endometrial stromal sarcoma†
Poorly differentiated endometrial sarcoma
Miscellaneous sarcomas
 Rhabdomyosarcoma
 Angiosarcoma
 Malignant fibrous histiocytoma
 Neurogenic sarcoma
 Alveolar soft part sarcoma
 Others
Mixed müllerian tumors
 Müllerian adenosarcoma
 Malignant müllerian mixed tumor (carcinosarcoma)
 Uterine tumor resembling ovarian sex cord tumor‡

*Not a true sarcoma but is included here because occasional cases have been fatal (see text).
†Reasons for rare use of this category are explained in the text.
‡Exhibits epithelial differentiation but most likely of endometrial stromal cell origin.

194

almost always less circumscribed than leiomyomas and cannot be shelled out as easily from the adjacent myometrium. The cut surface is typically bulging, soft, fleshy, and focally necrotic and hemorrhagic (Figure 15–1).[5] In 90% of cases, the leiomyosarcoma is either the only mass or, when associated with leiomyomas (as they often are), the largest mass. Rarely, a leiomyosarcoma arises in a leiomyoma.

On microscopic examination, tumors are usually hypercellular and composed of long fascicles of spindle-shaped cells (Figure 15–2) that exhibit at least moderate and, usually, focally severe nuclear atypia, including bizarre tumor giant cells in some cases. Hypocellular regions may be seen focally in otherwise characteristically hypercellular neoplasms, while myxoid tumors (see below) are commonly hypocellular. The tumors almost always have a high mitotic rate (10 or more mitotic figures [MFs]/10 high-power fields [HPFs]; 90% have > 15 MFs/10 HPFs) (see Figure 15–2), including atypical mitoses. Despite the atypia, the cytologic features can still usually be seen, at least focally, to be characteristic of smooth muscle cells with cigar-shaped nuclei and eosinophilic tapering cytoplasm.[6,7] Vascular invasion is present in 10 to 20% of tumors. Tumor cell necrosis, which is highly characteristic of leiomyosarcomas, is common and is characterized by an abrupt transition from viable areas to eosinophilic zones of necrosis without an interposed zone of granulation tissue or fibrous tissue (Figure 15–3). Preserved nuclei with marked pleomorphism and hyperchromasia can still be seen focally within the necrotic areas, and perivascular

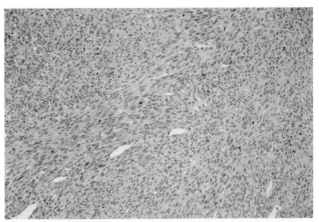

Figure 15–2. Leiomyosarcoma. Typical growth of long fascicles of spindled cells with brisk mitotic activity.

tumor cells are often preserved in the necrotic areas, as well as ghost outlines of dead tumor cells.[8] This appearance contrasts with the infarct-type necrosis that is common in leiomyomas, in which tumor cells and vessels are mummified, frequently associated with recent hemorrhage and separated from the viable tumor by a rim of granulation or fibrous tissue. Leiomyosarcomas almost always have irregular infiltrating margins (Figure 15–4), but sometimes they invade as rounded masses or tongues, which occasionally can simulate the typical invasive pattern of endometrial stromal sarcomas (see below). The great majority of tumors are grade 2 or 3 (out of 3), but an occasional tumor is grade 1.

Although, as noted, most leiomyosarcomas are easy to diagnose as smooth muscle tumors, in some instances, immunohistochemical stains may be help-

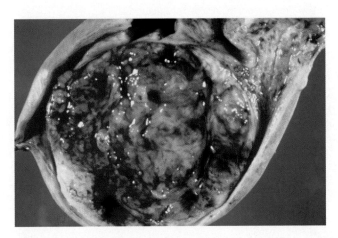

Figure 15–1. Leiomyosarcoma. The tumor has a fleshy, hemorrhagic, and focally necrotic cut surface.

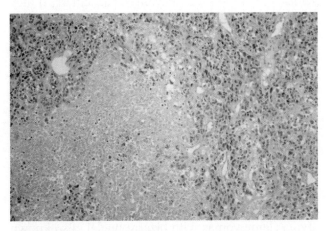

Figure 15–3. Leiomyosarcoma. There is extensive tumor cell necrosis.

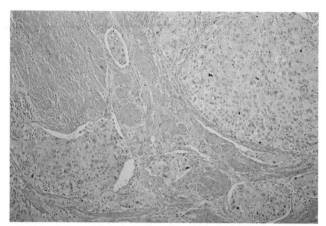

Figure 15–4. Leiomyosarcoma. Irregular infiltrative margins and lymphovascular invasion are typical features.

ful in establishing their smooth muscle origin. The most specific markers are desmin (Figure 15–5) and h-caldesmon, but it is important to remember that leiomyosarcomas may also be positive for epithelial markers, including cytokeratins and epithelial membrane antigen.[9–12] Electron microscopy can be used but is rarely employed now because of the aid provided by immunohistochemistry.

The differential diagnosis of a conventional leiomyosarcoma includes variants of benign smooth muscle tumors that, on gross or microscopic examination, may cause concern for malignancy. Leiomyomas may be extensively necrotic (due to infarction) or focally hemorrhagic ("apoplectic") in patients taking oral contraceptives or in pregnant patients.[13,14] Additionally, leiomyomas from pregnant patients often have a diffusely beefy sectioned surface due to the so-called red (or carneous) degeneration.[14] Some serosal or subserosal leiomyomas, particularly if they are hydropic, may produce striking masses protruding from the external aspect of the specimen, which, to the inexperienced, may be alarming.[15] It should also be noted that uterine leiomyomas may be associated with leiomyomas in the broad ligament or numerous peritoneal leiomyomas (so-called diffuse peritoneal leiomyomatosis).[16]

Several problematic microscopic findings may be seen in benign smooth muscle tumors which may potentially lead to the misdiagnosis of sarcoma. These are the presence of degenerative-type nuclear atypia (leiomyomas with bizarre nuclei, also known as symplastic leiomyomas), increased cellularity

(cellular and highly cellular leiomyomas), increased mitotic activity (mitotically active leiomyomas), infiltrative growth (dissecting and cotyledonoid leiomyomas), and vascular permeation (leiomyoma with vascular invasion and intravenous leiomyomatosis).[17–26] All these leiomyoma variants, except the first, generally lack significant cytologic atypia and also lack tumor cell necrosis, which are important microscopic features when evaluating the benign or malignant nature of a smooth muscle tumor. A benign diagnosis is aided in cases of leiomyomas with bizarre nuclei by the usual focality of atypical nuclei with intervening areas of typical leiomyoma. Even when the bizarre nuclei are diffusely distributed, as they occasionally are, benign-appearing interposed cells can be appreciated on careful scrutiny. Furthermore, the cytologic atypia of this variant of leiomyoma is not matched by a comparable degree of mitotic activity, provided care is taken not to mistake karyorrhectic nuclei for normal or atypical mitotic figures.[17]

Leiomyosarcomas also have to be distinguished from smooth muscle tumors of uncertain malignant potential. This term is used for smooth muscle tumors that have at least one, or usually two or more, worrisome features, but fall short of meeting the criteria for leiomyosarcoma. Some of these tumors may have tumor cell necrosis but lack cytologic atypia and the brisk mitotic activity of leiomyosarcomas. Other smooth muscle tumors in this category may exhibit other combinations of worrisome findings, including more than 15 MFs/10 HPFs without sig-

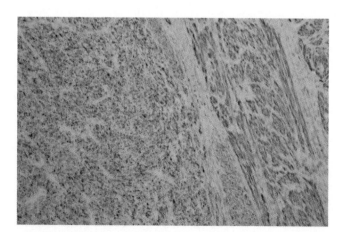

Figure 15–5. Leiomyosarcoma. There is diffuse desmin positivity of the neoplastic smooth muscle cells.

nificant cytologic atypia or hypercellularity, the presence of abnormal mitotic figures, or severe cytologic atypia associated with borderline mitotic counts (8 or 9 MFs/10 HPFs).[8,27,28]

The differential diagnosis of a conventional spindle cell leiomyosarcoma can include other uterine sarcomas, particularly low-grade endometrial stromal sarcoma and "endometrial sarcoma not otherwise specified." The typical growth pattern of stromal sarcomas, described below, and their typical vasculature readily distinguish these tumors from a leiomyosarcoma. Rare leiomyosarcomas have striking tongue-like growth and vascular invasion that, on low power, can suggest a stromal sarcoma; however, on high-power scrutiny, they have tumor cells that are more spindled than the fusiform cells of stromal sarcoma and lack the classic vasculature of that neoplasm.[28] If needed, immunohistochemical stains for muscle markers usually help.[9] Muscle markers may also help in the differential diagnosis with endometrial sarcoma not otherwise specified. The latter tumors, considered below, have features of a nonspecific sarcoma because they lack smooth muscle differentiation and the typical growth of low-grade endometrial stromal sarcoma, and cannot be classified as any other variant of sarcoma.[29]

Leiomyosarcoma Variants

Myxoid Leiomyosarcoma

This is a rare variant of leiomyosarcoma that can create diagnostic problems because its myxoid appearance and low mitotic rate can lead to a misdiagnosis of a benign smooth muscle tumor. These tumors are usually large and have a gelatinous cut surface (Figure 15–6). They frequently are well circumscribed on gross examination.[30–32]

On microscopic examination, however, the tumors typically infiltrate the myometrium in irregular tongues, in some cases filling the lumens of myometrial veins. The tumors are defined by an abundant paucicellular myxoid matrix (Figure 15–7) that is strongly positive with alcian blue and colloidal iron staining. The tumor cells may be uniformly distributed throughout the myxoid stroma (see Figure

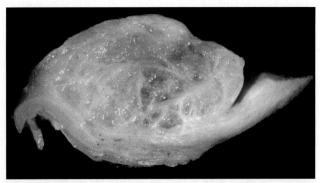

Figure 15–6. Myxoid leiomyosarcoma. The tumor is grossly well circumscribed with a gelatinous cut surface.

15–7), arranged in fascicles, or may surround cavities filled with myxoid material. Most of the tumor cells are oval or spindle shaped and have scant cytoplasm. In the initial report describing this tumor, nuclei were usually small with focal mild to moderate nuclear pleomorphism and inconspicuous nucleoli. Most of the tumors had a low mitotic rate.[32] However, in a recent study, there was evidence of greater cytologic atypia.[33] This finding facilitated the diagnosis when present; in its absence, tumor cell necrosis warranted a diagnosis of myxoid leiomyosarcoma, as did a mitotic index > 2 MFs/10 HPFs.[33] Nonmyxoid areas, which are present to a variable degree (Figure 15–8), exhibit greater degrees of nuclear pleomorphism and mitotic activity and architectural and cytologic features that help establish the malignant smooth muscle nature of the neoplastic cells. Tumor recurrence and distant metastases are frequent. In some cases, the recurrent tumor in the abdominal

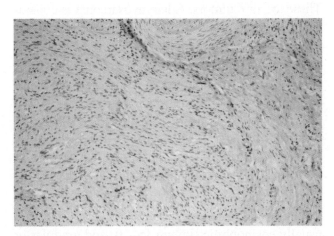

Figure 15–7. Myxoid leiomyosarcoma. Spindle cells with scant cytoplasm are uniformly distributed in a paucicellular myxoid matrix.

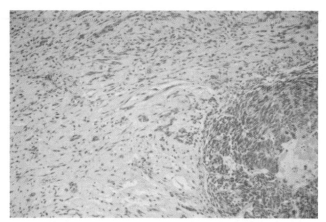

Figure 15–8. Hypocellular myxoid area in a myxoid leiomyosarcoma merging with a more typical spindled component.

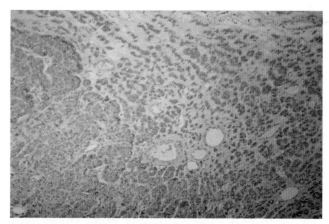

Figure 15–9. Epithelioid leiomyosarcoma. The tumor grows in nests and cords surrounded by scanty hyalinized stroma.

cavity has mimicked the appearance of pseudomyxoma peritonei. In contrast to typical leiomyosarcoma, the postoperative interval to recurrence or metastases involving the abdomen, liver, lungs, or brain may be as long as 10 years.[30–32]

The main differential diagnosis is with the rare myxoid leiomyoma. Myxoid degeneration in leiomyomas is more commonly seen in pregnant patients.[14] Although these tumors may have infiltrative margins, they are often well circumscribed. They do not have tumor cell necrosis and mitotic counts are < 2 MFs/10 HPFs.[34] The distinction between myxoid leiomyoma and myxoid leiomyosarcoma may be difficult in curettage specimens, due to the limited amount of material sampled and the inability to assess the border of the tumor with the myometrium.

Epithelioid Leiomyosarcoma

These are rare tumors. A leiomyosarcoma is considered to be epithelioid when at least 50% of the tumor is composed of epithelioid cells. Grossly, they cannot be distinguished from conventional leiomyosarcoma. On microscopic examination, they most frequently show a diffuse growth of tumor cells, but they can also form nests, cords, or trabeculae (Figure 15–9) and, occasionally, pseudoglandular spaces. The background stroma may be edematous or myxoid or show variable degrees of hyalinization that may result in a plexiform pattern. The cells are definitionally round to polygonal, with abundant, usually eosinophilic (Figure 15–10) and granular or vacuolated cytoplasm. In up to 25% of tumors, the

cytoplasm is clear. In some instances, the cells may have a rhabdoid appearance imparted by the presence of intracytoplasmic eosinophilic globules. The nuclei are round, with one or more prominent nucleoli (see Figure 15–10).[6]

Criteria for predicting malignant behavior are less well established for epithelioid smooth muscle tumors than for spindle cell smooth muscle tumors. Overall, recent studies have shown that epithelioid tumors with marked cytologic atypia and mitotic activity higher than 3 to 5 MFs/10 HPFs or tumor cell necrosis alone behave in a malignant fashion.[34–37]

The differential diagnosis of epithelioid leiomyosarcomas includes primary high-grade endometrial carcinomas, carcinomas metastatic to the uterus, and, rarely, other tumors whose cells have appreciable eosinophilic or clear cytoplasm, such as malignant melanoma, placental site trophoblastic tumor, epithe-

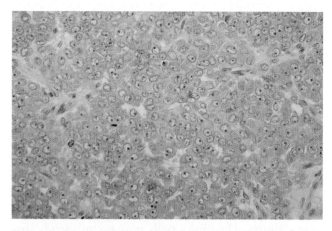

Figure 15–10. Epithelioid leiomyosarcoma. The neoplastic cells have abundant eosinophilic cytoplasm, round nuclei, and prominent nucleoli.

lioid trophoblastic tumor, and the recently described "PEComa" (considered in "Miscellaneous Rare Sarcomas of Soft Tissue Type" to follow). A minor typical fascicular growth is present in many epithelioid leiomyosarcomas and is helpful in differential diagnosis. Focal glandular or squamous differentiation in cases of high-grade carcinoma is often a helpful diagnostic feature, although care must be taken to distinguish glandular spaces of the carcinoma from pseudoglandular spaces of some epithelioid leiomyosarcomas. In some cases, immunohistochemical or ultrastructural studies may be needed to establish the diagnosis.

Other Variants

Rare leiomyosarcomas contain a prominent component of osteoclastic-type giant cells. In some cases, the giant cell component of the tumor has resembled a benign or malignant giant cell tumor of bone.[38,39] These cells are considered to be of histiocytic origin and they are more frequently seen near areas of hemorrhage or necrosis. Rare leiomyosarcomas, which can be focally or diffusely yellow, contain large xanthomatous cells with abundant cytoplasm containing lipid vacuoles and multiple or multilobulated nuclei, sometimes in a wreath-like arrangement.[40] The xanthomatous cells are disposed in solid sheets or are intimately admixed with smooth muscle cells and frequently with acute inflammatory cells.

Natural History

Leiomyosarcomas are aggressive tumors. The survival rates range from 15 to 30%, with a median survival ranging from 13 to 43 months (see Chapter 16).[6] In a large Gynecology Oncology Group (GOG) study, the recurrence rate was 71%. As the primary mode of spread of leiomyosarcoma is hematogenous, the first recurrence was in the lung in 40% of cases and in the pelvis in only 13%.[2] There has been no consistency among various studies with respect to a correlation between survival and patient age (and menopausal status), clinical stage, or gross or microscopic features.[1,2,41] However, some studies have shown that postmenopausal women have a poorer prognosis and a higher frequency of metasta-

sis than premenopausal women. Epithelioid or myxoid variants were more often associated with metastases in one study.[3]

INTRAVENOUS LEIOMYOMATOSIS

Intravenous leiomyomatosis is defined as the presence of intravenous proliferations of benign-appearing smooth muscle in the absence of, or outside the confines of, a leiomyoma.[6] Although histologically benign, this tumor may behave in an aggressive fashion and, for this reason, is considered in this chapter.

The clinical presentation is usually similar to that of the ordinary uterine leiomyoma, but extrauterine venous involvement occurs in approximately 30% of these cases.[42] Although frequently confined to the pelvis, the tumor may extend into the inferior vena cava and reach to the right side of the heart, sometimes with a fatal outcome. In rare cases, patients with intact uteri and no pelvic manifestations present with cardiac involvement. Occasional patients have had solitary metastases (lungs, pelvic lymph nodes).[26,42] Rarely, spread to these sites can be seen without intravenous growth of a morphologically benign smooth muscle tumor (so-called benign metastasizing leiomyoma).

On gross examination, the uterus is usually enlarged, with multiple, rubbery, gray-white myometrial masses, some of which form worm-like plugs of tumor within myometrial veins (Figure 15–11). On microscopic examination, the intravascular tumor may resemble a typical leiomyoma but, most often, has a somewhat distinctive appearance characterized by clefts and a lobulated contour of an intravascular tumor, extensive hydropic change or hyalinization, and a content of numerous thick-walled vessels (Figure 15–12). Occasionally, the appearance is that of a leiomyoma variant, including cellular leiomyoma (Figure 15–13), leiomyoma with bizarre nuclei, lipoleiomyoma, myxoid leiomyoma, or epithelioid leiomyoma.[26]

The differential diagnosis includes leiomyoma with vascular invasion and low-grade endometrial stromal sarcoma. The former shows limited microscopic vascular growth confined to the tumor.[43] Endometrial stromal sarcomas may show a similar intravascular growth pattern but usually lack thick-

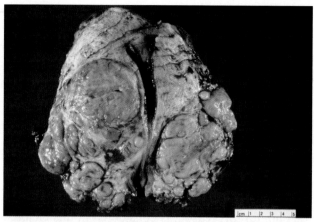

Figure 15–11. Intravenous leiomyomatosis. Multiple worm-like plugs of tumor are distending the myometrial veins.

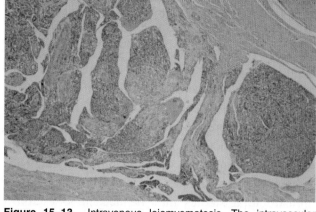

Figure 15–13. Intravenous leiomyomatosis. The intravascular tumor resembles a cellular leiomyoma.

walled vessels and lobulation and involve the endometrium as well as the myometrium.

Rare patients experience pelvic or cardiac recurrences, as many as 15 years after hysterectomy, from continued growth of residual intravascular tumor. In such cases, an initial diagnosis of a primary cardiac tumor is made, especially in women in whom the diagnosis of intravenous leiomyomatosis was missed in the hysterectomy specimen. Progesterone therapy or gonadotropin-releasing hormone (GnRH)–agonists may be useful in controlling unresectable tumor.[44]

ENDOMETRIAL STROMAL SARCOMAS

Until recently, these tumors (often referred to as endolymphatic stromal myosis in the older literature) were divided into low-grade and high-grade

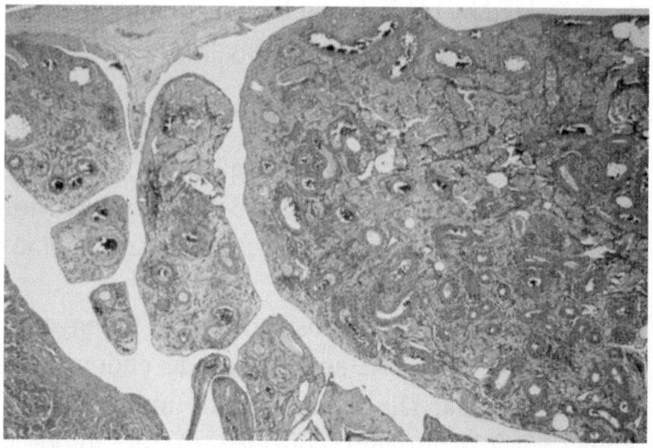

Figure 15–12. Intravenous leiomyomatosis. The intravascular tumor has thick-walled vessels, a common finding in intravenous leiomyomatosis. Note the lobulated contours and clefts.

categories based on mitotic rate.[45] However, mitotic rate does not reliably divide these tumors into two different prognostic groups, and the current convention is to reserve the diagnosis of endometrial stromal sarcoma for tumors with obvious stromal differentiation by their pattern and cell type and without division into low- and high-grade groups. Most tumors that were formerly classified as high-grade endometrial stromal sarcomas are now placed in the category of poorly differentiated endometrial sarcoma.[29] However, we believe that the diagnosis of high-grade endometrial stromal sarcoma is still occasionally appropriate when a tumor has the typical pattern of low-grade endometrial stromal sarcoma but has unequivocal nuclear atypia and other ominous morphologic features. Some such tumors arise on a background of typical low-grade endometrial stromal sarcoma.

On gross examination, endometrial stromal sarcomas are characterized by single or multiple yellow-to-tan soft masses that may project into the endometrial cavity, usually accompanied by nodular or diffuse permeation of the myometrium, often with worm-like plugs of tumor filling and distending the myometrial veins (Figure 15–14).[14,18,46,47] Some tumors, however, may be well circumscribed on gross examination. The tumors may have areas of necrosis and hemorrhage; cystic degeneration is seen rarely.

On microscopic examination, the tumors characteristically show irregular tongues or rounded masses of tumor cells infiltrating the myometrium (Figure 15–15). Myometrial (Figure 15–16) as well

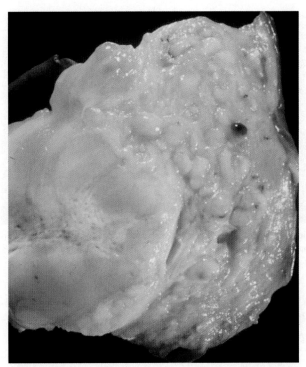

Figure 15–14. Endometrial stromal sarcoma. Several small tan nodules are present in the myometrium adjacent to a large dominant mass. Some of the small nodules distend the myometrial veins.

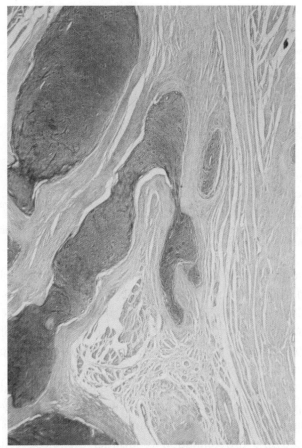

Figure 15–15. Endometrial stromal sarcoma. There is the typical permeative growth pattern of irregular islands of darkly staining tumor in the myometrium.

as extrauterine veins are frequently invaded.[14,18,46,47] Although most tumors show an overtly infiltrative pattern, in some tumors the margin may be focally infiltrative. For this reason, it is very important to sample extensively the interface between the tumor and the surrounding myometrium to ascertain this infiltrative growth, which is crucial to the distinction from an endometrial stromal nodule (see above). Most tumors show a conspicuous component of small arterioles that may be hyalinized. Although most tumors are densely cellular, some of them are hypocellular secondary to the presence of abundant intercellular collagen, myxoid change, or extensive areas of hyalinization that may be either diffuse or, more commonly, in the form of small regular hyaline plaques.[48]

Tumor cells resemble normal endometrial stromal cells that are often focally disposed in a whorled pattern around the arterioles (Figure 15–17). They are small, oval to spindle, with scant amounts of cytoplasm, and round to oval nuclei with inconspicuous or small nucleoli and evenly dispersed chromatin. Cytoplasm is typically scant but is rarely abundant and even oxyphilic, sometimes even having a rhabdoid

appearance.[49–51] Significant nuclear atypia is usually absent or mild. Mitotic activity is usually low (< 3 MFs/10 HPF), but higher mitotic rates do not exclude the diagnosis if the tumor cells resemble normal endometrial stromal cells and the tumor shows the characteristic tongue-like growth.[18,46,47] Other associated findings include (1) histiocytes that may be seen scattered throughout the tumor or forming sheets frequently associated with cholesterol clefts, (2) broad areas of necrosis due to infarction, (3) smooth muscle differentiation, and (4) epithelial differentiation. The latter two phenomena are now discussed in more detail.

Smooth muscle differentiation may occur as discrete islands (sometimes erroneously suggesting epithelial differentiation) in a background of neoplastic endometrial stroma or may exhibit a characteristic "starburst pattern," in which nodules have a central area of hyalinization from which collagen fibrils radi-

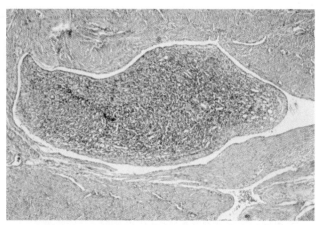

Figure 15–16. Endometrial stromal sarcoma. A plug of tumor is present within a vessel.

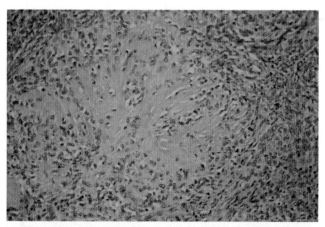

Figure 15–18. Endometrial stromal sarcoma with smooth muscle differentiation. A central hyalinized area is associated with radiating bands of collagen that surround small neoplastic cells ("starburst" pattern).

ate toward the periphery (Figure 15–18). Embedded in their outermost portion are cells with more cytoplasm than typical endometrial stromal cells. These areas merge with small and disorganized fascicles of smooth muscle that, in turn, may merge with more mature fascicles of smooth muscle.[52]

Occasionally, areas with an unequivocal epithelial appearance are seen in stromal sarcomas. The epithelial differentiation most commonly resembles the sex cord–like differentiation of ovarian granulosa cell and Sertoli cell tumors in the form of anastomosing cords of one to two cells, broad trabeculae, small nests, sertoliform or retiform tubular structures, or Call-Exner–like bodies; diffuse sheets may also be seen.[18,46,50,53] The epithelial-like cells may vary from small, round, and regular with scanty cytoplasm to large with abundant eosinophilic, clear, or foamy cytoplasm. The nuclei are usually small and regular

with little pleomorphism and indistinct nucleoli. Nuclear grooves are rare or absent, and mitotic figures are typically scarce.

Another less common form of epithelial differentiation is endometrioid-like glands (Figure 15–19). These glands may vary from scant to prominent and may be cytologically benign, atypical, or have malignant nuclear features, resembling an endometrioid adenocarcinoma.[54] Endometrioid-type glands may be particularly confusing when seen in extrauterine foci of disease. In the past, such foci have sometimes been misinterpreted as "aggressive endometriosis." The endometrioid glands in primary endometrial stromal sarcoma may also cause confusion with müllerian adenosarcoma, but the latter tumors do not usually have the typical growth pattern or infiltration of stromal sarcomas. Stromal sarcomas lack the periglandu-

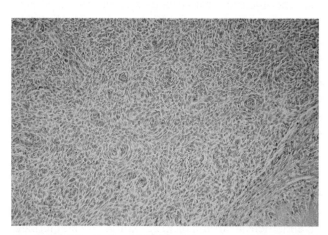

Figure 15–17. Endometrial stromal sarcoma. Closely packed small round to oval cells with scanty cytoplasm focally whorling around arterioles.

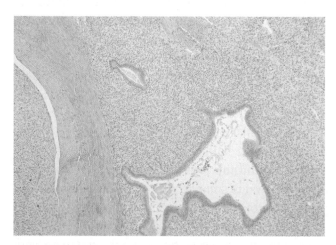

Figure 15–19. Endometrial stromal sarcoma. Scattered endometrioid glands in a background of otherwise typical tumor.

lar cuffing and polypoid-papillary projections that are typically present within the gland lumens of many adenosarcomas.[55]

The differential diagnosis of endometrial stromal sarcoma includes mostly the benign variant of endometrial stromal tumor, the endometrial stromal nodule, and a variant of leiomyoma, the highly cellular leiomyoma. The microscopic appearance of an endometrial stromal nodule is identical to that of endometrial stromal sarcoma; however, an endometrial stromal nodule has a noninfiltrative, expansile border on microscopic examination, although it is allowed to have focal irregularities in the form of lobulated or finger-like projections into the adjacent myometrium that do not exceed 3 mm. No vascular invasion should be seen.[56,57] For that reason, the differential diagnosis between an endometrial stromal nodule and a low-grade endometrial stromal sarcoma can only be made when evaluation of the margins of the tumor is possible, a distinction that usually requires a hysterectomy specimen.

The features of highly cellular leiomyomas that may cause confusion with endometrial stromal sarcomas are dense cellularity, prominent vascularity, and irregularity of the tumor margins.[19] Distinctive helpful microscopic features seen in highly cellular leiomyomas are the presence of numerous large, thick-walled blood vessels, merging of tumor cells with more conventional smooth muscle neoplasia, and an immunoprofile that supports the smooth muscle nature of the tumor, including positivity for smooth muscle markers. Cluster designation 10 (CD10), a recently described marker of endometrial stromal tumors (Figure 15–20), however, is positive in 40% of highly cellular leiomyomas and accordingly is not reliable in the differential diagnosis of endometrial stromal sarcoma and highly cellular leiomyoma.[9]

Endometrial stromal sarcomas are sometimes confused with intravenous leiomyomatosis, particularly its cellular variant. The intravascular tumor in intravenous leiomyomatosis usually shows foci of hydropic change and thick-walled blood vessels, which, respectively, are absent or infrequent in endometrial stromal sarcomas. Also, extravascular tumor in intravenous leiomyomatosis does not have the typical growth of stromal sarcoma.[26] If necessary,

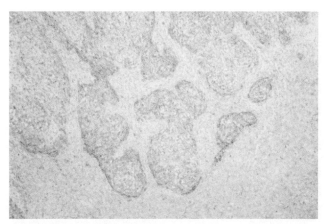

Figure 15–20. Endometrial stromal sarcoma. The neoplastic cells are immunoreactive for CD10.

immunohistochemistry may be helpful in the differential diagnosis, but this rarely should be needed.

POORLY DIFFERENTIATED ENDOMETRIAL SARCOMAS

These tumors do not show evidence of endometrial stromal differentiation on microscopic examination. They are very aggressive and carry a poor prognosis.[29] They have no distinctive gross features that set them apart from other malignant mesenchymal tumors. They lack the typical growth patterns and vascularity of low-grade endometrial stromal sarcomas (Figure 15–21) and, in contrast, show destructive myometrial invasion, marked cellular pleomorphism, and brisk mitotic activity (Figure 15–22)[29] It has been suggested that poorly differentiated endometrial sarcomas are closely related to MMMTs, as they show considerable histologic resemblance to the sarcomatous component of these tumors ("monophasic MMMTs").[6] Thus, these tumors should be diagnosed only after extensive sampling has excluded foci of carcinoma, as well as foci of smooth or skeletal muscle differentiation, which would allow a pure high-grade sarcoma to be classified as either a leiomyosarcoma or rhabdomyosarcoma.

RHABDOMYOSARCOMAS

These are rare tumors and should only be diagnosed after thorough sampling has ruled out a minor malignant epithelial component, which would place the

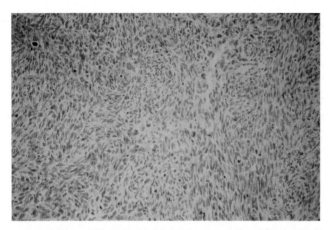

Figure 15–21. Poorly differentiated endometrial sarcoma. Intersecting fascicles of neoplastic cells have a nonspecific growth pattern.

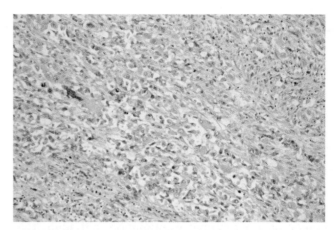

Figure 15–23. Pleomorphic rhabdomyosarcoma. Haphazardly oriented pleomorphic cells are admixed with typical rhabdomyoblasts with abundant eosinophilic cytoplasm.

tumor in the category of MMMT as noted above. Most uterine rhabdomyosarcomas are actually primary in the cervix, only rare neoplasms are primary in the corpus.[58,59] The great majority of endometrial rhabdomyosarcomas are of the pleomorphic subtype.[60,61] They typically occur in elderly patients and frequently present as polypoid intracavitary masses that are soft and fleshly, with frequent hemorrhagic necrosis. On microscopic examination, they consist of haphazardly oriented pleomorphic cells admixed with aggregates of large rhabdomyoblasts identified by their abundant, dense eosinophilic cytoplasm with focal cytoplasmic cross striations (Figure 15–23). Frequently, necrosis and hemorrhage occur. Direct extension of the tumor into adjacent organs as well as distant metastasis are frequent. Despite aggressive treatment, these tumors are associated with a very poor prognosis, and most patients die within 15 months after presentation.[60,61]

ANGIOSARCOMAS

These are rare aggressive tumors that occur predominantly in peri- and postmenopausal women. On gross examination, they are large masses with extensive areas of hemorrhage and necrosis, usually showing extensive myometrial invasion.[62]

On microscopic examination, tumors have an infiltrative border with well- to poorly developed, sometimes anastomosing, vascular channels. Some of these channels show focal papillary architecture, a lining of highly atypical cells with nuclear hyperchromasia, and brisk mitotic activity. Some angiosarcomas may display an epithelioid morphology. Two tumors have been described arising within a leiomyoma.[63] These tumors are positive for endothelial markers, including factor VIII, CD31, and CD34.

ALVEOLAR SOFT PART SARCOMA

About 20 cases of this variant of soft tissue tumor have been primary in the uterus, but only about one-third of them have arisen in the uterine corpus.[64–66] They have more commonly occurred in younger patients than other rare forms of uterine sarcoma. Gross examination typically reveals a well-circumscribed, solid endometrial or myometrial tumor that is often yellow-to-tan or white. Microscopic examination shows the typical nested pattern and other features of this tumor as seen in soft tissues elsewhere (Figure 15–24). The differential diagnosis includes a primary carcinoma with an unusual pattern and

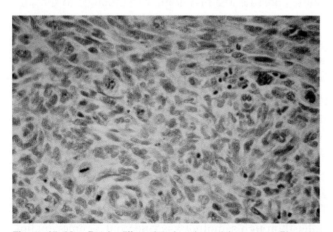

Figure 15–22. Poorly differentiated endometrial sarcoma. Pleomorphic cells are associated with brisk mitotic activity and apoptotic bodies.

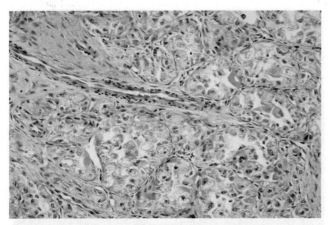

Figure 15–24. Alveolar soft sarcoma. Nests of cells with abundant cytoplasm that, in some cells, is markedly eosinophilic.

metastatic carcinoma to the uterus, such as renal cell carcinoma. These tumors have had a favorable prognosis in the limited experience to date. In rare cases, cytogenetic studies may be helpful as these tumors are associated with a specific chromosomal abnormality, that is, der(17)t(X;17)(p11;p25).[67]

MISCELLANEOUS RARE SARCOMAS OF SOFT TISSUE TYPE

The most common tumor in this category is the so-called malignant fibrous histiocytoma.[68] The tumors have usually occurred in middle-aged to elderly patients and are typically large polypoid masses with extensive hemorrhagic necrosis. Microscopic examination shows a spindle cell tumor with overt cytologic atypia, often with a storiform pattern, sometimes including tumor giant cells. The prognosis is poor.[68]

Almost every type of soft tissue–type sarcoma has been described rarely in the uterine corpus and each is classified according to the criteria used for those outside the uterus.[6] One of these, the so-called malignant rhabdoid tumor, can potentially be confused with undifferentiated carcinoma or even an endometrial stromal sarcoma in which some of the tumor cells have a rhabdoid appearance.[50,51,69] A true malignant rhabdoid tumor does not exhibit epithelial differentiation or epithelial markers on immunohistochemical evaluation, and it does not have the distinctive growth pattern of endometrial stromal sarcoma.[69]

A newly described mesenchymal tumor of low-grade malignancy of the soft tissues and uterus is the

tumor considered to arise from perivascular epithelioid cells and is designated "PEComa." The clinical presentation is similar to other uterine tumors, presenting as a pelvic mass. On gross examination, the tumors may be either well circumscribed or show infiltrative margins, and they have a white-to-gray-to-tan cut surface. On microscopic examination, these tumors may have a smooth tumor-myometrium interface, but frequently, they infiltrate the myometrium in a tongue-like manner similar to that seen in low-grade endometrial stromal sarcomas. The tumors are, however, composed of cells with abundant, clear to eosinophilic cytoplasm (in contrast to most low-grade endometrial stromal sarcomas) and have round to oval, medium-sized nuclei that are arranged in broad sheets or small solid nests separated by scant hyalinized stroma. They may also contain a spindled cell component, although this is not prominent. These cells are positive for HMB-45 and may express other melanocytic as well as smooth muscle markers; they are negative for S-100 and cytokeratins. Some of these tumors may be associated with lymphangioleiomyomatosis and the tuberous sclerosis syndrome.[70] The main differential diagnosis is with an epithelioid smooth muscle tumor with which they have probably been previously confused. The latter frequently shows a spindled cell component and is nonreactive with HMB-45. The long-term prognosis of these tumors is not well established, as experience is very limited. However, some of these tumors have shown an aggressive behavior.[71,72]

MIXED MÜLLERIAN TUMORS

These tumors are classified into three categories: (1) the müllerian adenofibroma, a clinically benign lesion, which will not be further considered; (2) the müllerian adenosarcoma, a low-grade malignant lesion in most cases; and (3) MMMT, a highly malignant neoplasm. The müllerian adenosarcoma differs from MMMT, by definition, in having an epithelial component that is usually benign or atypical in appearance but may range up to adenocarcinoma in situ. Additionally, the stromal component of the müllerian adenosarcoma is, with rare exceptions, less atypical than that of MMMT.

Müllerian Adenosarcoma

These tumors predominantly occur in post-menopausal patients, but more occur in pre-menopausal patients (approximately 30%) than is the case with MMMT. The usual presentation is abnormal vaginal bleeding and an enlarged uterus. The tumor frequently protrudes through the external os (Figure 15–25). Some tumors are initially misdiagnosed as recurrent endometrial "polyps."[55,73] Occasional patients have had a history of pelvic radiation or are on tamoxifen therapy.[74] The neoplasms are almost always confined to the uterus (stage I) at presentation.[55]

On gross examination, the endometrial cavity is typically involved by a polypoid, often villous, broad-based mass (see Figure 15–25). Varying degrees of myometrial invasion are present in a minority of cases (Figure 15–26). Rare tumors are exclusively myometrial in location. The sectioned surface of the neoplasms is often spongy (see Figure 15–26) with cystic spaces filled with a watery or mucoid fluid surrounded by white-to-tan tissue.[55,75]

Low-power microscopic examination typically shows a periglandular condensation of the sarcomatous stroma (Figure 15–27); the glands usually

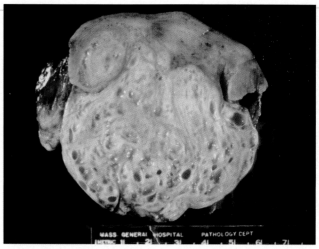

Figure 15–26. Müllerian adenosarcoma. The tumor has a spongy cut surface and focally infiltrates the myometrium.

exhibit some degree of cystic dilatation and often contain papillary to polypoid intraluminal fronds of the sarcomatous component (Figure 15–28). The glands are lined with a variety of benign to atypical müllerian epithelia, most commonly of the endometrioid type (Figure 15–29). Metaplastic epithelium of mucinous, hobnail, or squamous type may be seen. The sarcomatous component is usually low grade (see Figure 15–29), typically resembling endometrial stromal sarcoma, fibrosarcoma, or combinations thereof. As noted, the sarcomatous stroma is typically more cellular around the glands; in these areas, mitotic figures are usually evident. Away from the periglandular foci, the stroma is often relatively acellular and sometimes extensively hyalinized with a deceptively benign appearance.

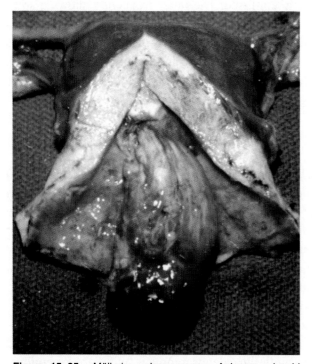

Figure 15–25. Müllerian adenosarcoma. A large, polypoid broad-based mass protrudes through the cervical os.

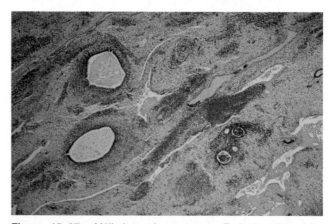

Figure 15–27. Müllerian adenosarcoma. Typical periglandular condensation of the sarcomatous component.

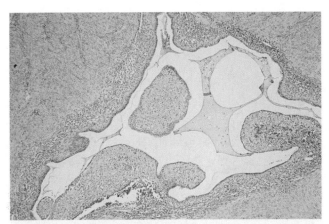

Figure 15–28. Müllerian adenosarcoma. The sarcomatous stroma forms polypoid intraluminal projections.

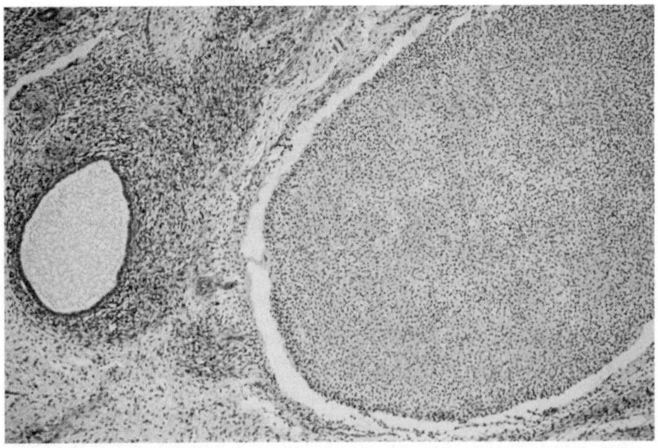

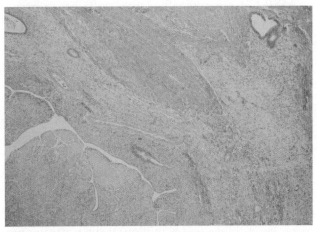

Figure 15–30. Müllerian adenosarcoma with cartilage as a heterologous element.

Occasional tumors contain heterologous elements in the form of fat, cartilage (Figure 15–30), and rhabdomyoblasts. In occasional cases, the stromal component shows sex cord–like differentiation.[76] Only a minority of tumors invade the myometrium (Figure 15–31), and the invasion is usually superficial. The invasive front of the tumor is typically well circumscribed, but occasionally the neoplasm invades in irregular tongues. Approximately 10% of tumors exhibit overgrowth of the sarcomatous component, the so-called "müllerian adenosarcoma with sarcomatous overgrowth."[77]

The differential diagnosis of these tumors is mainly with endometrial polyps containing cellular stroma. Although these polyps may show some mitotic activity, they lack any significant degree of cytologic atypia, and they do not show the typical

architecture of a müllerian adenosarcoma.[78] Some endometrial polyps may be associated with atypical (bizarre) stromal cells, a frequent finding in fibroepithelial polyps of the female lower genital tract. The atypical stromal cells are scattered throughout the polyp, but mitotic figures, as well as stromal cellularity, periglandular cuffing, and polypoid intraluminal projections of the stroma are lacking.[79]

These tumors are typically of low malignant potential with vaginal or abdominal pelvic recurrence in about 25% of the cases, often at intervals of 5 years or more after hysterectomy. Hematogenous spread occurs in less than 5% of the cases. The risk of recurrence is greater with myoinvasive tumors (46%) than with noninvasive tumors (12.7%).[55,77,80] These tumors have recurred as pure sarcoma in 70% of cases, adenosarcoma in almost 30%, and carci-

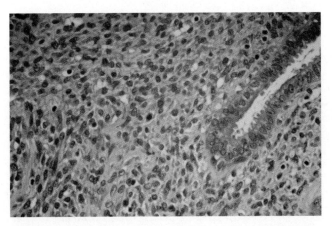

Figure 15–29. Müllerian adenosarcoma. A benign endometrioid gland is surrounded by plump mitotically active neoplastic stromal cells.

Figure 15–31. Müllerian adenosarcoma with irregular myometrial invasion.

nosarcoma very rarely. Sarcomatous overgrowth is associated with recurrence, hematogenous metastasis, and death from tumor in 70%, 40%, and 60% of patients, respectively.

Malignant Müllerian Mixed Tumor

These tumors almost always occur in postmenopausal patients. Risk factors are similar to those of patients with endometrial adenocarcinoma. A history of pelvic radiation is occasionally present, as it is in some patients with müllerian adenosarcoma. The patients typically present with abnormal vaginal bleeding, and the uterus is almost always enlarged. Pelvic or abdominal pain is frequent. Extrauterine spread is present at the time of diagnosis in up to one-third of cases. We consider these tumors distinct from sarcomatoid carcinomas in contrast to some authors who have recently written on this topic.[81] These tumors derive from epithelial cells, and indeed, for many years they have been considered to ultimately derive from endometrioid epithelial cells. However, they should be classified, like tumors in general, according to their morphologic features, rather than their histogenesis, particularly when their morphology is associated with relatively consistent clinical features, such as an aggressive clinical course in this instance. Some endometrial adenocarcinomas have spindled cells that retain an epithelial phenotype, whereas in the MMMT the spindled cells are sarcomatous. This issue is further considered in the context of sarcomatoid carcinomas in Chapter 5.

MMMTs are typically large, soft, broad-based polypoid tumors that occupy much, sometimes all, of the endometrial cavity and may protrude through the external os. There is often obvious myometrial invasion. The sectioned surface is fleshy, with areas that may show hemorrhage, necrosis, and cystic degeneration (Figure 15–32).[82,83]

On microscopic examination, MMMTs by definition have an intimate admixture of carcinomatous and sarcomatous components that are usually high grade, although focally, one component may predominate. The carcinomatous component takes the form of a high-grade müllerian-type carcinoma (Figure 15–33), most often high-grade endometri-

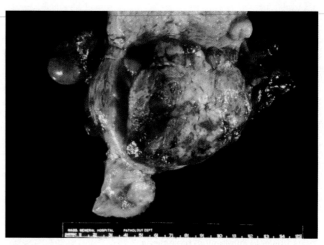

Figure 15–32. Malignant müllerian mixed tumor. There is a polypoid, fleshy mass with extensive necrosis and hemorrhage.

oid carcinoma or serous carcinoma, but sometimes high-grade clear cell carcinoma or a nonspecific carcinoma. Squamous differentiation and foci of undifferentiated carcinoma, including small cell undifferentiated carcinoma, may be seen. The sarcomatous component typically resembles high-grade endometrial sarcoma (see Figure 15–33) but may resemble fibrosarcoma, leiomyosarcoma, malignant fibrous histiocytoma, or undifferentiated sarcoma not otherwise specified. The sarcomatous component may be focally hypocellular and not strikingly atypical cytologically. If such an area is sampled in a curettage, underdiagnosis as a benign lesion is possible. Heterologous elements are common and include benign or malignant appearing cartilage (see Figure 15–33), skeletal muscle differ-

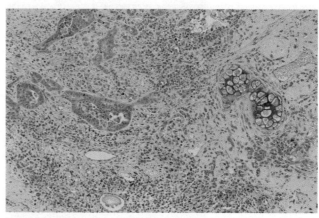

Figure 15–33. Malignant müllerian mixed tumor. Typical biphasic growth of highly malignant epithelial and mesenchymal cells. Heterologous cartilage is present in the mesenchymal component.

entiation, and foci of osteoid. Hyaline droplets, both intracellular and extracellular, may be seen, especially in the sarcomatous component.[82–85] Rare types of differentiation include neuroectodermal tissue, yolk sac tumor, and foci resembling malignant rhabdoid tumor.

Myometrial invasion greater than the inner third is present in about 80% of cases, and in about 40% of cases there is deeper myometrial invasion.[82–85] Metastatic or recurrent tumor may be entirely carcinomatous (the most common), entirely sarcomatous, or contain both elements.

The 5-year survival ranges from 5 to 40%, with a median survival in most studies of under 2 years. The most important pathologic prognostic factors are stage, tumor size, and depth of invasion. Most survivors have tumors confined to the endometrium or superficial myometrial invasion.[82–84,86]

UTERINE TUMORS RESEMBLING OVARIAN SEX CORD TUMORS

This descriptive designation has been applied to rare uterine tumors, most of which are probably of endometrial stromal derivation. The terminology was selected because their cardinal microscopic feature is a resemblance to ovarian tumors of Sertoli or granulosa cell type. The patients are typi-

cally younger than those with adenosarcomas and MMMTs, with an average age of about 47 years. There are no unique clinical manifestations.[87]

On gross examination, they are usually solid, round, well-circumscribed myometrial masses that lack the worrisome gross features of other more malignant uterine tumors considered in this chapter. Sectioning typically shows a uniformly solid, fleshy, often yellow, but occasionally gray-to-tan, surface (Figure 15–34).[87]

On microscopic examination, a dominant epithelial pattern of growth in the form of tubules, trabeculae, cords, and nests imparts the required resemblance to ovarian sex cord tumors (Figure 15–35). Occasional tumors are associated with an appreciable intervening component of mature smooth muscle whose nature is unproven but may, in most cases, be entrapped myometrium incorporated within the slow-growing tumor. The margins of the neoplasm may be somewhat irregular, a feature without proven adverse prognostic significance. The tumor cells vary from small with scant cytoplasm to large with abundant eosinophilic or pale, even lipid-rich cytoplasm. The nuclei are generally small and regular with little pleomorphism, and mitotic figures are generally infrequent.[87] Most of these tumors are clinically benign, although rare tumors have been clinically malignant.

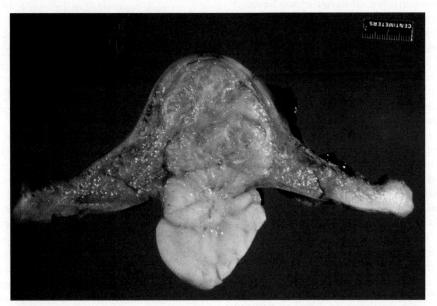

Figure 15–34. Uterine tumor resembling an ovarian sex cord tumor. A large polypoid mass within a white-to-tan cut surface protrudes into the endometrial cavity.

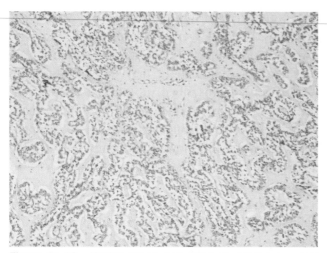

Figure 15–35. Uterine tumor resembling an ovarian sex cord tumor. Anastomosing trabeculae of neoplastic cells are embedded in a hyalinized stroma.

REFERENCES

1. Barter JF, Smith EB, Szpak CA, et al. Leiomyosarcoma of the uterus: clinicopathologic study of 21 cases. Gynecol Oncol 1985;21:220–7.

2. Major FJ, Blessing JA, Silverberg SG, et al. Prognostic factors in early-stage uterine sarcoma. A Gynecologic Oncology Group study. Cancer 1993;71:1702–9.

3. Jones MW, Norris HJ. Clinicopathologic study of 28 uterine leiomyosarcomas with metastasis. Int J Gynecol Pathol 1995;14:243–9.

4. Burns B, Curry RH, Bell ME. Morphologic features of prognostic significance in uterine smooth muscle tumors: a review of eighty-four cases. Am J Obstet Gynecol 1979; 135:109–14.

5. Clement PB. The pathology of uterine smooth muscle tumors and mixed endometrial stromal-smooth muscle tumors: a selective review with emphasis on recent advances. Int J Gynecol Pathol 2000;19:39–55.

6. Clement PB, Young RH. Mesenchymal and mixed epithelial-mesenchymal tumors of the uterine corpus and cervix. In: Atlas of gynecologic surgical pathology. Philadelphia: W. B. Saunders Company; 2000. p. 177–210.

7. Wilkinson N, Rollason TP. Recent advances in the pathology of smooth muscle tumours of the uterus. Histopathology 2001;39:331–41.

8. Bell SW, Kempson RL, Hendrickson MR. Problematic uterine smooth muscle neoplasms. A clinicopathologic study of 213 cases. Am J Surg Pathol 1994;18:535–58.

9. Oliva E, Young RH, Amin MB, Clement PB. An immunohistochemical analysis of endometrial stromal and smooth muscle tumors of the uterus: a study of 54 cases emphasizing the crucial importance of using a panel because of overlap in immunoreactivity for individual antibodies. Am J Surg Pathol 2002;26:403–12.

10. Nucci MR, O'Connell JT, Huettner PC, et al. h-Caldesmon expression effectively distinguishes endometrial stromal tumors from uterine smooth muscle tumors. Am J Surg Pathol 2001;25:455–63.

11. Rush DS, Tan J, Baergen RN, Soslow RA. h-Caldesmon, a novel smooth muscle-specific antibody, distinguishes between cellular leiomyoma and endometrial stromal sarcoma. Am J Surg Pathol 2001;25:253–8.

12. Iwata J, Fletcher CD. Immunohistochemical detection of cytokeratin and epithelial membrane antigen in leiomyosarcoma: a systematic study of 100 cases. Pathol Int 2000;50:7–14.

13. Myles JL, Hart WR. Apoplectic leiomyomas of the uterus. A clinicopathologic study of five distinctive hemorrhagic leiomyomas associated with oral contraceptive usage. Am J Surg Pathol 1985;9:798–805.

14. Norris HJ, Hilliard GD, Irey NS. Hemorrhagic cellular leiomyomas ("apoplectic leiomyoma") of the uterus associated with pregnancy and oral contraceptives. Int J Gynecol Pathol 1988;7:212–24.

15. Clement PB, Young RH, Scully RE. Diffuse, perinodular, and other patterns of hydropic degeneration within and adjacent to uterine leiomyomas. Problems in differential diagnosis. Am J Surg Pathol 1992;16:26–32.

16. Tavassoli FA, Norris HJ. Peritoneal leiomyomatosis (leiomyomatosis peritonealis disseminata): a clinicopathologic study of 20 cases with ultrastructural observations. Int J Gynecol Pathol 1982;1:59–74.

17. Downes KA, Hart WR. Bizarre leiomyomas of the uterus: a comprehensive pathologic study of 24 cases with long-term follow-up. Am J Surg Pathol 1997;21:1261–70.

18. Hart WR, Billman JK Jr. A reassessment of uterine neoplasms originally diagnosed as leiomyosarcomas. Cancer 1978;41:1902–10.

19. Oliva E, Young RH, Clement PB, et al. Cellular benign mesenchymal tumors of the uterus. A comparative morphologic and immunohistochemical analysis of 33 highly cellular leiomyomas and six endometrial stromal nodules, two frequently confused tumors. Am J Surg Pathol 1995; 19:757–68.

20. Perrone T, Dehner LP. Prognostically favorable "mitotically active" smooth-muscle tumors of the uterus. A clinicopathologic study of ten cases. Am J Surg Pathol 1988; 12:1–8.

21. O'Connor DM, Norris HJ. Mitotically active leiomyomas of the uterus. Hum Pathol 1990;21:223–7.

22. Prayson RA, Hart WR. Mitotically active leiomyomas of the uterus. Am J Clin Pathol 1992;97:14–20.

23. Roth LM, Reed RJ, Sternberg WH. Cotyledonoid dissecting leiomyoma of the uterus. The Sternberg tumor. Am J Surg Pathol 1996;20:1455–61.

24. Roth LM, Reed RJ. Dissecting leiomyomas of the uterus other than cotyledonoid dissecting leiomyomas: a report of eight cases. Am J Surg Pathol 1999;23:1032–9.

25. Norris HJ, Parmley T. Mesenchymal tumors of the uterus. V. Intravenous leiomyomatosis. A clinical and pathologic study of 14 cases. Cancer 1975;36:2164–78.

26. Clement PB, Young RH, Scully RE. Intravenous leiomyomatosis of the uterus. A clinicopathological analysis of 16 cases with unusual histologic features. Am J Surg Pathol 1988;12:932–45.

27. Longacre TA, Hendrickson MR, Kempson RL. Predicting clinical outcome for uterine smooth muscle neoplasms with a reasonable degree of certainty. Adv Anat Pathol 1997;4:95–104.

28. Kempson RL, Hendrickson MR. Smooth muscle, endometrial stromal, and mixed müllerian tumors of the uterus. Mod Pathol 2000;13:328–42.

29. Evans HL. Endometrial stromal sarcoma and poorly differentiated endometrial sarcoma. Cancer 1982;50:2170–82.

30. Schneider D, Halperin R, Segal M, et al. Myxoid leiomyosarcoma of the uterus with unusual malignant histologic pattern—a case report. Gynecol Oncol 1995;59:156–8.

31. Pounder DJ, Iyer PV. Uterine leiomyosarcoma with myxoid stroma. Arch Pathol Lab Med 1985;109:762–4.

32. King ME, Dickersin GR, Scully RE. Myxoid leiomyosarcoma of the uterus. A report of six cases. Am J Surg Pathol 1982;6:589–98.

33. Atkins K, Bell S, Kempson R, Hendrickson M. Myxoid smooth muscle tumors of the uterus. Mod Pathol 2001; 14:132A.

34. Atkins K, Bell S, Kempson R, Hendrickson M. Epithelioid smooth muscle tumors of the uterus. Mod Pathol 2001; 14:132A.

35. Prayson RA, Goldblum JR, Hart WR. Epithelioid smooth-muscle tumors of the uterus: a clinicopathologic study of 18 patients. Am J Surg Pathol 1997;21:383–91.

36. Oliva E, Nielsen PG, Clement PB, et al. Epithelioid smooth muscle tumors of the uterus. A clinicopathologic study of 80 cases [abstract]. Mod Pathol 1997;10:107A.

37. Kurman RJ, Norris HJ. Mesenchymal tumors of the uterus. VI. Epithelioid smooth muscle tumors including leiomyoblastoma and clear-cell leiomyoma: a clinical and pathologic analysis of 26 cases. Cancer 1976;37:1853–65.

38. Sieinski W. Malignant giant cell tumor associated with leiomyosarcoma of the uterus. Cancer 1990;65:1838–42.

39. Darby AJ, Papadaki L, Beilby JO. An unusual leiomyosarcoma of the uterus containing osteoclast-like giant cells. Cancer 1975;36:495–504.

40. Devaney K, Tavassoli FA. Immunohistochemistry as a diagnostic aid in the interpretation of unusual mesenchymal tumors of the uterus. Mod Pathol 1991;4:225–31.

41. Larson B, Silfversward C, Nilsson B, Pettersson F. Prognostic factors in uterine leiomyosarcoma. A clinical and histopathological study of 143 cases. The Radiumhemmet series 1936–1981. Acta Oncol 1990;29:185–91.

42. Mulvany NJ, Slavin JL, Ostor AG, Fortune DW. Intravenous leiomyomatosis of the uterus: a clinicopathologic study of 22 cases. Int J Gynecol Pathol 1994;13:1–9.

43. Canzonieri V, D'Amore ES, Bartoloni G, et al. Leiomyomatosis with vascular invasion. A unified pathogenesis regarding leiomyoma with vascular microinvasion, benign metastasizing leiomyoma and intravenous leiomyomatosis. Virchows Arch 1994;425:541–5.

44. Tresukosol D, Kudelka AP, Malpica A, et al. Leuprolide acetate and intravascular leiomyomatosis. Obstet Gynecol 1995;86:688–92.

45. Oliva E, Clement PB, Young RH. Endometrial stromal tumors: an update on a group of tumors with a protean phenotype. Adv Anat Pathol 2000;7:257–81.

46. Fekete PS, Vellios F. The clinical and histologic spectrum of endometrial stromal neoplasms: a report of 41 cases. Int J Gynecol Pathol 1984;3:198–212.

47. Chang KL, Crabtree GS, Lim-Tan SK, et al. Primary uterine endometrial stromal neoplasms. A clinicopathologic study of 117 cases. Am J Surg Pathol 1990;14:415–38.

48. Oliva E, Young RH, Clement PB, Scully RE. Myxoid and fibrous variants of endometrial stromal tumors of the uterus: a report of 10 cases. Int J Gynecol Pathol 1999; 18:310–9.

49. Oliva E, Clement PB, Young RH. Epithelioid endometrial stromal tumors: a report of three cases emphasizing their distinction from epithelioid smooth muscle tumors and other oxyphilic uterine tumors. Int J Gynecol Pathol 2002;21:48–55.

50. McCluggage WG, Date A, Bharucha H, Toner PG. Endometrial stromal sarcoma with sex cord-like areas and focal rhabdoid differentiation. Histopathology 1996;29:369–74.

51. Fitko R, Brainer J, Schink JC, August CZ. Endometrial stromal sarcoma with rhabdoid differentiation. Int J Gynecol Pathol 1990;9:379–82.

52. Oliva E, Clement PB, Young RH, Scully RE. Mixed endometrial stromal and smooth muscle tumors of the uterus: a clinicopathologic study of 15 cases. Am J Surg Pathol 1998;22:997–1005.

53. Baker RJ, Hildebrandt RH, Rouse RV, et al. Inhibin and CD99 (MIC2) expression in uterine stromal neoplasms with sex-cord-like elements. Hum Pathol 1999;30:671–9.

54. Clement PB, Scully RE. Endometrial stromal sarcomas of the uterus with extensive endometrioid glandular differentiation: a report of three cases that caused problems in differential diagnosis. Int J Gynecol Pathol 1992;11:163–73.

55. Clement PB, Scully RE. Müllerian adenosarcoma of the uterus: a clinicopathologic analysis of 100 cases with a review of the literature. Hum Pathol 1990;21:363–81.

56. Tavassoli FA, Norris HJ. Mesenchymal tumours of the uterus. VII. A clinicopathological study of 60 endometrial stromal nodules. Histopathology 1981;5:1–10.

57. Dionigi A, Oliva E, Clement PB, Young RH. Endometrial stromal nodules and endometrial stromal tumors with limited infiltration: a clinicopathologic analysis of 50 cases. Am J Surg Pathol 2002;26:567–81.

58. Daya DA, Scully RE. Sarcoma botryoides of the uterine cervix in young women: a clinicopathological study of 13 cases. Gynecol Oncol 1988;29:290–304.

59. Montag TW, D'Ablaing G, Schlaerth JB, et al. Embryonal rhabdomyosarcoma of the uterine corpus and cervix. Gynecol Oncol 1986;25:171–94.

60. Ordi J, Stamatakos MD, Tavassoli FA. Pure pleomorphic rhabdomyosarcomas of the uterus. Int J Gynecol Pathol 1997;16:369–77.

61. McCluggage WG, Lioe TF, McClelland HR, Lamki H. Rhabdomyosarcoma of the uterus: report of two cases, including one of the spindle cell variant. Int J Gynecol Cancer 2002;12:128–32.

62. Schammel DP, Tavassoli FA. Uterine angiosarcomas: a morphologic and immunohistochemical study of four cases. Am J Surg Pathol 1998;22:246–50.

63. Tallini G, Price FV, Carcangiu ML. Epithelioid angiosarcoma arising in uterine leiomyomas. Am J Clin Pathol 1993; 100:514–8.

64. Nielsen GP, Oliva E, Young RH, et al. Alveolar soft-part sarcoma of the female genital tract: a report of nine cases and review of the literature. Int J Gynecol Pathol 1995; 14:283–92.

65. Nolan NP, Gaffney EF. Alveolar soft part sarcoma of the uterus. Histopathology 1990;16:97–9.

66. Burch DJ, Hitchcock A, Masson GM. Alveolar soft part sarcoma of the uterus: case report and review of the literature. Gynecol Oncol 1994;54:91–4.

67. Sandberg A, Bridge J. Updates on the cytogenetics and molecular genetics of bone and soft tissue tumors: alveolar soft part sarcoma. Cancer Genet Cytogenet 2002;136:1–9.

68. Karseladze AI, Zakharova TI, Navarro S, Llombart-Bosch A. Malignant fibrous histiocytoma of the uterus. Eur J Gynaecol Oncol 2000;21:588–90.

69. Cho KR, Rosenshein NB, Epstein JI. Malignant rhabdoid tumor of the uterus. Int J Gynecol Pathol 1989;8:381–7.

70. Vang R, Kempson RL. Perivascular epithelioid cell tumor ("PEComa") of the uterus: a subset of HMB-45-positive epithelioid mesenchymal neoplasms with an uncertain relationship to pure smooth muscle tumors. Am J Surg Pathol 2002;26:1–13.

71. Pea M, Martignoni G, Zamboni G, Bonetti F. Perivascular epithelioid cell. Am J Surg Pathol 1996;20:1149–53.

72. Ruco LP, Pilozzi E, Wedard BM, et al. Epithelioid lymphangioleiomyomatosis-like tumour of the uterus in a patient without tuberous sclerosis: a lesion mimicking epithelioid leiomyosarcoma. Histopathology 1998;33:91–3.

73. Kerner H, Lichtig C. Müllerian adenosarcoma presenting as cervical polyps: a report of seven cases and review of the literature. Obstet Gynecol 1993;81:655–9.

74. Clement PB, Oliva E, Young RH. Müllerian adenosarcoma of the uterine corpus associated with tamoxifen therapy: a report of six cases and a review of tamoxifen-associated endometrial lesions. Int J Gynecol Pathol 1996;15:222–9.

75. Zaloudek CJ, Norris HJ. Adenofibroma and adenosarcoma of the uterus: a clinicopathologic study of 35 cases. Cancer 1981;48:354–66.

76. Clement PB, Scully RE. Müllerian adenosarcomas of the uterus with sex cord-like elements. A clinicopathologic analysis of eight cases. Am J Clin Pathol 1989;91:664–72.

77. Clement PB. Müllerian adenosarcomas of the uterus with sarcomatous overgrowth. A clinicopathological analysis of 10 cases. Am J Surg Pathol 1989;13:28–38.

78. Hattab EM, Allam-Nandyala P, Rhatigan RM. The stromal component of large endometrial polyps. Int J Gynecol Pathol 1999;18:332–7.

79. Tai LH, Tavassoli FA. Endometrial polyps with atypical (bizarre) stromal cells. Am J Surg Pathol 2002;26:505–9.

80. Kaku T, Silverberg SG, Major FJ, et al. Adenosarcoma of the uterus: a Gynecologic Oncology Group clinicopathologic study of 31 cases. Int J Gynecol Pathol 1992;11:75–88.

81. Bitterman P, Chun B, Kurman RJ. The significance of epithelial differentiation in mixed mesodermal tumors of the uterus. A clinicopathologic and immunohistochemical study. Am J Surg Pathol 1990;14:317–28.

82. Iwasa Y, Haga H, Konishi I, et al. Prognostic factors in uterine carcinosarcoma: a clinicopathologic study of 25 patients. Cancer 1998;82:512–9.

83. Gagne E, Tetu B, Blondeau L, et al. Morphologic prognostic factors of malignant mixed müllerian tumor of the uterus: a clinicopathologic study of 58 cases. Mod Pathol 1989; 2:433–8.

84. Nordal RR, Kristensen GB, Stenwig AE, et al. An evaluation of prognostic factors in uterine carcinosarcoma. Gynecol Oncol 1997;67:316–21.

85. Silverberg SG. Low-grade endometrial stromal sarcoma: a rare but often puzzling diagnostic problem. Pathol Case Rev 2000;5:173–80.

86. Silverberg SG, Major FJ, Blessing JA, et al. Carcinosarcoma (malignant mixed mesodermal tumor) of the uterus. A Gynecologic Oncology Group pathologic study of 203 cases. Int J Gynecol Pathol 1990;9:1–19.

87. Clement PB, Scully RE. Uterine tumors resembling ovarian sex-cord tumors. A clinicopathologic analysis of fourteen cases. Am J Clin Pathol 1976;66:512–25.

16

Treatment of Uterine Sarcomas

CAROLYN KRASNER, MD

MICHAEL V. SEIDEN, MD, PHD

Mesenchymal tumors of the uterus are a group of rare neoplasms, comprising only 3 to 5% of uterine cancers. On the basis of the SEER data (Surveillance, Epidemiology, and End Results program registries), the most common uterine sarcoma is the carcinosarcoma, or the malignant mixed müllerian tumor (MMMT), followed by leiomyosarcoma (LMS), and endometrial stromal sarcoma (ESS), with other sarcomas occurring less frequently.[1] Despite the low incidence of these tumors, they account for a high percentage of deaths from uterine malignancies, as much as 29% in one series.[2]

The literature that underpins the management of these tumors has several limitations, which, in turn, reduce confidence in the studies' conclusions. First, the evolving nomenclature and pathologic classification make it difficult, if not impossible, to compare studies that are often separated by decades. Indeed, single institutional experiences with these rare tumors often span several decades, during which time pathologic classification, surgical techniques, radiation therapy technologies, and chemotherapy have changed. Clinical studies often combine female patients with tumors of gynecologic origin together with both female and male patients with nongynecologic mesenchymal tumors. There are no randomized studies that contain enough patients to discriminate among competing therapies that might offer, at best, modest improvements in overall survival. Finally, within the field of mesenchymal tumors of the uterus, the three predominant histologies (MMMT, LMS, and ESS) have different natural histories and underlying biology, and there are few prospective clinical studies that focus

on individual histologic subtypes. The issue of randomized trials in rare tumors was the subject of an editorial in the *Journal of Clinical Oncology* addressing the state of knowledge in uterine sarcomas, in which the author argues that "rare tumors cannot undergo the same type of investigations as common ones."[3] Although that is certainly indisputable, this chapter attempts to approach the understanding of the treatment of these rare diseases with as much rigor and reliance on evidence-based medicine as is possible with what is available.

PRESENTATION

Most women with uterine sarcomas present with nonfunctional or postmenopausal vaginal bleeding (78% in a Finnish retrospective).[4] Other common presenting complaints include pelvic pain or pressure, vaginal discharge (which may be foul smelling), or a rapidly enlarging pelvic mass. They do not lend themselves to early detection by means of any specific screening test (see Chapter 14). Indeed, clinical studies evaluating women who present with "rapidly enlarging pelvic masses" most often report nonmalignant etiologies.[5] Rarely, an abnormal Pap smear result prompts a work-up. Endometrial biopsies are often unrevealing if the tumor does not involve the endometrium. On examination, these patients typically have an enlarged uterus, and sometimes the tumor may be seen protruding through the cervical os.

Patients will typically undergo a hysterectomy for what is presumed to be a benign leiomyoma (fibroid) or "central pelvic mass." The diagnosis of malignant gynecologic disease or sarcoma is often not anticipated preoperatively, or patients may have emergent surgical procedures due to bleeding, which may lead to surgical approaches that are sometimes inadequate for full staging procedures.

NATURAL HISTORY AND PATTERNS OF SPREAD

Developing therapeutic plans for women with mesenchymal tumors depends on an understanding of prognosis and the likelihood of local and distant disease recurrence, as well as the availability of a specific therapy to alter these outcomes. Surgical staging of sarcoma and careful pathologic review of these rare tumors (reviewed in Chapter 15) are important in the comprehensive care of these patients. The natural history and patterns of spread may be predicted, at least in part, by histology.

There have been a number of large retrospective reviews of uterine sarcoma elucidating the natural history and metastatic patterns of these diseases. Although there is some variation among the studies, it is clear that patients presenting with these mesenchymal tumors are at risk of both local (pelvis) and distant recurrences. Table 16–1 reviews three studies that included women with stage I (or stage I/II) disease treated with surgery alone.[6–8] First recurrences occurred with about equal frequency in the pelvis and at distant sites. Because these studies are all retrospective and these institutions all had radiotherapy departments, it might be reasonable to assume that patients included in the surgery-alone group were judged to be at "low risk" of recurrence. Thus, the risk of local recurrence may be higher in an unselected group of women with low-stage disease (Table 16–2).[9]

Distant recurrences are typically seen in the abdominal cavity (such as peritoneal or omental recurrences) or in the lung. Omental and peritoneal recurrences are not typically associated with ascites, as is the case with ovarian cancer, and metastatic disease in the upper abdomen tends not to be of the same miliary nature, as is seen in ovarian cancer. These patients may develop very large and, often, relatively asymptomatic recurrences in the upper abdomen. Hematogenous dissemination to the lungs is also common and is typically asymptomatic (initially) or may be associated with a cough. Other sites of metastatic disease include liver, bone, and brain. Soft tissue and scalp metastases as well as metastases to other visceral organs, such as the adrenals, are seen in a small subset of patients (Table 16–3).[10]

A randomized prospective trial conducted by the Gynecologic Oncology Group (GOG) evaluated the use of adjuvant Adriamycin versus no systemic therapy for patients with stage I or II tumors.[11] This study, begun in 1973 and completed in 1982, is useful to elucidate the natural history and patterns of spread in a prospectively collected group of women with early stage disease. This study (Table 16–4) showed that LMS was more likely to recur in the lungs, and MMMT recurred more often in the abdomen and pelvis.[9]

INITIAL SURGICAL MANAGEMENT OF SARCOMA

Overview

Surgery is the mainstay of treatment for uterine sarcomas. The extent of surgery may vary by histologic subtype. If the tumor is suspected preoperatively or diagnosed intraoperatively in consultation with the pathologist, an extended surgical staging, such as one used for endometrial adenocarcinoma with radical

Table 16–1.   LOCAL AND DISTANT RELAPSE RATES

Author	N	Local Relapse	Distant Relapse
Vongtama[6]*†	61	35	9
Major[7]*†	228	51	87
Echt[8]*‡	19	6	4
Total	308	92 (30%)	100 (32%)

*Site of first recurrence.
†Stage I and II.
‡Stage I only.

Table 16–2.   LOCAL RELAPSE RATE BY STAGE

Presenting Stage	Local Control Rate at 5 Years (n)
Stage I	94% (40)
Stage II	89% (9)
Stage III	55% (17)
Stage IV	0% (6)

Adapted from Knocke TH et al.[9]

Table 16–3. SITES OF DISTANT METASTASES	
Site	Frequency of Metastatic Disease
Lung	47%
Omentum/peritoneum	25%
Bone	24%
Para-aortic nodes	12%
Liver	12%
Brain	4%

Sites of distant recurrence in a collection of 45 cases of distant disease recurrence. Primary histology included 33 malignant mixed müllerian tumors, 7 leiomyosarcomas, 4 endometrial stromal sarcomas, 2 other. Note total equals more then 100% due to multiple sites of recurrence. Adapted From Salazar O et al.[10]

resection, bilateral salpingo-oophorectomy, peritoneal washings, para-aortic node resection, and visual inspection, is generally used. Though a survival benefit for surgical staging and lymphadenectomy has not been demonstrated, it is useful for prognosis and treatment planning. In addition, there is ample evidence that these tumors are relatively radiation and chemotherapy insensitive, and, hence, aggressive surgical cytoreduction, particularly of low-grade tumors, is appropriate. Patients with higher-grade tumors are much less likely to experience any benefit from surgical cytoreduction due to the rapid recurrence of distant disease. Thus, surgical judgment is key to deciding what is acceptable in terms of extensive surgical cytoreduction of nodal metastases or, in certain cases, peritoneal or even visceral disease. There are no controlled studies that measure the benefit of extensive surgical cytoreduction on survival of women with advanced-stage disease. There are clearly some patients for whom palliative or symptom-focused management makes the most sense and who should not be subjected to extensive surgery. That said, radiotherapy in place of surgical debulking has been consistently shown to lead to inferior survival.[12] A retrospective review of 73 patients, treated with either surgery, surgery and radiotherapy, or radiotherapy, as well as an extensive literature review of 900 patients, showed improved outcome with surgical treatment. No standardized trial of radiotherapy alone as primary treatment has been performed.

Carcinosarcoma

Patients with carcinosarcoma (MMMT) grossly confined to the uterus, International Federation of Gyne-

cology and Obstetrics (FIGO) stage I or II, are often upstaged at the time of laparotomy. A significant proportion of patients are upstaged by the finding of extrauterine disease if a full staging procedure is performed; this number ranges between 12 and 40%.[8,13,14] Dissemination and patterns of spread are similar to what may be found in poorly differentiated adenocarcinoma, that is, the epithelial component seems to dictate dissemination.[15] Common sites of metastatic disease include the serosal surfaces and the adnexae as well as intraperitoneal spread.

The GOG prospective staging study found that 17% of all patients with carcinosarcoma had lymph node involvement and, therefore, should undergo nodal sampling.[8] For a patient with obvious intraperitoneal spread, however, lymph node sampling is unlikely to change the prognosis. Similarly, for patients with disease spread within the pelvis or with extrapelvic extension, aggressive surgical debulking has not been shown to influence the outcome. Therefore, for advanced-stage tumors, palliative surgical efforts should be undertaken for the correction of obstruction and relief of pain.

Leiomyosarcoma

Leiomyosarcoma is seldom suspected prior to surgical exploration, and it is typically discovered during surgical resection of a presumed benign leiomyomata or postoperatively at the time of pathologic review. The standard operative procedure for a known LMS is total abdominal hysterectomy and bilateral salpingo-oophorectomy (BSO). In these patients, nodal metastases are uncommon, unless the disease clearly extends outside the uterus. Thus, routine node sampling or random biopsies in organ-confined disease is unlikely to demonstrate tumor. In contrast, both

Table 16–4. LOCAL RELAPSE RATE OF UTERINE SARCOMA BY HISTOLOGY	
Presenting Histology	Local Recurrence Rate at 5 Years (n)
LMS	76% (30)
ESS	91% (11)
MMMT	72% (28)

ESS = endometrial stromal sarcoma; LMS = leiomyosarcoma; MMMT = malignant mixed müllerian tumor.
Adapted from Knocke TH et al.[9]

Goff and colleagues and Leibsohn and colleagues reported that lymph node metastases in patients with advanced LMS were present when there was gross involvement of the nodes and/or obvious intra-abdominal disease.[16,17]

In the case of a postoperative diagnosis of LMS in a patient who has undergone a simple myomectomy with BSO, a completion hysterectomy should be performed because of risk of residual malignancy.[18,19]

Endometrial Stromal Sarcomas

Endometrial stromal sarcomas include both low-grade tumors and high-grade tumors, which should be considered as clinically separate entities. The surgical therapy of low-grade ESS, or endolymphatic stromal myosis, should aim to remove all disease, as this slow-growing disease may, in fact, be cured surgically, even in more advanced stages. Approximately 1 in 3 cases demonstrate node metastasis and pelvic lymph node resection is appropriate. The removal of all disease generally involves total abdominal hysterectomy, although radical hysterectomy is indicated if there is evidence of parametrial involvement. Occasionally, even more radical surgery may be performed, such as in the case of caval involvement. Surgical resection should include oophorectomy because these tumors are often hormonally sensitive. Thus, removal of the ovaries may serve to control any remaining disease, especially if the tumor is found to contain estrogen and/or progesterone receptors. One series that examined this question found a significantly lower recurrence rate, 43% versus 100%, in women who underwent oophorectomy at the time of their original surgery for low-grade ESS, although other studies have found that the addition of bilateral salpingo-oophorectomy did not decrease the rate of recurrence.[20,21] However, in view of the possible benefits, consideration of reoperation is reasonable in patients in whom the ovaries are not removed at the time of initial surgery. A reasonable, though unstudied, approach for patients for whom reoperation is not possible is treatment with an LHRH to reduce estrogen levels.

The surgical management of high-grade ESS generally follows the same principles as that for carci-nosarcoma. The tumor is initially grossly debulked. There is no evidence of a prognostic or therapeutic advantage for lymph node sampling.

ADJUVANT THERAPY

As described above, approximately 50 to 70% of women with stage I/II high-grade sarcomas can expect the recurrence of their disease in months to years from the time of their surgical resection.[19] Both local and systemic adjuvant therapies have been used in the context of clinical trials and, more commonly, as institutional standard practices that have been subsequently reviewed in retrospective studies. As discussed earlier, the lack of randomized studies makes it impossible to provide sound literature-based recommendations regarding the use of radiation therapy or chemotherapy.

Adjuvant Pelvic Radiation Therapy

Because at least 50% of patients with localized sarcoma will experience local recurrences, it is reasonable to hypothesize that radiation therapy could decrease the local recurrence rate. This theoretic benefit, however, is probably limited by the high incidence of distant recurrences. For example, a review of 235 cases of uterine sarcoma, in which both pelvic and distant recurrences were noted, demonstrated that while 67% of patients experienced pelvic recurrences, only 14% of women were described as having "pelvis-only" recurrences.[22] It is possible that improved regional control may ultimately lead to a lower incidence of systemic disease and death, but the improvement is likely to be limited to less than 14% of the group. Hence, it would require a very large trial to provide the power needed to demonstrate this modest effect (if, indeed, it exists). Randomized trials that specifically address this issue do not exist, and, thus, the only studies available for review are retrospective collections that suffer the obvious bias of selection.

The clinical trial GOG 20 randomized 225 sarcoma patients between no systemic chemotherapy and eight cycles of doxorubicin.[11,12] Even though not randomized, but instead delivered at the discretion of the individual investigators, it was at least prospectivly studied. In this study, 105 patients received radiation, and 51 patients did not. Multiple different techniques and radiation doses were used. The incidence of first recurrence in the pelvis was 54% in the nonradiated group and 23% in the radiated group ($p = .28$). In various analyses, such as investigation by any histology, there appeared to be no advantage in terms of disease-free survival to either chemotherapy or adjuvant radiation. The 77% pelvic control rate reported in this trial compares well with the 77.9% local control rate at 5 years as reported by Knocke and colleagues.[9] Specific control rates varied by stage and possibly with histology, with diseases other than LMS having a slightly better local control rate, although the size of the trial was such that this conclusion was not definitive.

The evaluation of overall survival and disease-free survival in nonrandomized retrospective series is not appropriate due to the obvious selection bias in these studies. Indeed, even evaluating pelvic failure rates is suspect due to potential bias of patient selection. Although these biases necessarily limit the veracity of the data, the bulk of the single-institution trials do demonstrate that pelvic irradiation is associated with a low incidence of locoregional relapse. Echt and colleagues retrospectively analyzed the outcome of 66 patients treated with surgery alone, radiation alone, or combined surgery and radiation and demonstrated that surgery plus radiation was associated with a lower incidence of pelvic failure, with those receiving surgery alone having a 33% chance of pelvic relapse (9/27) versus those treated with combined modality therapy not experiencing a single pelvic relapse (0/36).[7] Hoffmann and colleagues also demonstrated a reduction in local recurrences in a retrospective study of 54 patients.[23] This review included 22 patients treated with surgery alone and 32 receiving both surgery and radiation and demonstrated fewer pelvic recurrences in women who had surgery and radiation. The European Organization for Research and Treatment of Cancer (EORTC) trial 55874 is an important randomized trial directly addressing the benefit of adjuvant pelvic irradiation. In this study, patients with early-stage uterine sarcoma were randomized to receive either surgery alone or surgery followed by adjuvant irradiation. The results of this study are currently pending.

There is a discrepancy as to whether patients with all stages of disease benefit from radiation for improved local control. Three nonrandomized studies that address this arrive at different answers.[9,22,24] As would be expected, individuals with lower-stage disease and, therefore, a lower risk or burden of occult regional disease, have a higher chance of regional control with pelvic radiotherapy. A lower percentage of patients with stage I disease (56%) failed as compared with patients with higher-stage disease. These studies have also suggested that local control may be a little higher in patients with ESS, but the studies are not appropriately designed to make any definitive conclusions. Likewise, there is no convincing data that survival is positively or negatively impacted by radiation therapy.

Irradiation Technique

The approach to adjuvant pelvic irradiation of uterine sarcomas is similar to the management of other gynecologic malignancies. The four-field approach is most often used, aiming to cover all pelvic nodal drainage up to the bifurcation of the aorta. The proximal one-third of the vagina is included, but attempts to include all of the vagina result in significant morbidity involving the vagina and rectum, including acute diarrhea and pain and late stenosis and bleeding. Side effects may be significant in this group and must be considered in any palliative treatment decision. In Knocke and colleagues' series, acute side effects included 30.6% grade 1, 11.1% grade 2, and 6.9% grade 3 complications.[9] Late side effects consisted of chronic cystitis, enteritis, proctitis, and one case of small bowel necrosis, which resulted in death. The vagina was the most frequent site of late sequelae; 12 patients experienced grade 1 atrophy and 2 patients vaginal shortening or even obliteration; in all, 16% of patients had late sequelae grade 3 or higher, including cystitis, malabsorption, bowel necrosis and vaginal shortening, and atrophy. Doses in the range of 50 Gy in 1.8 to 2.0 Gy fractions are typically used. A comparison of 60 Gy with 50 Gy in patients with MMMT found an insignificant improvement in local control. However, currently, there are no data on an optimal radiation dose.[25]

Abdominal irradiation is also sometimes used as the entire peritoneal cavity is at risk of relapse.[26] It is not clear that this provides additional benefit over pelvic irradiation as abdominal recurrences are, in general, easier to manage surgically. When whole abdomen irradiation is used, the superior border must extend to the diaphragm and the inferior border to the inferior peritoneal reflection, with adequate margins superiorly and inferiorly as well as laterally. The total dose is generally 30 Gy, but care must be taken to localize the kidneys and shield them at 20 Gy, with liver shielding at 25 Gy. The pelvic irradiation is continued to a total of 50 Gy. The GOG is currently evaluating the role of adjuvant whole abdominal radiotherapy versus ifosfamide and cisplatin in women with surgical stage I to IV resected MMMT (GOG 150). Over 130 women have been enrolled on a study that was initiated in 1993. Results from this study are not yet reported.

Adjuvant Radiation Therapy: Conclusion

In summary, the decision to include adjuvant irradiation is based on the hypothesis that decreasing the local recurrence rate will provide benefit in quality of life gained through the reduction in risk of a pelvic relapse. Although this goal is laudable, there are no quality-of-life data or accurate estimates of risk reduction associated with pelvic radiotherapy. Thus, the judicious use of radiotherapy requires a careful discussion of the potential risks and possible benefits of radiotherapy in women with stage I/II sarcoma. There is little evidence to support the use of adjuvant radiotherapy in women with higher-stage disease. Randomized trials, currently in progress, may provide important information on the use of radiotherapy in the future.

ADJUVANT CHEMOTHERAPY

Given the extremely high risk of recurrence after local treatment, the rationale for adjuvant chemotherapy, namely, to eradicate micrometastases before overt recurrence as is done in other diseases, such as breast or colon cancer, is logical. The largest randomized trial evaluating the potential benefit of adjuvant chemotherapy in uterine sarcoma was performed by the GOG.[11] A total of 225 patients were enrolled, with 46 ineligible and 23 unevaluable, leaving 156 evaluable patients. They were stratified according to stage and whether they had received prior adjuvant radiotherapy, which was up to the discretion of the individual physician. Stage I/II patients were treated with doxorubicin at 60 mg/m^2 every 3 weeks with eight doses. Significantly, adjuvant radiation therapy prior to chemotherapy was allowed, at the discretion of the individual treating physicians. The results failed to show a statistically significant benefit to the use of doxorubicin as adjuvant therapy. Median survival with chemotherapy was 73.7 months, not statistically different from the control of 55 months. Similarly, the progression-free interval was not extended by the addition of this chemotherapy. When analyzed by histology, stage, and prior irradiation, no group showed a benefit. Compliance was suboptimal in one-third of patients randomized to the chemotherapy arm, but there was no survival difference between those receiving "optimal" treatment and those receiving "suboptimal" treatment. The study was powered to detect what most would consider an unobtainable benefit for systemic doxorubicin. The validity of this study was undermined by the many protocol deviations as well as the high dropout rate. Other criticisms include the heterogeneity of the patients and the fact that the study was not powered to look at individual histologies.

There are many small, nonrandomized trials employing multiple chemotherapeutic agents in the adjuvant setting. The lack of an appropriate randomized control arm makes interpretation impossible. Regimens included vincristine, dacarbazine, and cyclophosphamide; Adriamycin; cyclophosphamide, vincrisitine, Adriamycin, and dacarbazine (CyVADIC); cyclophosphamide, actinomycin D, and vincristine; ifosfamide; and cisplatin in combination with epirubicin or Adriamycin.[27–34] All these studies suggest that adjuvant therapy can be delivered safely, but none can evaluate the efficacy of the therapy. Despite the often favorable survival rates described in these small single-arm studies, the limited efficacy of these same drugs and/or combinations in metastatic disease makes it unlikely that any of these regimens would be demonstrated to be superior to a no-treatment arm in even a moderate-sized randomized trial.

Adjuvant Chemotherapy: Conclusion

There are no data that currently support the use of adjuvant chemotherapy in the management of sarcoma. This statement is tempered by the fact that there has never been a large enough randomized trial to detect the type of benefit that these drugs could most optimistically obtain. The fact that the randomized GOG study took 9 years to collect 156 evaluable patients highlights the need for international randomized trials to address this question or suggests waiting for the identification of dramatically more active systemic agents that could be capable of demonstrating a survival benefit in a small or moderate-sized randomized trial.

TREATMENT OF RECURRENT DISEASE

Surgery

There is a definite role for judicious surgical resection of recurrent uterine sarcoma. Due to the limited utility of both chemotherapy and radiation therapy in this collection of diseases, it is appropriate to consider the potential role of surgical resection in women with a solitary or limited recurrence of their sarcoma. As in the soft tissue sarcoma literature, some long-term survival is achieved by metastasectomy.[35] Decision points to be considered include time from initial diagnosis and the overall health of the individual. In one series of thoracotomy for isolated pulmonary recurrences, the most significant predictor of survival was unilateral versus bilateral metastasis. Five-year and 10-year survival rates after pulmonary resections were 43% and 35%, respectively.[36] Local and regional resections for recurrent disease may likewise be curative for late recurrence, especially in low-grade disease. At other times, it may be considered for palliative goals, such as relief of obstruction or of pain.

Resection of recurrent low-grade ESS may be curative, especially in the case of local recurrence. Some authors believe radical resection of locally recurrent disease as well as metastasectomy is jus-

tified in these patients, given their typically long disease-free intervals.[19]

Radiation Therapy

Palliative irradiation may be used for patients presenting with bulky, unresectable disease or with de novo presentation with metastatic disease. In this case, the irradiation is used to control pain and bleeding and/or to manage actual or potential obstruction of bowels, ureters, or bladder. The Radiation Therapy Oncology Group (RTOG) has designed a palliative schedule for treating bulky pelvic disease, shown in a phase II (RTOG 8502) trial to produce significant quality-of-life benefit by controlling symptoms while producing only minimal toxicity.[37] It is a split-course approach that allows for self-selection and dropout for those patients for whom other approaches, such as supportive care, may be more appropriate. It consists of multiple courses of 3.7 Gy twice a day for 2 days, followed by 2- to 4-week rest periods, with up to three repeats, for a total of 44.4 Gy, using shrinking fields. There was only 6% incidence of grade 3 or greater toxicity at 18 months.

Chemotherapy

The modest antitumor activity of chemotherapy in recurrent sarcoma can provide important palliation of symptoms, such as dyspnea or pain. Unfortunately, there exists no evidence that these interventions result in improved overall survival for women with these malignancies, although it is possible that this therapy does prolong the survival of a modest subset of women who respond to treatment. Because of the rarity of these diseases, most chemotherapy trials include patients with all histologies. Some trials attempt to evaluate the efficacy of particular drugs or drug combinations within histologic subgroups, but none of the studies is large enough to provide statistically meaningful results, although some trends do arise. The section below describes the results of single and combination chemotherapy trials for recurrent or persistent sarcomas. Additional information is also covered in the "Histologic Specific" section found following the "Chemotherapy" section of this chapter.

Table 16–5. AGENTS WITH ACTIVITY IN SOFT TISSUE SARCOMA

Agent	Range of Reported Response Rates (%)
Doxorubicin	16–34
Ifosfamide	18–35
Dacarbazine	18
Cisplatin	7–15
Methotrexate	0–37
Dactinomycin	17
Gemcitabine	17
Doxil	10
Vincristine	12

Adapted from Young JC et al[38]; Patel SR[39]; Judson I et al.[40]

Single-Agent Chemotherapy

A large number of agents have been evaluated in the treatment of women with soft tissue sarcomas. Table 16–5 lists the agents that have been evaluated in the treatment of soft tissue sarcoma of both gynecologic and nongynecologic origins.[38–40] Focusing on mesenchymal tumors of gynecologic origin, doxorubicin, ifosfamide, cisplatin, and paclitaxel have been studied most extensively and are reviewed in Table 16–6. Although no firm conclusions can be made, both the literature and our personal clinical experience suggest that MMMT and ESS are more chemotherapy sensitive than LMS (see Table 16–6).[41–55] In addition, most studies that have included patients with both chemotherapy-naive and chemotherapy-pretreated patients have demonstrated higher response rates in the chemotherapy-

naive population. Limited data also support the hypothesis that anthracyclines and ifosfamide may have better activity in LMS, whereas MMMT and ESS may be more sensitive to the taxanes and platinums. Newer drugs, such as liposomal doxorubicin, gemcitabine, and the marine product ET-743, all deserve further evaluation in the treatment of these diseases.[39,40,56,57] There are little data to support the idea that dose escalation of anthracyclines or alkylating agents (such as ifosfamide or cisplatin) is important in leading to meaningful clinical differences in response rates and no data suggesting that it improves survival. While there are no studies specifically targeting sarcomas of gynecologic origin, evaluation of high-dose single-agent ifosfamide in patients with LMS found only a 33% response, with significant toxicity and a duration of response of only 8 months.[58,59]

Combination Chemotherapy

Two-, three-, and even four-drug combinations have been evaluated in sarcoma, in both phase II and phase III trials. In general, combination regimens have demonstrated slightly higher response rates but no superior survival. Moderately large randomized trials in patients with a collection of nongynecologic and gynecologic soft tissue sarcomas comparing MAID (mesna, Adriamycin, ifosfamide, and dacarbazine) with simpler chemotherapy regimens have failed to

Table 16–6. SINGLE AGENT WITH ACTIVITY IN GYNECOLOGIC SARCOMAS

Agent	Dosage	MMMT % (n)	LMS % (n)	ESS % (n)	Reference
Adriamycin	60 mg/m² q21d	9 (41)	25 (28)		41
Ifosfamide	1.5 (1.2) g/m² x 5 d			33 (21)	42
Ifosfamide	1.5 (1.2) g/m² x 5 d	32 (28)			43
Ifosfamide	1.5 (1.2) g/m² x 5 d		17 (35)		44
Ifosfamide	1.5 g/m² x 5 d	36 (100)			45
Cisplatin		42 (18)			46
Cisplatin		19 (63)	3 (33)		47
Cisplatin*	50 mg/m² q21d	18 (34)			48
Paclitaxel	175 mg/m² q21d		9 (34)		49
Paclitaxel	170 (135) mg/m²	18.2 (44)			50
Etoposide	100 mg/m² x 3 d		0 (28)		51
Aminothiadiazole	125 mg/m² qw	4 (22)			52
Diaziquone (AZQ)	22.5–30 mg/ m² q21d	4 (23)			53
Trimetrexate	5 mg/m² bid x 5 q14d	5 (21)			54
Trimetrexate	5 mg/m² q/d x 5 q14d		4 (23)		55

*Second-line chemotherapy.
†Dose for patients with prior pelvic radiotherapy.
ESS = endometrial stromal sarcoma; LMS = leiomyosarcoma; MMMT = malignant mixed mullerian tumor.

Table 16–7.   COMBINATION TRIALS IN GYNECOLOGIC SARCOMAS

Combination	Dosage	MMMT % (n)	LMS % (n)	ESS % (n)	NS % (n)	Reference
Ifosfamide Adriamycin	5 g/m² over 24 h 50 mg/m²		30.3 (33)			62
Ifosfamide Adriamycin	5 g/m² over 24 h 50 mg/m²	30 (34)				60
Dacarbazine Adriamycin	250 mg/m²/d x 5 60 mg/m²	23 (31)	30 (20)			41
Cyclophosphamide Adriamycin	500 mg/m² 60 mg/m²				19 (26)	61
Ifosfamide Cisplatin	1.5 g/m²/d x 5 20 mg/m²/d x 5	54 (90)				43
Hydrea Dacarbazine Etoposide	500 mg q6h x 4 700 mg/m² 100 mg/m²/d x 3		18 (38)			63
Vincristine Actinomycin D Cyclophosphamide	1.5 mg/m²/wk 0.5 mg/m²/d x 5 300 mg/m²/d x 5	26 (27)	29 (14)	50 (2)		30

ESS = endometrial stromal sarcoma; LMS = leiomyosarcoma; MMMT = malignant mixed müllerian tumors; NS = not specified.

demonstrate a positive effect on survival.[60] Table 16–7 reviews the two-drug regimens reported in phase II trials or arms of phase III trials limited to gynecologic sarcomas.[30,41,43,60–63] All of these trials focus predominantly on MMMT or LMS because other histologic subtypes are too rare. The cyclophosphamide and doxorubicin regimen was given to women with a wide collection of gynecologic sarcomas, although most had MMMT and LMS.[61] Almost all published doublets contained doxorubicin, ifosfamide, or both; thus, response rates of 30% are not surprising nor significantly different from those reported for single-agent doxorubicin or ifosfamide. The ifosfamide and cisplatin doublet achieved the highest response rate of any chemotherapy used in the management of gynecologic sarcomas.[62] The phase III trial contained 224 patients, although 30 were declared either ineligible or nonevaluable; 92 women were randomly

allocated to ifosfamide-cisplatin, and had a response rate of 54%. Enthusiasm is tempered by the fact that only 20% of patients could complete the planned eight cycles of therapy. Grade 3 and 4 hematologic toxicity approached 90%. There were six treatment-related deaths and a case of acute myelogenous leukemia which developed after 8 cycles of chemotherapy, making the relationship between diagnosis and therapy uncertain. In total, 54% of patients discontinued this therapy due to toxicity, death, or withdrawal of consent.

Determining the merit of these more toxic combinations requires randomized trials that are appropriately powered to detect the modest survival benefit anticipated by the use of combination therapy. Three randomized trials with more than 100 patients have been reported (Table 16–8). The first two, reported by Omura and colleagues and Muss and

Table 16–8.   RANDOMIZED TRIALS IN GYNECOLOGIC SARCOMAS

Regimen	Treatment Arm (n)	Response Rate (%)	Progression-Free Survival (mo)	Overall Survival (mo)	Reference
Adriamycin	120	16		6.3	41
Adriamycin dacarbazine	106	24		5.8	
Adriamycin	50	19	5.1	11.6	60
Adriamycin cyclophosphamide	54	20	4.9	10.9	
Ifosfamide	102	36	4	7.6	43
Ifosfamide cisplatin	92	54*	6*	9.4	

*p < .05.

colleagues compared doxorubicin with either dacarbazine or cyclophosphamide.[41,61] Both studies included a mixed population of patients with MMMT and LMS. No statistical differences in survival or response were seen. The study by Sutton and colleagues demonstrates modestly superior response rates and progression-free survival rates for the ifosfamide and cisplatin doublet as compared with single-agent ifosfamide, although the overall survival is equivalent.[43] This study was restricted to women with MMMT, and it is possible that the higher response rates and slightly longer survivals in this study as compared with the Omura and colleagues' study are due to the greater chemotherapy sensitivity of MMMT as compared with LMS. A critical analysis of these studies suggests that none is large enough to definitively address if combination therapy is superior to single agents in improving survival in this patient population. For example, the comparison of ifosfamide to ifosfamide plus cisplatin was powered to have only a 50% chance of detecting a near doubling of overall survival (if one existed) in the ifosfamide/cisplatin arm of the trial.

Chemotherapy for MMMT

Malignant mixed müllerian tumors are the most common of uterine sarcomas and hence are the best represented in the literature. Controversy exists about the cell of origin of this malignancy, and while pathologic and therapeutic discussions of this malignancy have been characteristically reviewed within the larger body of sarcoma literature, evidence suggests this may actually be a de-differentiated epithelial malignancy (see Chapter 15). Regardless of the cell of origin, both distant and local metastases frequently occur. In the earlier literature, these tumors were divided into homologous and heterologous types, depending on whether the mesenchymal components of the tumor were composed of tissue types found within the uterine corpus (homologous) or outside the corpus (heterologous). This terminology is now outdated and has no identifiable genetic basis. Importantly, there does not seem to be a difference in response rates between the two subtypes. More useful in predicting response are performance status as well as prior radiation and prior chemotherapy status. Patients with normal performance status who are radiation and chemotherapy-naive have the best chance of response.

The malignancy demonstrates modest chemotherapy sensitivity to a variety of agents, most notably ifosfamide, cisplatin, and paclitaxel.[43,45,46,48,50] Ifosfamide-containing regimens are active but are typically associated with significant myelotoxicity and, in some cases, significant neurotoxicity, including serious central nervous system toxicity, particularly in the elderly. Also of note is the fact that responses do not tend to be durable, lasting only 1.5 to 8 months, as shown in the report by Sutton and colleagues.[43] Although prior therapy tends to reduce the chance of response, Thigpen and colleagues have demonstrated activity with moderate-dose cisplatin (50 mg/m^2 every 3 weeks) in this clinical setting, including some durable responses in excess of 1 year.[48] Likewise, the activity of paclitaxel in this malignancy raises the possibility that the combination of carboplatin and paclitaxel will be efficacious in these malignancies.[50] Indeed, this regimen has been demonstrated to be active in MMMT of the ovary, although this regimen still requires formal testing in MMMT of the uterus.[62,64]

Currently, the GOG is extending its study of the ifosfamide-cisplatin doublet in two randomized trials. The first compares this doublet with whole abdominal radiotherapy in individuals with small-volume or microscopic intraperitoneal disease (GOG 150). The second compares the ifosfamide-cisplatin doublet with ifosfamide and paclitaxel in women with bulkier disease (GOG 161).

Chemotherapy for LMS

Leiomyosarcoma is the second most common of the gynecologic malignancies and probably the least chemotherapy sensitive. Phase II studies evaluating single-agent activity in this disease demonstrate that only doxorubicin and ifosfamide have response rates in excess of 10%, although a few very durable responses have been reported with paclitaxel and dose-rate infusion gemcitabine.[39,41,44,49] Single agents with little response include etoposide, mitoxantrone, and trimetrexate.[51,54,55,65] As mentioned above, a randomized comparison of doxorubicin with doxorubicin plus darcarbazine demonstrated no difference in responses in the overall population or within the subgroup of 48 patients with LMS.[41]

Chemotherapy for ESS

Endometrial stromal sarcomas are made up of an interesting collection of neoplasms that have been referred to by several names, including, in the majority of older literature endolymphatic stromal myosis, (see Chapter 14). From a clinical perspective, the principal issue is whether an ESS is low or high grade because these malignancies behave in dramatically different ways. Although both types of ESS have a significant chance of recurrence, low-grade ESS has a natural history that often extends over a decade or more and is clearly hormonally sensitive and, thus, distinguished from the other gynecologic sarcomas. High-grade ESS is a rapidly progressive but often transiently chemotherapy-sensitive malignancy, which has a natural history that is similar to that of MMMT.

Low-grade ESS is a neoplasm derived from the endometrial stromal cell, and, as such, it should respond to hormonal manipulation. Steroid receptor analysis suggests that ovarian steroids may act as tropic agents for these tumors, and there are multiple reports documenting the presence of steroid receptors in low-grade ESS.[66–70] For example, Wade and colleagues examined hormone receptors in 60 uterine sarcomas, a significant proportion of which were positive for the estrogen receptor (48.3%) and progesterone receptor (30%).[69] In addition, as mentioned above, hysterectomy with concomitant oophorectomy seems to lower relapse rates as compared with procedures that preserve some or all of ovarian function.

The precise efficacy of hormonal therapy in this disease is controversial, although some authors have reported small series with response rates as high as 50% using progestational agents, with subsequent long-term survival.[66,68] A case report of an objective response to letrozole, an aromatase inhibitor, has recently been published, and these agents have certainly demonstrated a response in breast cancer resistant to progestins and tamoxifen, with a favorable side-effect profile.[71] In view of the relatively low morbidity involved in the treatment with hormones, it seems a reasonable approach in spite of the scanty

data. Whether this should be taken a step further and hormones used as adjuvant therapy has not yet been studied, although this is likely a widely accepted practice despite lack of clinical evidence.

Response of low-grade stromal tumors to chemotherapy has been dismal, possibly related to its generally low mitotic index. High-grade ESS has shown modest response to doxorubicin-based regimens, with up to a 50% response rate in one study.[20,69] Ifosfamide also demonstrated a response rate of 33% in a GOG phase II clinical trial.[42] A single case report of prolonged response to oral etoposide has been reported.[72]

New Agents

Ecteinascidin-743 (ET-743) is a marine product that has recently completed several phase II trials in the United States and Europe in patients with soft tissue sarcomas. Several different dosages and schedules are currently under evaluation. In two recently completed phase II studies, responses were noted in 14% of chemotherapy-naive patients and 8% of pretreated patients.[57,58] Responses were often very durable, with 12-month progression-free survival being 18% in chemotherapy-naive patients and 11 months in patients who had received prior chemotherapy. The median duration of response was 11 months. The drug is under regulatory review for approval in Europe and is undergoing further testing in the United States.

CONCLUSION

The treatment of sarcomas arising in the uterine corpus is partly guided by clinical trial results and partly by clinical experience. Surgical resection of the primary tumor and, in carefully selected cases, recurrent disease remains the cornerstone of current therapy. Patients are at risk of both local and distant relapses, and pelvic radiotherapy may decrease local recurrence rates but is unlikely to positively impact on overall survival due to the high incidence of systemic disease. There is no convincing evidence that chemotherapy improves median survivals in either the adjuvant or metastatic setting. The use of chemotherapy in patients with symptomatic metastatic disease offers the potential for palliation and perhaps extended survival in a small subset of responsive patients. Doxorubicin, ifosfamide, and cisplatin are the most active agents. Hormonal manipulations can provide prolonged responses in women with low-grade endometrial stromal sarcomas and should be considered prior to chemotherapy in this patient population. The relative rarity of these tumors and their relative radiation and chemotherapy resistance make progress in this field challenging. Better understanding of the biology that underpins these malignancies might provide the introduction of rational therapeutics that, in turn, might lead to improved patient outcomes.

REFERENCES

1. Harlow BL, Weiss NS, Lofton S. The epidemiology of sarcomas of the uterus. J Natl Cancer Inst 1986;76:399–402.

2. Nordal RR, Thoresen SO. Uterine sarcomas in Norway 1956-1992: incidence, survival and mortality. Eur J Cancer 1997;33(6):907–1.

3. Holland JF. Randomized trials in rare tumors [editorial]. J Clin Oncol 1985;3:1163–5.

4. Kahanpaa KV, Wahlstrom T, Grohn P, et al. Sarcomas of the uterus: a clinicopathologic study of 119 patients. Obstet Gynecol 1986;67(3):417–24.

5. Parker WH, Fu YS, Berek JS. Uterine sarcoma in patients operated on for presumed leiomyoma and rapidly growing leiomyoma. Obstet Gynecol 1994;83(3):414–8.

6. Vongtama V, Karlen JR, Piver S, et al. Treatment, results and prognostic factors in stage I and II sarcoma of the corpus uteri. Am J Roentgenol Radium Ther Nucl Med 1976; 126:139–470.

7. Echt G, Johnson J, Steel J, et al. Treatment of uterine sarcomas. Cancer 1990;66:35–9.

8. Major FJ, Blessing JA, Silverberg SG, et al. Prognostic factors in early-stage uterine sarcoma. A Gynecologic Oncology Group study. Cancer 1993;71 4 Suppl:1702–9.

9. Knocke TH, Kucera H, Dorfler D, et al. Cancer results of postoperative radiotherapy in the treatment of sarcoma of the corpus uteri. Cancer 1998;83(9):1972–9.

10. Salazar O, Bonfiglio TA, Patten SF, et al. Uterine sarcomas, natural history, treatment and prognosis. Cancer 1978;42: 1161–70.

11. Omura G, Blessing J, Major F, et al. A randomized clinical trial of adjuvant Adriamycin in uterine sarcomas: a Gynecologic Oncology Group study. J Clin Oncol 1985;3: 1240–5.

12. Hornback NB, Omura G, Major FJ. Observations on the use of adjuvant radiation therapy in patients with stage I and II uterine sarcoma. Int J Radiat Oncol Biol Phys 1986; 12(12):2127–30.

13. Dinh TV, Slavin RE, Bhagavan BS, et al. Mixed müllerian tumors of the uterus: a clinicopathologic study. Obstet Gynecol 1989;74(3 Pt 1):388–92.

14. Silverberg SG, Major FJ, Blessing JA, et al. Carcinosarcoma (MMMT) of the uterus: a GOG pathologic study of 203 cases. Int J Gynecol Pathol 1990;9:1–9.

15. Podczaski FS, Noomert CA, Steven CH Jr, et al. Management of malignant mixed müllerian tumor of the uterus. Gynecol Oncol 1989;32:240.

16. Goff BA, Rice LW, Fleischbaker D, et al. Uterine leiomyosarcoma and endometrial stromal sarcoma: lymph node metastases and sites of recurrence. Gynecol Oncol 1993;50:105–9.

17. Leibsohn S, d'Ablaing G, Mishell PR, Schaerth JB. Leiomyosarcoma in a series of hysterectomy specimens performed for presumed uterine leiomyomas. Am J Obstet Gynecol 1990;162:968–74.

18. Berchuck A, Rubin S, Hoskins W, et al. Treatment of uterine leiomyosarcoma. Obstet Gynecol 1988;71:845–50.

19. O'Connor DM, Norris HJ. Mitotically active leiomyomas of the uterus. Hum Pathol 1990;21(2):223–7.

20. Berchuck A, Rubin SC, Hoskins WJ, et al. Treatment of endometrial stromal tumors. Gynecol Oncol 1990;36(1): 60–5.

21. Norris HJ, Taylor HB. Mesenchymal tumors of the uterus. I. A clinical and pathological study of 53 endometrial stromal tumors. Cancer 1966;19(6):755–66.

22. Salazar OM, Bonfiglio TA, Patten SE, et al. Uterine saromas: analysis of failures with special emphasis on use of adjuvant radiation. Cancer1978;42:1152–60.

23. Hoffman W, Schmandt S, Kortmann RD, et al. Radiotherapy in the treatment of uterine sarcoma: a retrospective analysis of S4. Gynecol Oncol Invest 1996;42:49–57.

24. Sorbe B. Radiotherapy and/or chemotherapy as adjuvant therapy of uterine sarcomas. Gynecol Oncol 1985;20:281–9.

25. Perez CA, Askin F, Baglan RJ, et al. Effects of irradiation on mixed müllerian tumors of the uterus. Cancer 1979; 43(4):1274–84.

26. Fleming WP, Peters WA III, Kumar NB, Morley GW. Autopsy findings in patients with uterine sarcoma. Gynecol Oncol 1984;19(2):168–72.

27. Van Nagell J, Hanson M, Donaldson E, Gallion H. Adjuvant vincristine, dactinomycin, and cyclophosphamide therapy in stage I uterine sarcoma. A pilot study. Cancer 1986;57:1451–4.

28. Piver MS, Barlow JJ, Lele SB, Yazigi R. Adriamycin in localized and metastatic uterine sarcomas. J Surg Oncol 1979; 12(3):263–5.

29. Hannigan EV, Freedman RS, Rutledge FN. Adjuvant chemotherapy in early uterine sarcoma. Gynecol Oncol 1983;15(1):56–64.

30. Piver MS, DeEulis TG, Lele SB, Barlow JJ. Cyclophosphamide, vincristine, Adriamycin, and dimethyltriazeno imidazole carboxamide (CYVADIC) for sarcomas of the female genital tract. Gynecol Oncol 1982; 14(3):319–23.

31. Hannigan EV, Freedman RS, Elder KW, Rutledge FN. Treatment of advanced uterine sarcoma with vincristine, actinomycin D, and cyclophosphamide. Gynecol Oncol 1983; 15(2):224–9.

32. Kushner D, Webster K, Belinson J, et al. Safety and efficacy of adjuvant single-agent ifosfamide in uterine sarcoma. Gynecol Oncol 2000;78(2):221–7.

33. Manolitsas TP, Wain GV, Williams KE, et al. Multimodality therapy for patients with clinical stage I and II malignant

mixed müllerian tumors of the uterus. Cancer 2001; 15;91(8):1437–43.

34. Peters WA III, Rivkin SE, Smith MR, Tesh DE. Cisplatin and Adriamycin combination chemotherapy for uterine stromal sarcomas and mixed mesodermal tumors. Gynecol Oncol 1989;34(3):323–7.

35. Mountain CF, McMurtrey MJ, Hermes RF. Surgery for pulmonary metastases: 20 year experience. Am Thorac Surg 1984:38:323–30.

36. Levenback C, Rubin SC, McCormack PM, et al. Resection of pulmonary metastases from uterine sarcomas. Gynecol Oncol 1992;45:202–5.

37. Spanos W Jr, Guse C, Perez C, et al. Phase II study of multiple daily fractionations in the palliation of advanced pelvic malignancies: preliminary report of RTOG 8502. Int J Radiat Oncol Biol Phys 1989;17(3):659–61.

38. Young JC, Glatstein CJ, Rosenberg SA, Antman KH. Sarcomas of soft tissues. In: DeVita VT, Hellman S, Rosenberg SA, editors. Cancer principles and practice of oncology. 4th ed. Philadelphia (PA): JB Lippincott Co.; 1993.

39. Patel SR, Gandhi V, Jenkins J, et al. Phase II clinical investigation of gemcitabine in advanced soft tissue sarcomas and window evaluation of dose rate on gemcitabine triphosphate accumulation. J Clin Oncol 2001;19(15):3483–9.

40. Judson I, Radford JA, Harris M, et al. Randomised phase II trial of pegylated liposomal doxorubicin (DOXIL/CAELYX) versus doxorubicin in the treatment of advanced or metastatic soft tissue sarcoma: a study by the EORTC Soft Tissue and Bone Sarcoma Group. Eur J Cancer 2001;37(7):870–7.

41. Omura GA, Major FJ, Blessing JA, et al. A randomized study of Adriamycin with and without dimethyl triazenoimidazole carboxamide in advanced uterine sarcomas. Cancer 1983;52(4):626–32.

42. Sutton G, Blessing JA, Park R, et al. Ifosfamide treatment of recurrent or metastatic endometrial stromal sarcomas previously unexposed to chemotherapy: a study of the Gynecologic Oncology Group. Obstet Gynecol 1996;87(5 Pt 1): 747–50.

43. Sutton G, Brunetto VL, Kilgore L, et al. A phase III trial of ifosfamide with or without cisplatin in carcinosarcoma of the uterus: a Gynecologic Oncology Group study. Gynecol Oncol 2000;79(2):147–53.

44. Sutton GP, Blessing JA, Barrett RJ, McGehee R. Phase II trial of ifosfamide and mesna in leiomyosarcoma of the uterus: a Gynecologic Oncology Group study. Am J Obstet Gynecol 1992;166(2):556–9.

45. Sutton GP, Blessing JA, Rosenshein N, et al. Phase II trial of ifosfamide and mesna in mixed mesodermal tumors of the uterus (a Gynecologic Oncology Group study). Am J Obstet Gynecol 1989;161:309–12.

46. Gershenson DM, Kavanagh JJ, Copeland LJ, et al. Cisplatin therapy for disseminated mixed mesodermal sarcoma of the uterus. J Clin Oncol 1987;5(4):618–21.

47. Thigpen JT, Blessing JA, Beecham J, et al. Phase II trial of cisplatin as first-line chemotherapy in patients with advanced or recurrent uterine sarcomas: a Gynecologic Oncology Group study. J Clin Oncol 1991;9(11):1962–6.

48. Thigpen JT, Blessing JA, Orr JW, DiSaia PJ. Phase II trial of cisplatin in the treatment of patients with advanced or

recurrent mixed mesodermal sarcomas of the uterus: a Gynecologic Oncology Group study. Cancer Treat Rep 1986;70:271–4.

49. Sutton G, Blessing J, Ball H. Phase II trial of paclitaxel in leiomyosarcoma of the uterus: a Gynecologic Oncology Group study. Gynecol Oncol 1999;74:346–9.

50. Curtin JP, Blessing JA, Soper JT, DeGeest K. Paclitaxel in the treatment of carcinosarcoma of the uterus: a Gynecologic Oncology Group study. Gynecol Oncol 2001;83(2):268–70.

51. Thigpen T, Blessing JA, Yordan E, et al. Phase II trial of etoposide in leiomyosarcoma of the uterus: a Gynecologic Oncology Group study. Gynecol Oncol 1996;63(1):120–2.

52. Asbury R, Blessing JA, Moore D. A phase II trail of aminothiadiazole in patients with mixed mesodermal tumors of the uterine corpus: a Gynecologic Oncology Group study. Am J Clin Oncol 1996;19(4):400–2.

53. Slayton RE, Blessing JA, Clarke-Pearson D. A phase II trial of diaziquone (AZQ) in mixed mesodermal sarcomas of the uterus. A Gynecologic Oncology Group study. Invest New Drugs 1991;9(1):93–4.

54. Fowler JM, Blessing JA, Burger RA, Malfetano JH. Phase II evaluation of oral trimetrexate in mixed mesodermal tumors of the uterus: a Gynecologic Oncology Group study. Gynecol Oncol 2002;85(2):311–4.

55. Smith HO, Blessing JA, Vaccarello L. Trimetrexate in the treatment of recurrent or advanced leiomyosarcoma of the uterus: a phase II study of the Gynecologic Oncology Group. Gynecol Oncol 2002;84(1):140–4.

56. Demetri GD. ET-743: the US experience in sarcomas of soft tissues. Anticancer Drugs 2002;13(1):S7–9.

57. Delaloge S, Yovine A, Taamma A, et al. Ecteinascidin-743: a marine-derived compound in advanced, pretreated sarcoma patients—preliminary evidence of activity. J Clin Oncol 2001;19(5):1248–55.

58. Sutton G, Blessing JA, Malfetano JH. Ifosfamide and doxorubicin in the treatment of advanced leiomyosarcomas of the uterus: a Gynecologic Oncology Group study. Gynecol Oncol 1996;62(2):226–9.

59. Le Cesne A, Judson I, Crowther D, et al. Randomized phase III study comparing conventional-dose doxorubicin plus ifosfamide versus high-dose doxorubicin plus ifosfamide plus recombinant human granulocyte-macrophage colony-stimulating factor in advanced soft tissue sarcomas: a trial of the European Organization for Research and Treatment of Cancer/Soft Tissue and Bone Sarcoma Group. J Clin Oncol 2000;18(14):2676–84.

60. Antman K, Crowley J, Balcerzak SP, et al. An intergroup phase III randomized study of doxorubicin and dacarbazine with or without ifosfamide and mesna in advanced soft tissue and bone sarcomas. J Clin Oncol 1993;11(7):1276–85.

61. Muss HB, Bundy BN, Adcock L, Beecham J. Mitoxantrone in the treatment of advanced uterine sarcoma. A phase II trial of the Gynecologic Oncology Group. Am J Clin Oncol 1990;13(1):32–4.

62. Sit AS, Price FV, Kelley JL, et al. Chemotherapy for malignant mixed müllerian tumors of the ovary. Gynecol Oncol 2000;79(2):196–200.

63. Muss HB, Bundy B, DiSaia PJ, et al. Treatment of recurrent or advanced uterine sarcoma. A randomized trial of doxorubicin versus doxorubicin and cyclophosphamide (a

phase III trial of the Gynecologic Oncology Group). Cancer 1985;55(8):1648–53.

64. Duska LR, Garrett A, Eltabbakh GH, et al. Paclitaxel and platinum chemotherapy for malignant mixed müllerian tumors of the ovary. Gynecol Oncol 2002;85(3):459–63.

65. Currie J, Blessing JA, Muss HB, et al. Combination chemotherapy with hydroxyurea, dacarbazine (DTIC), and etoposide in the treatment of uterine leiomyosarcoma: a Gynecologic Oncology Group study. Gynecol Oncol 1996;61(1):27–30.

66. Sabini G, Chumas JC, Mann WJ. Steroid hormone receptors in endometrial stromal sarcomas. A biochemical and immunohistochemical study. Am J Clin Pathol 1992;97(3):381–6.

67. Katz L, Merino MJ, Sakamoto H, Schwartz PE. Endometrial stromal sarcoma: a clinicopathologic study of 11 cases with determination of estrogen and progestin receptor levels in three tumors. Gynecol Oncol 1987;26(1):87 97.

68. Baker VV, Walton LA, Fowler WC Jr, Currie JL. Steroid receptors in endolymphatic stromal myosis. Obstet Gynecol 1984;63 3 Suppl:72S–4S

69. Wade K, Quinn MA, Hammond I, et al. Uterine sarcoma: steroid receptors and response to hormonal therapy. Gynecol Oncol 1990;39(3):364–7.

70. Piver MS, Rutledge FN, Copeland L, et al. Uterine endolymphatic stromal myosis: a collaborative study. Obstet Gynecol 1984;64(2):173–8.

71. Maluf FC, Sabbatini P, Schwartz L, et al. Endometrial stromal sarcoma: objective response to letrozole. Gynecol Oncol 2001;82(2):384–8.

72. Lin YC, Kudelka AP, Tresukosol D, et al. Prolonged stabilization of progressive endometrial stromal sarcoma with prolonged oral etoposide therapy. Gynecol Oncol 1995;58(2):262–5.

Index

Page numbers followed by f indicate figure. Pages numbers followed by t indicate table.